Roberto De Ponti
From Signals to Colours
A Case-based Atlas of Electroanatomic Mapping in
Complex Atrial Arrhythmias

**Roberto De Ponti**

# From Signals to Colours

## A Case-based Atlas of Electroanatomic Mapping in Complex Atrial Arrhythmias

Based on the experience of the Project of ElectroAnatomic mapping in Complex arrhythmia Evaluation (PEACE)

Springer

Roberto De Ponti
Department of Heart Sciences
University of Insubria-Varese
Ospedale di Circolo and Macchi Foundation
Varese, Italy

ISBN 978-88-470-0648-5 Springer Milan Berlin Heidelberg New York
e-ISBN 978-88-470-0649-2

Library of Congress Contro Number 2007931631

Springer is part of Springer Science+Business Media
springer.com
© Springer-Verlag Italia 2008
I reprint: January 2008; II reprint: March 2008; III reprint: May 2008

This work is subject to copyright. All rights are reserved, whether the whole or part of the material is concerned, specifically the rights of translation, reprinting, reuse of illustrations, recitation, broadcasting, reproduction on microfilm or in any other way, and storage in data banks. Duplication of this publication or parts thereof is permitted only under the provisions of the Italian Copyright Law in its current version, and permission for use must always be obtained from Springer. Violations are liable to prosecution under the Italian Copyright Law.

The use of general descriptive names, registered names, trademarks, etc. in this publication does not imply, even in the absence of a specific statement, that such names are exempt from the relevant protective laws and regulations and therefore free for general use.
Product liability: The publishers cannot guarantee the accuracy of any information about dosage and application contained in this book. In every individual case the user must check such information by consulting the relevant literature.

Cover layout: Simona Colombo, Milan, Italy
Typesetting: Compostudio, Cernusco s/N (Milan), Italy
Printing and binding: Grafiche Porpora, Segrate (MI), Italy

Springer-Verlag Italia S.r.l., Via Decembrio 28, I-20137 Milan, Italy
*Printed in Italy*

*To my wife Cristina and to our son Riccardo.
... I am just wondering how life would have been without them.*

# Foreword

*The diagnosis and treatment of arrhythmias are major commitments of our School of Cardiology. Indeed, the field of cardiac arrhythmias is broad and often difficult; time and dedication are required to yield the necessary expertise. Since the early days, technology has made essential contributions to the study of cardiac arrhythmias and, over the years, electrophysiology has progressed from intracavitary signals recorded on seemingly endless printouts to computer-generated maps that three-dimensionally reconstruct the electrical activity of the heart. I remember when, at the end of 1970s, our department received its first multi-channel computerised mapping system, developed as a prototype by an Italian company. It was nearly 2 m tall, had a tiny black and green screen and an entire afternoon was often required to elaborate and transfer data it acquired. Nevertheless, it was a valuable support to our work and crucial to our effort to start the program of mapping-guided antiarrhythmic surgery. At that time, intraoperative maps were printed out on a white sheet of paper and consisted of rectangles filled by dots, numbers, and lines, from which the three-dimensional shape of the mapped heart chamber was hard to imagine. Nonetheless, while in those days the technology was limited, all the basic concepts needed for signal analysis and arrhythmia diagnosis were already known. The relationship between technology and knowledge has been a mutually reinforcing one, and, at that time, resulted in our ability to cure many forms of arrhythmias by surgical ablation. Although in the early phases, intraoperative mapping followed by computation and elaboration of the map were time-consuming to the surgeon, the urgent desire to proceed with the intervention and to cure the patient was usually satisfied within minutes by the provision of accurate and useful information.*

*Over the last decade, new technologies have been widely introduced in the field of interventional electrophysiology. Mapping technology is now so sophisticated that three-dimensional reconstruction of a heart chamber by electroanatomic mapping, which combines spatial and electrical information, is possible with an accuracy of less than 1 mm. This has become even more attractive with imaging integration, in which a three-dimensional rendering of a magnetic resonance or computed tomography image is superimposed onto the electroanatomic mapping. This process allows real-time navigation of the mapping catheter based on a high-resolution image of the heart. How should we react to this unparalleled and explosive evolution of technology? In the literature, there is a wide body of evidence that electroanatomic mapping has improved the outcome of the ablation procedure for several arrhythmias and it has led to new and "non-conventional" procedures. Nonetheless, further progress will not be possible if we expect that the diagnosis and treatment of arrhythmias can be relegated to stand-alone computers acting as "autopilots" for electrophysiology. As technology increases, our knowledge must increase as well. The enormous amount of data provided by new technologies has to be analysed and interpreted to provide new answers to new questions.*

*This is the approach taken in this book by Roberto De Ponti, with whom, after having shared some of the earlier days of electrophysiology, I have observed and experienced the impressive developments that have been made in this field over the past several years. This book is an example of how technology and knowledge can merge to advance the frontiers in the study of cardiac arrhythmias. I have been overwhelmed by the enthusiasm of those who have joined our group, and by their willingness to discuss and interpret electroanatomic mapping data of complex arrhythmias. Let us hope that this is just the beginning and that the best is still to come.*

July 31, 2007

*Jorge A. Salerno-Uriarte*
*Department of Heart Sciences*
*University of Insubria-Varese*
*Ospedale di Circolo and Macchi Foundation*
*Varese, Italy*

# Preface

*What is a complex case? Although the concept of what is complex may be personal, there is a common sense of complexity in electrophysiology. In most cases, a complex case involves a patient who comes or is referred after a single or multiple unsuccessful procedures in other centres and is still suffering from the same or a similar arrhythmia. Some other cases are expected to be complex prior to the first procedure, because the patient has an acquired or a congenital heart disease and previously underwent complex cardiac surgery. Yet, in other circumstances, the case becomes complex directly before our eyes, when, for example, during the electrophysiology procedure we realise that what was expected to be a typical atrial flutter based on surface electrocardiogram turns out to be not dependent on cavotricuspid isthmus conduction and requires solid mapping data in order to be successfully treated. Only in a few cases, very rarely to be honest, is the arrhythmia less complex than expected. In these cases, the main difficulty often arises from the fact that the operator has to stick to the evidence and not be prejudiced by the belief that the case has to be necessarily complex, based on the pre-procedural evaluation.*

*In 2003, the Project of ElectroAnatomic mapping for Complex Arrhythmia Evaluation (PEACE) was initiated in Italy and coordinated by our Center. This book represent the result of this experience. The aim of the project and therefore of this book was to obtain as much information as possible from electroanatomic mapping in order to obtain a correct diagnosis and define a rational ablation strategy in a "learning before burning" process. In this book, the reader will find very few conventional electrophysiology signal recordings–only those that were deemed necessary. There are many other books and papers, written by brilliant authors, including pioneers in this field, showing conventional tracings in complex arrhythmias. What we want to present in "From Signals to Colours" is the outstanding and unparalleled contribution of electroanatomic mapping in the muddy field of complex atrial arrhythmias. This does not mean that conventional electrophysiology has been forgotten or abolished. Far from being in conflict with what is considered conventional in electrophysiology, electroanatomic mapping is, in fact, based on conventional recordings, and black and white conventional signals are embedded and integrated in a colour-coded electroanatomic map to obtain a more complete and more intuitive display of the electrical activation of a given heart chamber during a given arrhythmia. Some of the results obtained by this project are shown in the 25 cases presented in this book. Basically, this project's major achievements have been procedure simplification and increased success rate, obtained widely and in a replicable way among centres, when complex arrhythmias are approached.*

*The project could not have been developed and, consequently, the book could not have been written without the personal and active contribution of all participants. Their names and centres are listed below.*

- *Department of Heart Sciences, University of Insubria – Ospedale di Circolo and Macchi Foundation, Varese: Raffaella Marazzi, Fabrizio Caravati, Luigi Addonisio, Lucia De Luca, Valerio De Sanctis, Luigi Di Biase, Gianluca Gonzi, Luca Panchetti and Jorge A. Salerno-Uriarte. Department of Radiology of the same Institution: Domenico Lumia and Carlo Fugazzola*

- *Interventional Cardiology Unit, Circolo Hospital, Busto Arsizio, Varese: Giulia Filippini and Ettore Petrucci*

- *Diagnostic and Interventional Electrophysiology Unit, Civile Hospital, Camposampiero, Padua: Piero Turrini, Stella Baccilieri and Roberto Verlato*

- *Department of Cardiology, Villa Pini d'Abruzzo Hospital, Chieti: Raffaele Luise*

- *Cardiology Unit, Conegliano Veneto Hospital, Conegliano Veneto, Treviso: Leonardo Corò, Luigi Sciarra and Pietro Delise*

- *Electrophysiology Unit, Department of Cardiology, S. Carlo Hospital, Milan: Daniele Malaspina and Massimo Pala*

- *Cardiology Department, Civile Hospital, Mirano, Venice: Franco Zoppo, Francesca Zerbo and Emanuele Bertaglia*

- *Departmant of Cardiology, C.C. dott. Pederzoli, Presidio Ospedaliero ULSS22, Peschiera del Garda, Verona: Antonio Fusco and Alfredo Vicentini*

- *Arrhythmia Unit, Cardio-Thoracic Department, University of Pisa, Pisa: Giuseppe Arena, Ezio Soldati and Maria Grazia Bongiorni*

- *Interventional Cardiology Unit, S. Maria Nuova Hospital, Reggio Emilia: Fabio Quartieri, Nicola Bottoni and Carlo Menozzi*

- *Institute of Cardiology, Department of Cardiovascular Medicine, Catholic University of the Sacred Heart, Rome: Antonio Dello Russo, Michela Casella and Gemma Pelargonio*

- *Department of Pediatric Cardiology, Bambino Gesù Hospital, Rome: Massimo Stefano Silvetti and Fabrizio Drago*

- *Electrophysiology Laboratory, Cardiology Unit, S. Chiara Hospital, Trento: Massimiliano Marini and Maurizio Del Greco. Department of Radiology of the same Institution: Maurizio Centonze*

*I feel personally very much in debt with Gabriele Fischetto and Andrea Lenzi for ideating, developing and supporting the PEACE.*

*Being formatted as an atlas, this book focuses on images. For each case, a brief presentation is given and the narrative of the procedure is oriented towards a complete understanding of images. Among them, electroanatomic maps obviously represent the vast majority and they are left as they are generated by the system, with the addition of some asterisks or arrows in a very few cases. This has been made on the assumption that they are or, however, should become self-explanatory and in this process reading of the initial chapter on methodology is of crucial importance. A brief commentary completes each case, underlining what we have learned from the procedure and making correlations with other cases presented in the book. Only essential references are reported, since in-depth discussion of each topic possibly brought up by each case is beyond the aims of this book.*

*Comparison of different experiences and constructive discussion have always been the fundamentals of this project. Therefore, anyone willing to join the group should feel free to access the open forum at peaceonline@libero.it for further discussion and feed-back. On my side, I would be very satisfied if this experience could minimally contribute in rendering less challenging the approach to complex cases in some other center, as it did in ours.*

*April 30, 2007*

*Roberto De Ponti*
*Department of Heart Sciences*
*University of Insubria-Varese*
*Ospedale di Circolo and Macchi Foundation*
*Varese, Italy*

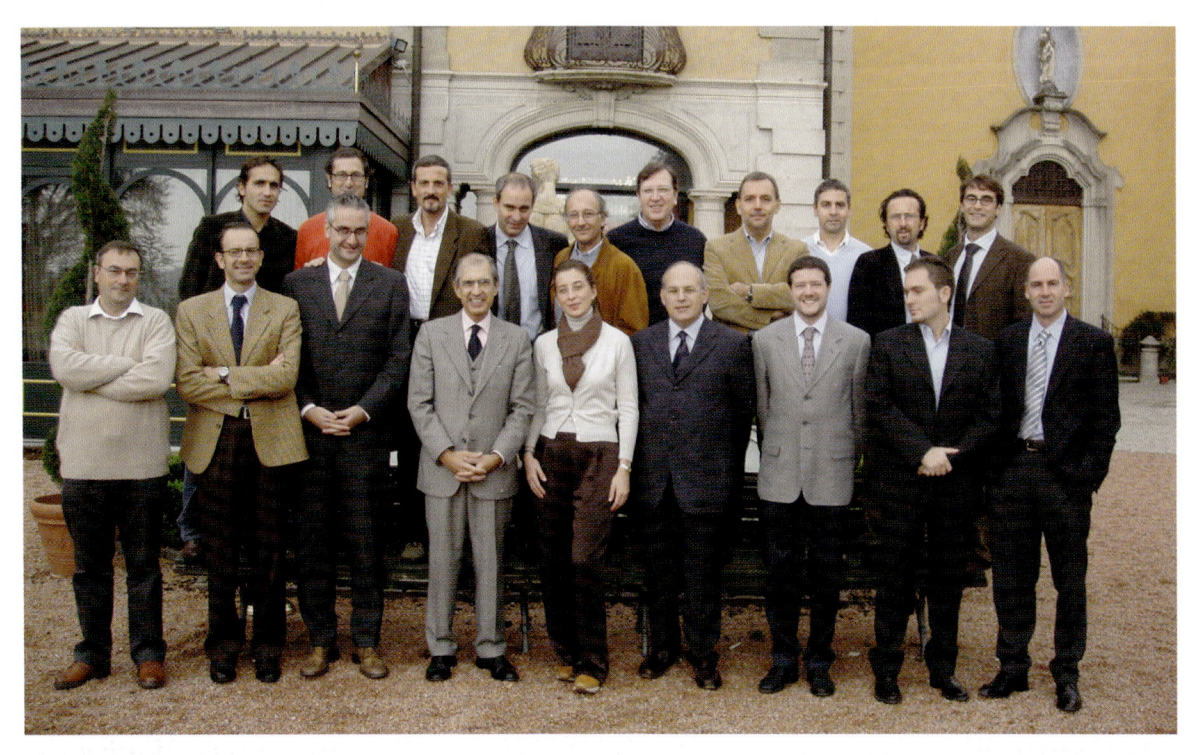

*Some of the members of the "Project of ElectroAnatomic mapping in Complex arrhythmia Evaluation" (PEACE) during a break in the meeting on October 22, 2005 at the Villa Porro Pirelli, Varese, Italy*

# Contents

Electroanatomic Mapping in Evaluation of Complex Atrial Arrhythmias .................................... 1

**Part I.** **Focal Atrial Arrhythmias** .................................................................................................. 13
    Case 1.   Focal Atrial Tachycardia in the Right Atrium in a Postsurgical Patient: Rare but Possible ..... 15
    Case 2.   Focal Atrial Tachycardia in an Enlarged Right Atrium after Rastelli's Operation:
             Ambiguous Mapping Data in Conflict with the Orthodoxies ................................. 21
    Case 3.   Focal Atrial Tachycardia Associated with a Macroreentrant Tachycardia: Two Arrhythmias
             with Different Mechanisms and Similar Morphologies in a Non-surgical Left Atrium
             with Electrically Silent Areas ............................................................................. 27
    Case 4.   Focal Atrial Tachycardia From the Right Superior Pulmonary Vein with Irregular Cycle
             and P Wave Morphology: the Missing Link in the Chain Connecting Organized and
             Disorganized Atrial Arrhythmias? ....................................................................... 37
    Case 5.   Focal Atrial Tachycardia from the Right Superior Pulmonary Vein with Stable
             P Wave Morphology and Cycle Length: the Problem of Discriminating between a
             Right and Left Origin ........................................................................................ 45

**Part II.** **Macroreentrant Atrial Tachycardia/Flutter** ........................................................................ 57
    Case 6.   Counter-clockwise Atrial Flutter in the Donor's Right Atrium After Heart Transplantation:
             a Peculiar Example of Single-Loop Right Atrial Reentry ...................................... 59
    Case 7.   Single-loop Macroreentry in the Left Atrium in an "Atrial Cardiomyopathy":
             Discrimination between Right and Left Circuits and the Paradox of Proximal-to-distal
             Coronary Sinus Activation in a Left-sided Arrhythmia ......................................... 65
    Case 8.   Double-loop Reentry in the Right Atrium with a Shared Mid-Diastolic Isthmus
             in a Postsurgical Patient: Identifying and Targeting the Shared Isthmus ................ 73
    Case 9.   Double-loop Reentry in the Left Atrium with a Shared Mid-Diastolic Isthmus in a
             Non-surgical Patient with Left Atrial Scarring: a More Common than Expected
             Arrhythmia? ................................................................................................... 79
    Case 10. Macroreentrant Atrial Tachycardia in a Left Atrium With a Prosthetic Mitral Valve
             (Example 1): a Reentrant Circuit Confined to the Left Atrial Roof and the Need for
             Reconstruction of the Entire Reentrant Circuit ................................................... 87
    Case 11. Macroreentrant Atrial Tachycardia in a Left Atrium With a Prosthetic Mitral Valve
             (Example 2): the Problem of Minimal Amplitude Potentials .................................. 95
    Case 12. Counter-clockwise Isthmus-dependent Peritricuspid Reentry with an Atypical
             Electrocardiographic Pattern: what Should Be Complex is not Always Actually Complex ..... 103

Case 13. Recurrence of Typical Counter-clockwise Atrial Flutter in a Postsurgical Patient: an Unexpected Trap .................................................................................. 111

Case 14. Two Macroreentrant Tachycardias in a Patient after Fontan Surgery: the Difference between "Isthmic" and "Rotational" Atrial Macroreentry ..................................... 119

Case 15. Organised Atrial Arrhythmias after Atrial Fibrillation Ablation in the Left Atrium (Example 1): an Arrhythmogenic Incomplete Linear Lesion with Modified Left-to-right Atrial Propagation ................................................................................. 129

Case 16. Organised Atrial Arrhythmias after Atrial Fibrillation Ablation in the Left Atrium (Example 2): Association of Multiple Potentially Pro-arrhythmogenic Factors Resulting in a Tachycardia with a Longer Cycle Length ................................................. 137

Case 17. Organised Atrial Arrhythmias after Atrial Fibrillation Ablation in the Left Atrium (Example 3): do Lesions in the Left Atrium Have a Mid-term Evolution? .................... 145

Case 18. A Non-clinical Macroreentrant Right Atrial Tachycardia with Two Independent Loops: the Exception to the Rule of a Shared Mid-diastolic Isthmus in Double-loop Reentry ........ 151

Case 19. A Peculiar Clockwise Peritricuspid Atrial Flutter: the Exception to the Rule of Aiming at the Mid-diastolic Isthmus ........................................................... 157

## Part III. Atrial Ablation Based on Substrate Mapping in Sinus Rhythm ................................. 163

Case 20. Non-inducible Atrial Flutter in a Patient with Prior Surgery for Congenital Heart Disease (Example 1): Ablation Based on Substrate Mapping in Sinus Rhythm ....................... 165

Case 21. Non-inducible Atrial Flutter in a Patient with Prior Surgery for Congenital Heart Disease (Example 2): Substrate Mapping in Sinus Rhythm with the Help of Imaging Integration .... 173

## Part IV. Peculiar Anatomies .................................................................................. 181

Case 22. Isolated Congenital Unilateral Absence of the Right Pulmonary Artery and Left Atrial Flutter: Are they Related? ....................................................................... 183

Case 23. Left Atrial Ablation of Atrial Fibrillation in a Patient with Dextrocardia: the Complexities of an Inverted Anatomy ............................................................................ 189

Case 24. Uncommon Anatomy of the Pulmonary Veins (Example 1): Common Trunk of the Inferior Pulmonary Veins ................................................................................... 193

Case 25. Uncommon Anatomy of the Pulmonary Veins (Example 2): the "Roof Pulmonary Vein" ...... 197

# Electroanatomic Mapping in Evaluation of Complex Atrial Arrhythmias

Electroanatomic mapping was introduced into clinical practice more than 10 years ago and its use has become increasingly widespread. The principles [1] and basics [2] of the Carto system have been the subject of many publications and we assume that they are well-known to the reader. In the following pages, the electroanatomic mapping method used to approach the cases reported in this book is described. Since some of the concepts and settings are innovative, it is important to refer to these pages for a complete understanding of the method used for diagnosis and treatment in the 25 cases presented here.

## Setting the Window of Interest

The window of interest is the part of the tachycardia cycle analysed by the system to identify the electrical signal that is annotated for activation mapping and evaluated for voltage mapping. The duration of the window of interest should be set at the beginning of the procedure, before point acquisition. The window of interest comprises the backward and forward intervals, which precede and follow, respectively, the reference signal. Since the catheter in the coronary sinus is usually stable even in a prolonged procedure, a coronary sinus atriogram is most often chosen, with an atrial deflection prevailing over the ventricular one. The mechanism (focal vs macroreentrant) of the arrhythmia will determine how the window of interest is set.

In focal arrhythmias, the window of interest is usually easily set, since its duration must exceed the duration of the surface P wave by 100 ms. In fact, the window of interest onset is set 70–80 ms before the P-wave onset and it usually terminates 20–30 ms after the termination of the surface P wave. It is important not to unnecessarily increase the value of the window of interest in order to avoid, as much as possible, (1) having two atrial deflections in the window of interest in focal atrial tachycardia with a very short cycle length (200–250 ms); (2) including ventricular deflections in the limits of the window of interest, as these can be erroneously computed for automatic calculation of voltage amplitude, with the subsequent need for site by site off-line re-analysis. However, when a long interval between the bipolar signal at the earliest activated site and the P wave onset is expected, especially in patients exhibiting major atrial conduction disturbances, the duration of the backward interval of the window of interest may be increased, so that its onset is 100–120 ms before the onset of the surface P wave.

For macroreentrant arrhythmias, there are two options to set the window of interest. In both, the length of the window of interest should span no more than 90–95% of the tachycardia cycle length to avoid, due to minimal variations of the tachycardia cycle length, the presence of two deflections within the limits of the window of interest.

In the first option, the setting is standardised, so that both the backward and forward intervals correspond to roughly 45% of the tachycardia cycle length. In this way, the rainbow of colours in the activation map expresses the activation sequence. Nonetheless, none of the colours is indicative of a given chronology, since using this setting the chronology of the onset of the window in the tachycardia cycle is random.

The second option involves a specific setting for each tachycardia morphology such that the onset of the window is fixed in mid-diastole, as identified on the surface electrocardiogram. For this setting, the following formulas should be used to calculate the backward and forward intervals:

$$\text{Backward interval} = \frac{\text{TCL} - \text{DUR}^{PW}}{2} + \text{Interval}^{PWonset\text{-}ref}$$

Forward interval = (TCL − Backward interval) · 0.90

where TCL is the tachycardia cycle length, $\text{DUR}^{PW}$ is the duration of the surface P wave during tachycardia (interval "a" in Fig. 1), and interval$^{PWonset\text{-}ref}$ is the interval between the onset of the P wave and the reference signal (interval "b" in Fig. 1), which has a negative value when the reference signal precedes the P wave onset. Using this method, not only does the rainbow of colours in the activation map identify the activation sequence, but each colour is also indicative of a given chronology. Therefore, as shown in Fig. 1 by the colour-coded scale in relation to the window of interest and the surface tracing, red and yellow identify mid- and late-diastolic activation, respectively, and dark blue and purple identify early- and mid-diastolic activation, respectively. The remaining colours identify areas of systolic activation. With this setting, the isthmus of

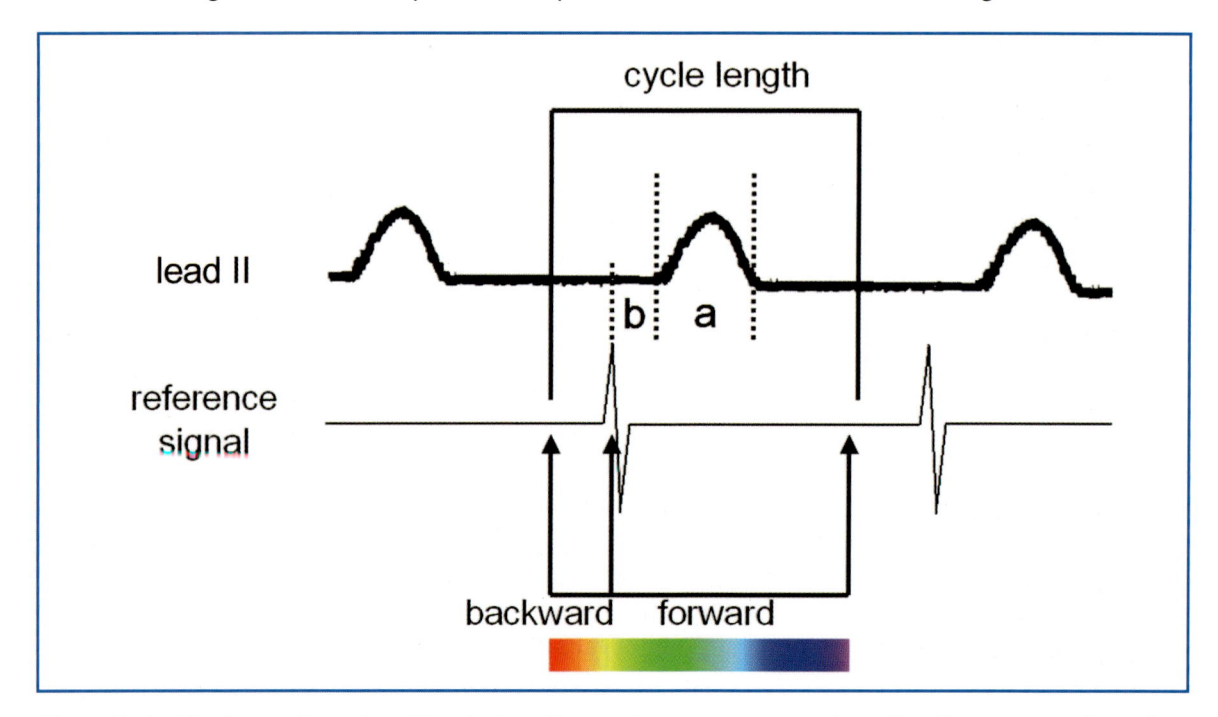

**Fig. 1.** Method for the specific setting of the window of interest in macroreentrant tachycardias. The *top tracing* shows the P wave on lead II; the *second tracing* is a schematic representation of the reference signal. The window of interest extends from mid-diastole to the mid-diastole of the next cycle; the backward interval is from the mid-diastole to the reference signal and the forward interval from the reference signal to 95% of the tachycardia cycle. Interval *a* is the duration of the P wave during tachycardia, and interval *b* is measured from P wave onset to the reference signal. Using this method, each colour is indicative of a given chronology, as indicated by the colour bar at the bottom of the figure

mid-diastolic activation is easily identified by the interface between the red and purple areas, once activation along the entire macroreentrant circuit has been reconstructed. P wave onset and duration are measured on the 12-leads synchronously displayed, usually at a sweep speed of 100 mm/s. This sweep speed aims to be an optimal compromise between lower and higher speeds, since these can make definition of the surface P wave duration more difficult or less accurate. Since clear identification of the surface P wave is the key point when using this method, carotid sinus massage or intravenous adenosine bolus are used to obtain a temporary atrioventricular conduction block.

When this setting is used, additional information can be gathered from the electroanatomic map that allows, in particular, identification of the mid-diastolic isthmus independently of entrainment mapping, as demonstrated in our pilot experience [3]. Therefore, this setting has been used systematically in all the cases of macroreentrant tachycardia/flutter presented in this book.

In case the nature of the arrhythmia (focal or macroreentrant) is not clear at the beginning of the procedure, the window of interest can be set as for a macroreentrant arrhythmia using this method. In our experience, this does not compromise the accuracy of annotation when, during mapping, the arrhythmia turns out to be focal.

## Mapping

Mapping is usually commenced in the right atrium and continues in the left, if a right-sided arrhythmia is excluded. Mapping of the right atrium, when the surface P wave morphology clearly predicts a left arrhythmogenic substrate, may be time-consuming. However, even in these cases, right atrial mapping may be very useful and a considerable amount of time will be spared if mapping is limited to 30-40 points. Right atrial mapping during a left-sided arrhythmia may identify a wide range of right atrial by-stander activation patterns, from the more typical (as in Case 10) to the more complex (as in Cases 7, 9, 11 and 15) depending on the underlying heart disease, prior surgery or prior ablation. Moreover, in particular cases, it can identify an unexpected right-sided arrhythmia, in spite of the surface P wave morphology (as in Case 12), thereby avoiding unnecessary transseptal catheterisation.

At the beginning of mapping, acquired sites should be homogeneously distributed to reconstruct the cardiac chamber. Only regions with a bipolar signal amplitude <0.05 mV and not distinguishable from baseline noise are defined as electrically silent and, therefore, are not annotated and tagged by grey dots. As pointed out in Cases 2 and 11, every effort should be made to analyse the electrical signal also in sites with minimal but still-discernible bipolar deflections, in order not to miss the target area for ablation. In the presence of multicomponent or fragmented potentials, the first sharp deflection is annotated. In focal arrhythmias, the analysis of unipolar deflection is crucial, since the site of origin of the tachycardia is associated with a rapid downstroke in unipolar signals, although this general rule has exceptions (Cases 2, 3 and 4). In macroreentrant arrhythmias, signals inscribed in the part of the tachycardia cycle outside the limits of the window of interest (which spans 90–95% of the tachycardia cycle length) are annotated, with respect to the reference signal, as "early" if the first sharp deflection precedes the window of interest limits or "late" if it follows. Sites with double potentials separated by ≥50 ms are indicative of conduction block with activation detour and are tagged with blue dots. In the right atrium, the site of His-bundle recording is usually tagged by an orange dot, while in the left atrium the pulmonary veins can be tagged by tubular icons when their electrical activation is not expected to contribute to clarification of the arrhythmia mechanism. When they are crucial for a correct diagnosis, as in Cases 4 and 5, they are reconstructed as separate chambers and their electrical signals are annotated. They are also reconstructed as separate chambers when the electroanatomic map is used to register a three-dimensional computed tomography or magnetic resonance image imported in the electroanatomic system, as in Cases 5, 17, 24 and 25. In these situations, it is crucial to acquire only proximal sites and to avoid distortion of the pulmonary vein anatomy by extreme catheter deflections or torsions.

In the final phase, high-density mapping may be required in some areas, such as the earliest activated area in focal arrhythmias or the mid-diastolic isthmus in macroreentrant tachycardias, to better clarify the arrhythmogenic substrate and plan the ablation strategy. Throughout the entire mapping phase, it is important that the tachycardia does not vary. Arrhythmia variations may be detected by monitoring the surface P wave morphology, the tachycardia cycle and the intracavitary activation sequence. In macroreentrant forms, the cycle length should be very stable, but beat-to-beat variations not exceeding 10% of the cycle length and 30 ms are acceptable. Moreover, in these forms, it is possible that catheter manipulation and positioning on the mid-diastolic isthmus prolong the tachycardia cycle or even terminate the tachycardia due to the catheter bumping sites in this area, which may be particularly sensitive. If the tachycardia cycle is significantly prolonged, mapping should be terminated, since acquisition of the new mapping sites with the old setting of the window of interest alters the activation map. Acquisition of new sites is possible only with the re-map option, after the window of interest has been reset. The consequences of tachycardia cycle length prolongation or termination with non-inducibility due to catheter bumping in the mid-diastolic area can be limited in terms of map completeness by mapping this area of the chamber last.

## Activation Map

In focal arrhythmias, activation mapping is completed when a site of early activation surrounded by a circle of sites, all with a later activation time, is identified. In macroreentrant forms, activation mapping is completed when the mapped activation in a given heart chamber spans ≥90% of the tachycardia cycle length. To calculate the percentage of the cycle length reconstructed by electroanatomic mapping, the following formula should be used:

$$\% \text{ of TCR} = \frac{\text{mapped activation}}{\text{TCL}}$$

where % of TCR is the percentage of the tachycardia cycle reconstructed in the electroanatomic map, mapped activation is the sum of the values appearing at the limits of the colour bar and TCL is the tachycardia cycle length. To correctly determine the mapped activation, the values appearing at the limits of the colour bar should be summed when they are of opposite sign; when both are negative, the value appearing at the top has to be subtracted from the one appearing at the bottom.

Interpretation of the activation map is intuitive in focal arrhythmias, since the colour distribution identifies a centrifugally spreading pattern, from the earliest activated site to the latest one. Ideally, these two sites are located in diametrically opposite areas of the considered heart chamber, although this pattern may be modified by the presence of conduction disturbances, electrically silent areas and sites of prior surgical atriotomy.

In macroreentrant arrhythmias, the colour distribution identifies the reentrant circuit, with the course of reentry moving from red to purple. According to the above-described method for setting the window of interest, the red area encounters the purple one in a "head-meets-tail" pattern in the mid-diastolic isthmus. This region is magnified by a dark red band that appears

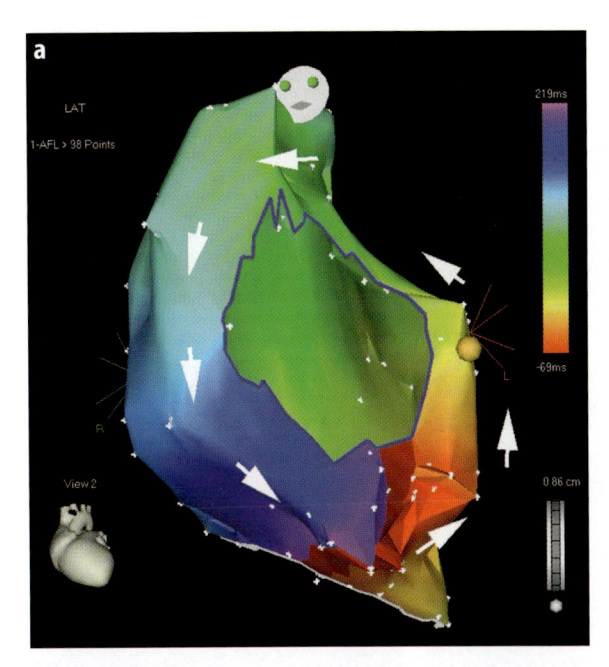

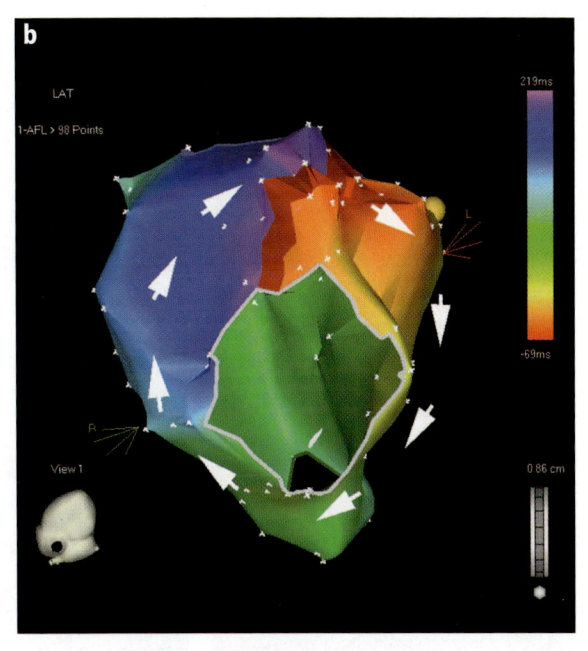

**Fig. 2a, b.** Activation map of the right atrium during typical counter-clockwise isthmus-dependent atrial flutter with a cycle length of 290 ms in left anterior oblique (LAO) (**a**) and inferior (**b**) views. In (**a**), the distribution of the rainbow of colours around the tricuspid annulus indicates the reentry course in the direction indicated by the *arrows*. Equal colour distribution around the tricuspid annulus and the inferior vena cava (**b**) indicates the presence of a double-loop reentry, counter-clockwise around the tricuspid annulus and clockwise around the inferior vena cava os. The mid-diastolic isthmus is where the "head" (in *red*) of the circuit encounters its "tail" (in *purple*) in a classic "head-meets-tail" pattern. Here, as expected, the mid-diastolic isthmus is located in the cavotricuspid isthmus. It is highlighted by the *dark red band*, which is automatically interposed between the red and purple colours when the "early meets late" option is active. The sum of the absolute values at the top and at the bottom of the colour band is 288 ms and indicates that 99.3% of the tachycardia cycle has been mapped

when the "early meets late" option is active. An example of a macroreentry activation map is shown in Fig. 2, where the electroanatomic activation pattern of a typical counter-clockwise isthmus-dependent atrial flutter sustained by double-loop reentry (one counter-clockwise around the tricuspid annulus and one clockwise around the inferior vena cava os) is shown. After high-density mapping in the area of the mid-diastolic isthmus to accurately define its boundaries, the isthmus extension between the two boundaries is calculated–a step that is of crucial importance for ablation.

## Propagation Map

Although the propagation map is derived from the activation map, the progression of the red band in the animated videoclip created in this type of map allows a better and more intuitive way to analyse the wavefront in a single- or double-chamber view. Usually, the size of the red band expressing propagation is manually set at 20 ms.

In a focal arrhythmia, the propagation map clearly shows a centrifugally spreading propagation pattern, beginning at the earliest activated site. In this type of arrhythmia, it may be of interest to analyse propagation in the first 10–15 ms in order to determine the size of the focal rhythm's site of origin, which may not be clearly displayed by the fusion of red-orange colours in the activation map. Differences in the early phase of propagation from two different structures, such as a perisinus focal atrial tachycardia and the sinus node, are described in Case 1.

In macroreentrant tachycardias, the propagation map allows careful analysis of the reentry course, from the mid-diastolic isthmus (identified by the dark red band) along its circuit until it

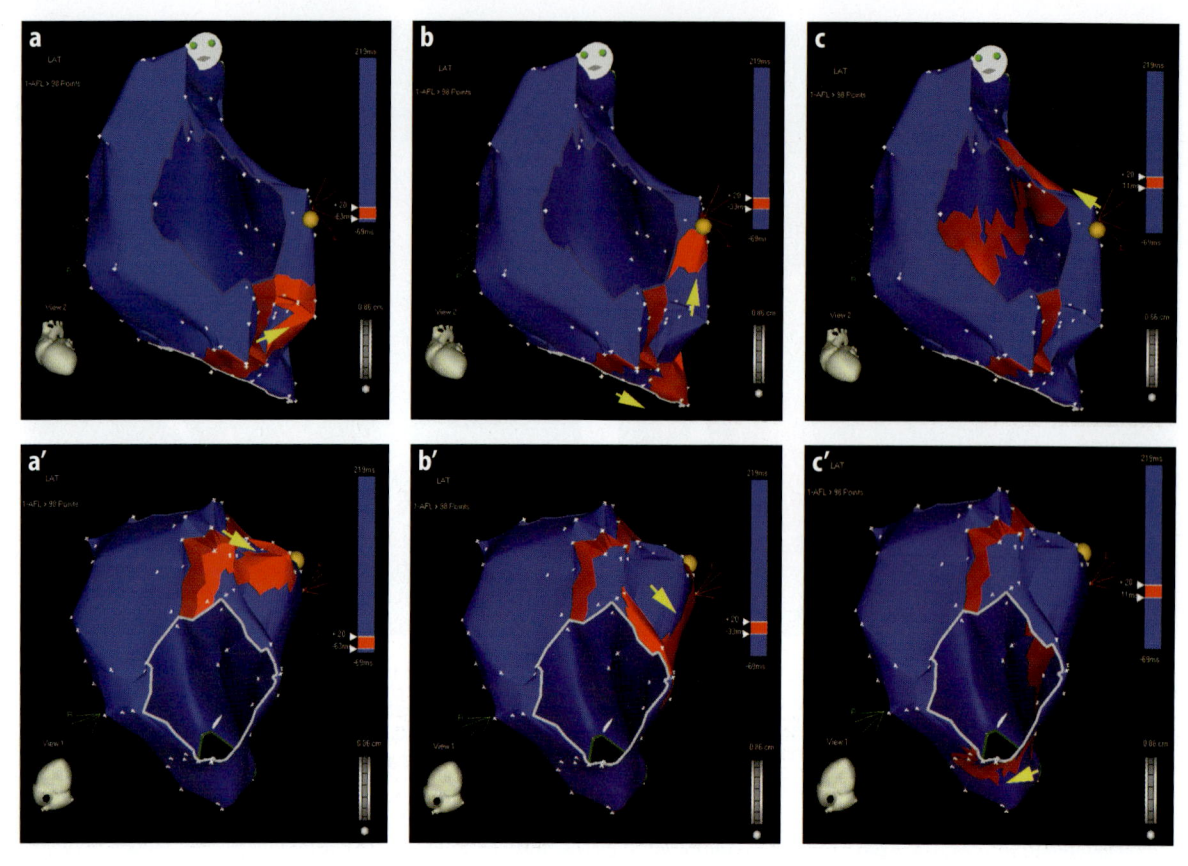

**Fig. 3a–f'.** Sequential frames of the propagation map of the right atrium during typical counter-clockwise isthmus-dependent atrial flutter, already shown in Fig. 2 as an activation map, in LAO (**a–f**) and inferior (**a'–f'**) views. The site of the mid-diastolic isthmus is still shown by the fixed *dark red band*. The propagation is visualised by the moving *light red band*, indicated by ▶

returns to the mid-diastolic area. When multiple reentrant loops are suspected, careful evaluation of the wavefront upon its exit from the mid-diastolic isthmus is required to detect splitting of the loops, as discussed in a case of right double-loop reentry (Case 8) and in a case of left double-loop reentry (Case 9). A double-loop reentry is present when activation along each loop spans >90% of the tachycardia cycle length. An example of the propagation map in the same counter-clockwise isthmus-dependent atrial flutter presented in Fig. 2 is given in Fig. 3, where the presence of the two loops (counter-clockwise around the tricuspid annulus and clockwise around the inferior vena cava) is very clearly shown.

## Use of Entrainment

Reports on the use of transient entrainment [4] with evaluation of the post-pacing interval [5] have been seminal in the study of reentrant rhythms. However, the systematic use of entrainment mapping to define the reentry course and the ablation target in macroreentrant atrial tachycardia and flutter has several limitations and thus has not been widely employed in highly qualified centres [6–9]. In fact, since entrainment stimulation may cause arrhythmia termination or degeneration into atrial fibrillation, or cannot be performed because of the lack of electrical capture in the tested site, this technique may not be able to correctly define the critical isthmus. Moreover, chronic antiarrhythmic drug therapy can alter electrical conduction properties and

the *arrows*. Counter-clockwise and clockwise propagation around the tricuspid annulus and the os of the inferior vena cava, respectively, is evident

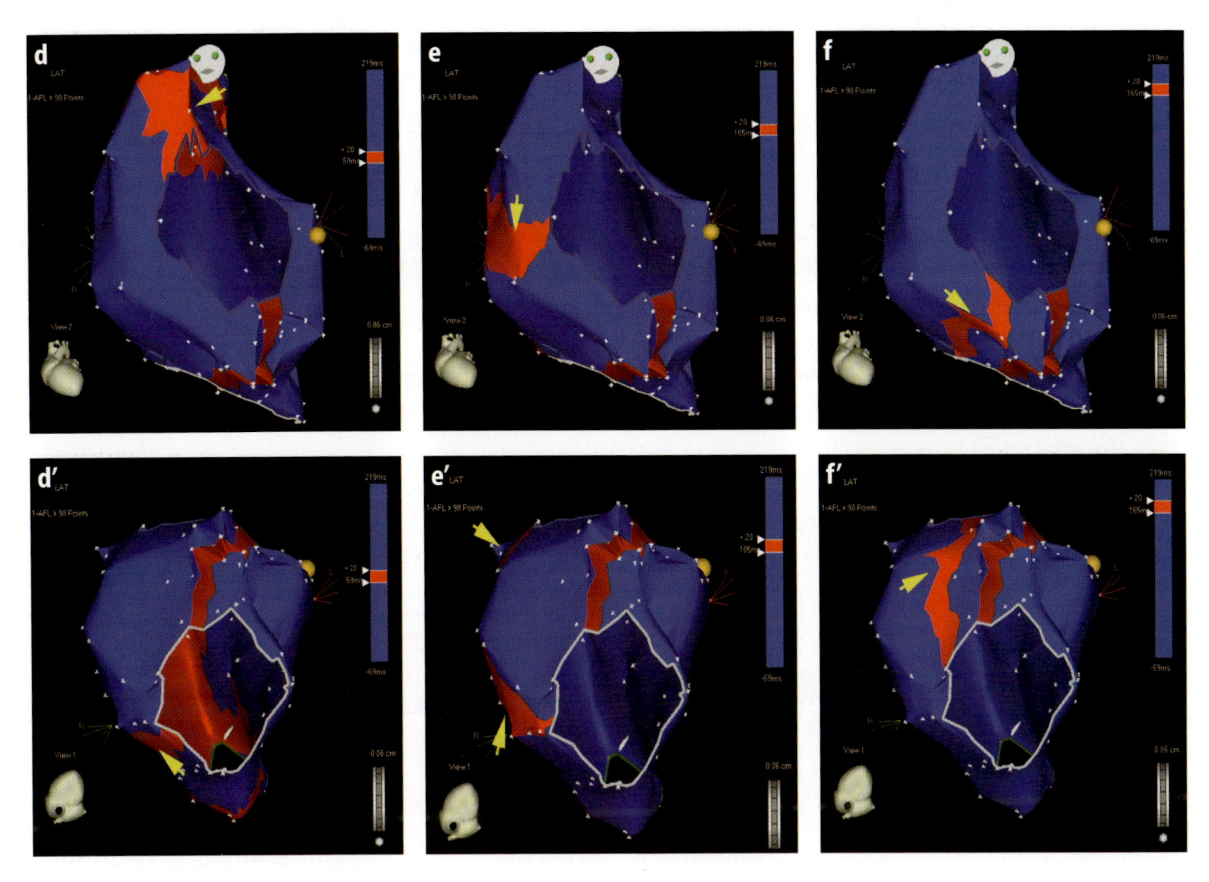

thus the response to entrainment. In fact, in patients with typical isthmus-dependent atrial flutter receiving amiodarone [10], entrainment in the cavo-tricuspid isthmus resulted in a post-pacing interval exceeding the atrial flutter cycle length by > 20 ms in 37% of the cases; the maximum value was 65 ms. Finally, due to the extension of the critical isthmus, entrainment mapping "per se" has a low positive predictive value for defining a single successful ablation site [11].

In our recently published paper [3], 81 morphologies of atrial macroreentrant tachycardia were electroanatomically mapped using the above-described setting of the window of interest. Entrainment mapping confirmed the critical role of the isthmus identified by electroanatomic mapping in all the cases in which this approach could be tested, accounting for 51% of the morphologies. In the remaining morphologies, electrical stimulation resulted in no capture (15%) or arrhythmia termination (6%), or was not performed (28%) due to the risk of arrhythmia degeneration or tachycardia cycle-length instability after catheter positioning in the mid-diastolic isthmus. Nevertheless, the ablation results were independent from entrainment mapping validation. Even in patients not subjected to entrainment mapping, the mid-diastolic isthmus could be identified based on electroanatomic mapping alone by using the specific setting of the window of interest and was successfully ablated with tachycardia termination in the vast majority of cases.

Based on this experience and previous considerations, entrainment mapping was not systematically used to define the target area for ablation in the cases reported in this book. The results of the sporadic use of entrainment mapping are reported for the respective cases.

## Voltage Map

Only bipolar voltage maps are shown in this book and they serve to discriminate areas of low voltage from areas of preserved voltage. Since unipolar recordings are more susceptible to far-field electrical activity, in accordance with previously published data [12], they were considered not suitable for this purpose. Based on our previous experience, corroborated by recently published reports [13, 14], the cut-off value between low voltage and preserved voltage was fixed at 0.5 mV. Areas with values between 0.1 and 0.05 mV, although of very low voltage, were still considered electrically active and, consequently, their activation was annotated. Every effort was made to precisely define the border between an electrically silent area (voltage < 0.05 mV) and the surrounding, still-viable tissue, although the Carto system tends to magnify the size of the area annotated as scar.

In some of the cases reported in this book, the voltage in the area targeted for ablation was taken into account. Usually, areas with voltages > 1.5–2.0 have been found, both in our experience and in previous reports [15], to be more resistant to ablation, even when an irrigated-tip catheter is used.

## Conduction Velocity and Measurement of the Length of the Reentrant Pathway

As recently reported [16], the wavefront propagation velocity in electroanatomic maps can be accurately calculated using a novel algorithm; however, it is not yet available in the present software version. Nevertheless, a qualitative and quantitative estimate of the conduction velocities on the electroanatomic map can still be obtained. According to previous studies [16, 17], normal conduction velocity ranges between 60 and 115 cm/s, whereas values below 40 cm/s definitively identify areas of slow conduction.

Qualitatively, areas of slow conduction are depicted by the crowding of isochronal lines in the activation map or by narrowing of the 20 ms red band in the propagation map. Quantitatively, the conduction velocity can be estimated by dividing the distance by the activation time interval between two points. However, great care should be used in choosing these points, and only adjacent points (less than 20 mm apart) in line with the propagation wavefront and in a non-curvilinear part of the heart chamber should be considered. If two points located in an oblique or perpendicular direction with respect to one of the propagation wavefronts are considered, this will cause overestimation of the actual conduction velocity, since the activation times of these two points reflect their almost simultaneous activation rather than being the result of sequential activation by the propagating wavefront. The direction of the propagating wavefront can by visualised on the electroanatomic map by evaluating the direction of the 20-ms red band in the propagation map or the course of the 5 to 10 ms isochronal lines in the activation map. If an area in the heart chamber with a marked curvature is considered, the true conduction velocity will be underestimated, since the Carto system underestimates the actual distance by giving the direct distance between the two points and does not consider the curvilinear surface. In the section of this book dealing with macroreentrant tachycardia, conduction velocity was calculated both in the mid-diastolic isthmus and in three segments of the outer loop. In spite of the above-mentioned methodological limitations, these data can well-estimate the real values in these cases. It is interesting to note that, in our experience, very slow conduction is present in the mid-diastolic isthmus in the vast majority of patients, whereas higher/normal conduction velocities are found along the outer loop.

Estimates of the length of the reentrant circuit can be obtained by using the area measure-

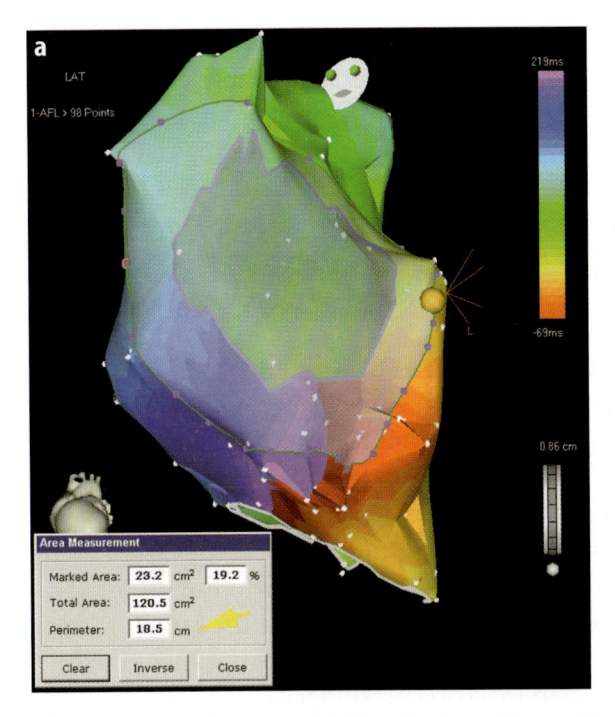

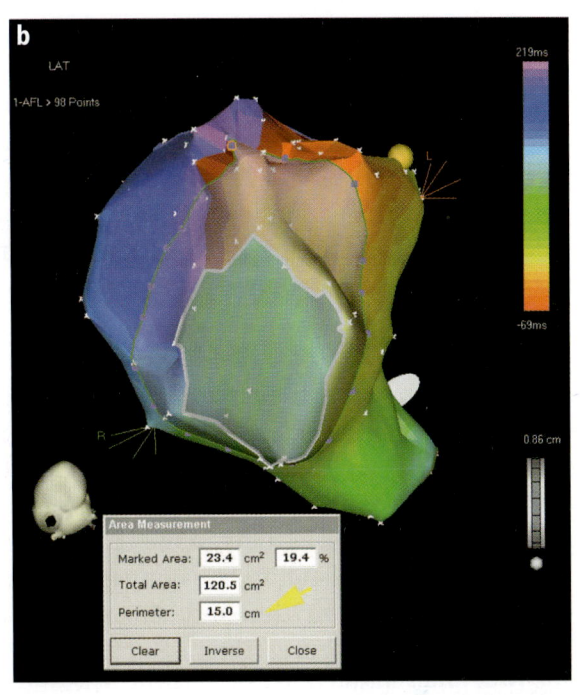

**Fig. 4a, b.** Activation map, with 12-ms isochronal lines, of the right atrium during the same atrial flutter shown in the previous figures, in caudal LAO (**a**) and inferior (**b**) views. To estimate the length of the reentrant pathway, points are distributed for each of the rainbow of colours to create a line that perpendicularly crosses the isochronal lines, both around the tricuspid annulus (**a**) and the inferior vena cava os (**b**), in this double-loop reentry. As evident in (**a**) and (**b**), the length of the reentrant pathway is not necessarily the shortest anatomical route around the central obstacle. The *arrow* indicates the length of the pathway for each loop, as automatically calculated by the software

ment option, which automatically calculates the perimeter of a given area demarcated by multiple points. As shown in Fig. 4, on the activation map with 10- to 15-ms isochronal lines, the points are distributed for each colour, so that the shortest course of the reentrant pathway can be calculated by using the line connecting the points, that is perpendicular to the isochronal lines. In the case of the double-loop reentry shown in Fig. 4, as well as in other cases presented in this book, differences in the length of the reentrant pathway may be observed between the two loops. Accordingly, different conduction velocities along the two loops are a key element in their synchronisation to create the classic "figure-of-eight" pattern.

## Ablation Strategy

Most of the cases presented in this book involve the use of an open-circuit irrigated-tip catheter for ablation. This is not surprising considering the predominance of left atrial arrhythmias and complex substrates. Both for safety and for efficacy reasons, the use of non-irrigated-tip catheters in the left atrium and in enlarged atrial chambers is strongly discouraged. In this book, the power and duration of ablation varied from case to case; therefore, the respective values have been specified in each case. Conversely, the irrigation flow rate was set for each case at 20 ml/s for power settings below 30 W and 30 ml/s for power settings between 30 and 50 W.

In extrapulmonary focal forms of arrhythmia, the ablation strategy was aimed at the earliest activated area after its accurate definition. In focal atrial tachycardia located inside a pulmonary vein (Cases 4 and 5), the latter was electrically disconnected by circumferential ostial ablation, with the disappearance/dissociation of the pulmonary vein's electrical activity.

In macroreentrant arrhythmias, the mid-diastolic isthmus was the ablation target. In our experience [3] this site is the weakest part of the reentrant circuit, generally exhibiting low-amplitude potentials and slow conduction velocities. When an irrigated-tip catheter is used, the number of applications–and, hence, the difficulty in arrhythmia ablation–correlates with isthmus extension, the value of which is significantly higher in the subset of patients undergoing unsuccessful ablation than in those with successful ablation [3]. On occasion (Case 19), targeting the mid-diastolic isthmus may not be the most convenient strategy. In these exceptional cases an alternative strategy is required. Thus, in this book the ablation strategy is indicated for each case and widely discussed when necessary.

Based on previous data [15], the ablation end-point in macroreentrant arrhythmias is conduction block across the target isthmus. However, especially in cases involving the left atrium, this may not be easily demonstrated. In some patients, a clear uninterrupted line of double potentials (Case 8) and/or modification of the activation at electroanatomic mapping consistent with a line of conduction block (Case 13) can be demonstrated. In others, only the disappearance of the electrical activity in the target area is observed in relation to: (1) the location of the isthmus, (2) the possibility of having an activation wavefront perpendicular to the line of ablation either in sinus rhythm or during pacing, and (3) the very low voltage of the target isthmus and the surrounding area. Interestingly, in one of these cases (Case 3) demonstration of the conduction block along the mid-diastolic isthmus of a left macroreentrant tachycardia was possible only during a focal atrial tachycardia originating from the left atrial roof, induced after successful ablation of the reentrant form.

After arrhythmia has been interrupted and ablation completed, induction of arrhythmia by programmed electrical stimulation with multiple extrastimuli and bursts is attempted. This is done with the aim of checking the inducibility of: (1) the index form, if the procedural end-point is not clearly achieved, and (2) a new tachycardia morphology. If an organised arrhythmia is not inducible 30 min following the termination of ablation, the procedure is terminated and considered acutely successful. If a new morphology with stable cycle length is reproducibly inducible, the arrhythmia is usually mapped and considered for ablation.

## References

1. Gepstein L, Hayam G, Ben-Haim SA. A novel method for nonfluoroscopic catheter-based electroanatomic mapping of the heart. In vitro and in vivo accuracy results. Circulation 1997; 95: 1611-1622
2. Kautzner J, Pedersen AK, Peichl P. Basic principles of electro-anatomic mapping. In: Kautzner J, Pedersen AK, Peichl P (eds) Electro-anatomic mapping of the heart: an illustrated guide to the use of the CARTO system. Remedica, London, 2006; pp. 2-30
3. De Ponti R, Verlato R, Bertaglia E et al. Treatment of macroreentrant atrial tachycardia based on electroanatomic mapping: identification and ablation of the mid-diastolic isthmus. Europace 2007; 9: 1449-457
4. Waldo AL. From bedside to bench: entrainment and other stories. Heart Rhythm 2004; 1: 94-106
5. Stevenson WG, Khan H, Sager P et al. Identification of reentry circuit sites during catheter mapping and radiofrequency ablation of ventricular tachycardia late after myocardial infarction. Circulation 1993; 88: 1647-1670
6. Jaïs P, Shah DC, Haïssaguerre M et al. Mapping and ablation of left atrial flutters. Circulation 2000; 101: 2928-2934
7. Shah D, Jaïs P, Takahashi A et al. Dual-loop intra-atrial reentry in humans. Circulation 2000; 101: 631-639
8. Stevenson IH, Kistler PM, Spence SJ et al. Scar-related right atrial macroreentrant tachycardia in patients without prior atrial surgery: electroanatomic characterization and ablation outcome. Heart Rhythm 2005; 2: 594-601
9. Magnin-Poull I, De Chillou C, Miljoen H et al. Mechanism of right atrial tachycardia occurring late af-

ter surgical closure of atrial septal defects. J Cardiovasc Electrophysiol 2005; 16: 681-687
10. Fatemi M, Mansourati J, Rosu R, Blanc JJ. Value of entrainment mapping in determining the isthmus-dependent nature of atrial flutter in the presence of amiodarone. J Cardiovasc Electrophysiol 2004; 15: 1409-1415
11. Triedman JK, Alexander ME, Berul CI et al. Electroanatomic mapping of entrained and exit zones in patients with repaired congenital heart disease and intra-atrial reentrant tachycardia. Circulation. 2001; 103: 2060-2065
12. De Groot NMS, Schalij MJ, Zeppenfeld K et al. Voltage and activation mapping: how the recordings technique affects the outcome of catheter ablation preprocedures in patients with congenital heart disease. Circulation 2003; 108: 2099-2106
13. Sanders P, Morton JB, Kistler PM et al. Electrophysiological and electroanatomic characterization of the atrial in sinus node disease: evidence of diffuse atrial remodeling. Circulation 2004; 109: 1514-1522
14. Marcus GM, Yang Y, Varosy PD et al. Regional left atrial voltage in patients with atrial fibrillation. Heart Rhythm 2007: 4: 138-144
15. Ouyang F, Ernst S, Vogtmann T et al. Characterization of reentrant circuits in left atrial macroreentrant tachycardia: critical isthmus block can prevent atrial tachycardia recurrence. Circulation 2002; 105: 1934-1942
16. Kojodjojo P, Kanagaratnam P, Markides V et al. Age-related changes in human left and right atrial conduction. J Cardiovasc Eletrophysiol 2006; 17: 120-127
17. Harrild DM, Henriquez CS. A computer model of normal conduction in the human atria. Circ Res 2000; 87: e25-e36

# Part I

# Focal Atrial Arrhythmias

# Case 1
# Focal Atrial Tachycardia in the Right Atrium in a Postsurgical Patient: Rare but Possible

## Case Presentation

This is a 43-year-old male patient who, at the age of 15, underwent surgery for tetralogy of Fallot and tricuspid valvuloplasty for associated Ebstein disease. Ten years later, he began complaining of palpitations, which became more frequently recurrent and drug refractory, so that in 1999 he underwent an electrophysiology procedure in our institution. At the time of our initial observations, a description of the surgical intervention was unavailable. However, clinical atrial tachycardia at a cycle length of 440 ms was reproducibly inducible and it was diagnosed as an intraatrial macroreentrant tachycardia, with the critical isthmus of slow conduction located between the coronary sinus os and the inferior vena cava. Limited radiofrequency energy delivery in that region suppressed the tachycardia. No other tachycardia was inducible thereafter. Of interest, conventional mapping during sinus rhythm showed two vertical lines of double potentials along the septum and the anterolateral right atrium, likely related to surgical incisions/sutures. Moreover, during programmed atrial stimulation, conduction delay over the anterolateral right atrial wall, where a 20-pole catheter had been placed, was observed. In this area, preserved voltage amplitude was present at that time. The patient remained asymptomatic until February 2004, when recurrence of the palpitations was documented at electrocardiogram as the arrhythmia shown in Fig. 1. Since the QRS complex was superimposable with the one recorded on sinus rhythm, the supraventricular origin of the arrhythmia was clear; however, the wide QRS complex due to right bundle branch block did not allow analysis of P wave morphology. Adenosine injection reproducibly terminated the tachycardia, so that the surface electrocardiogram did not facilitate determination of its origin. During subsequent hospital admission, the patient experienced multiple drug-refractory recurrences of the arrhythmia and therefore underwent electrophysiologic evaluation.

## Procedure

At baseline, a non-sustained form of the clinical tachycardia with 1:1 atrioventricular conduction was present; it became sustained, with a cycle length of 290 ms, during isoprenaline infusion. Based on the arrhythmia's presentation and its response to isoprenaline infusion, a focal origin of the tachycardia was expected; therefore, the window of interest was set accordingly. Electroanatomic mapping was performed during atrial tachycardia and re-mapped during transient sinus rhythm, with a coronary sinus atriogram as reference signal. Surprisingly, early in

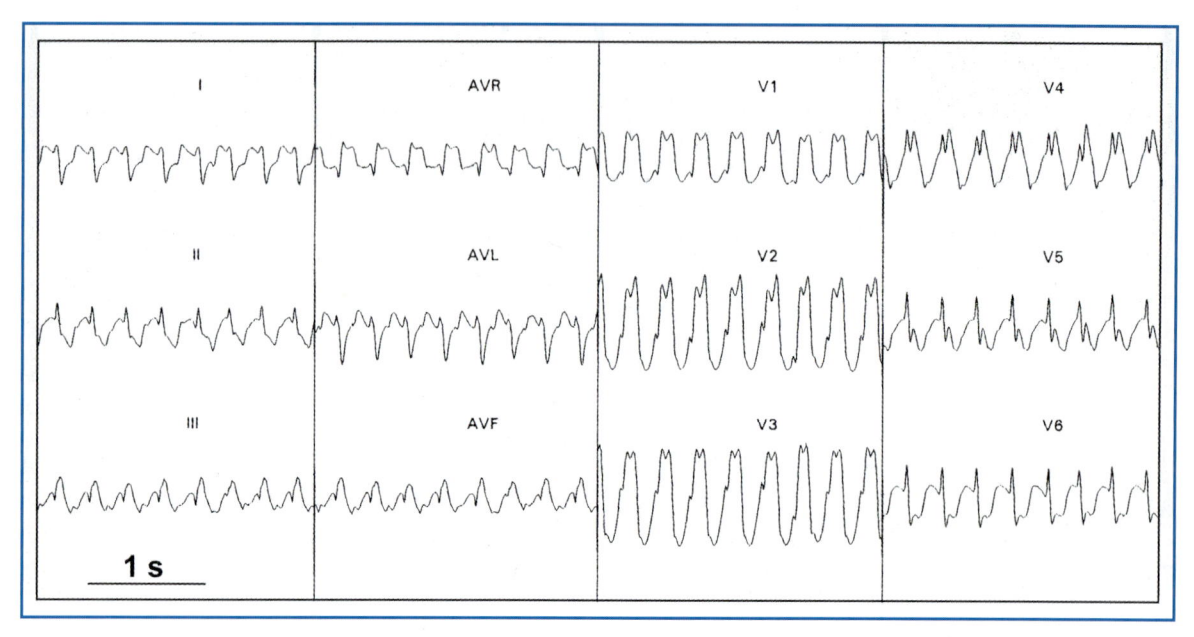

**Fig. 1.** Twelve-lead electrocardiogram of the clinical atrial tachycardia. The cycle length was 290 ms. The wide QRS complex with a right bundle branch block is superimposible on that in sinus rhythm and does not allow visualisation of the P wave

the mapping procedure, the complete absence of electrical activity in a wide area of the right atrium, which included the anterolateral wall, the cavotricuspid isthmus, and part of the posterior wall, became apparent (Fig. 2a). While a line of double potentials was still recorded along the atrial septum (Fig. 2b), in the anterolateral area, where the second line of double potentials was recorded at conventional mapping five years earlier, electrical activity was completely absent. Analysis of the evidence obtained from activation mapping showed that, during tachycardia, right atrial activation lasted 148 ms, equal to 51% of the tachycardia cycle length. In addition, a centrifugally spreading activation pattern originated from the earliest site, which was located on the crest of the right appendage, where the bipolar recording preceded the coronary sinus atriogram by 252 ms and the unipolar one showed a rapid downstroke. Even in the absence of identification of P wave onset, this finding confirmed that the focal tachycardia originated from this site. As shown in Fig. 2b, a later activation of the atrial septum and of the insertion of Bachmann's bundle in the right atrium excluded a left-to-right atrial propagation, as is the case in a left-sided arrhythmia. Analysis of the voltage mapping during tachycardia (Fig. 3) evidenced that the tachycardia focus was located in an area of low voltage (<0.5 mV), at the border zone between the area with preserved voltage and the scar tissue. Electroanatomic mapping on sinus rhythm (Fig. 4) allowed measurement of the distance between the tachycardia focus and the sinus node to assess possible damage to sinus-node function due to ablation. In this case, the distance was 16 mm; therefore, the ablation was considered safe. Although the tachycardia focus was adjacent to the sinus-node area, analysis of propagation mapping of the two rhythms yielded two distinct patterns. In fact, as shown in Fig. 5a-c, in the first 20 ms of activation, the tachycardia focus propagated from a single spot of very limited extension, with a clear centrifugally spreading pattern. Conversely, activation during sinus rhythm (Fig. 5a'-c') showed a "multispot" pattern, with multiple distinct sites exhibiting similarly early activation times, which resulted in a larger area activated in a shorter time than was the case for the tachycardia focus. Radiofrequency energy delivery at the earliest activated site using an irrigated-tip catheter (maximum power 40 Watts, cut-off temperature 43°C, duration 45 s) produced early and sudden tachycar-

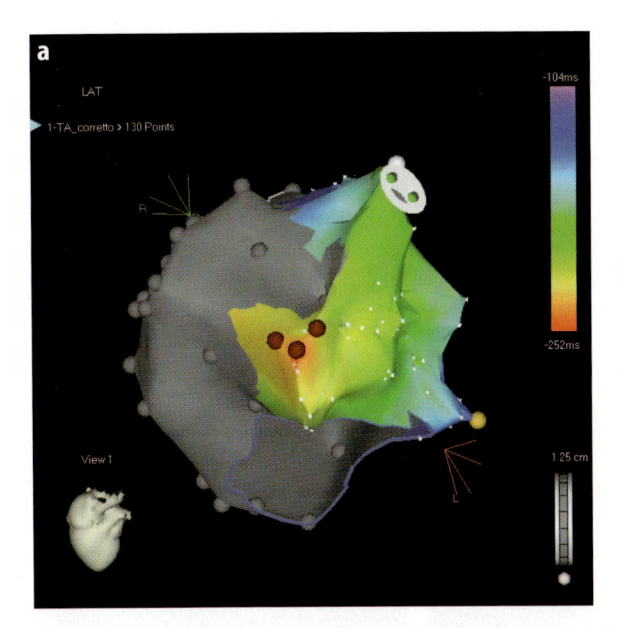

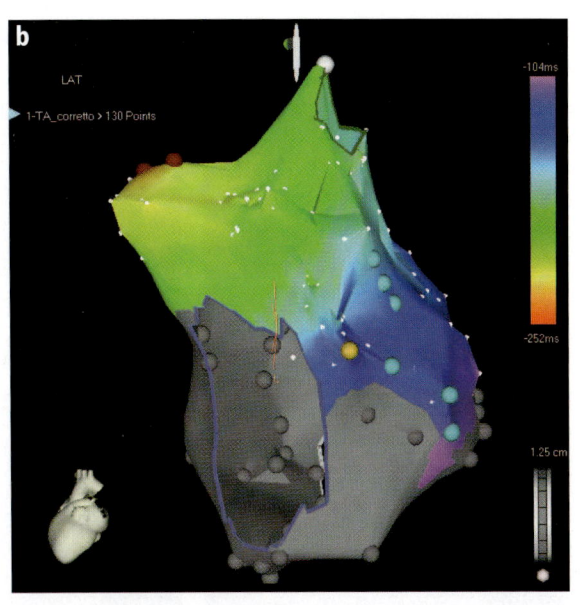

**Fig. 2a, b.** Activation mapping of the right atrium during atrial tachycardia in a cranial left anterior oblique (LAO) projection (**a**) and a left lateral view (**b**). The electrically silent areas are marked in *grey*; the *orange dot* identifies the His-bundle area. The earliest activated site (*in red*) is at the crest of the right appendage, where ablation was performed (central *red dot* corresponds to the effective application; the other two dots indicate bonus applications on sinus rhythm). Moreover, in *b*, prior atriotomy is evident as a vertical line of double potentials (*blue dots*) along the atrial septum

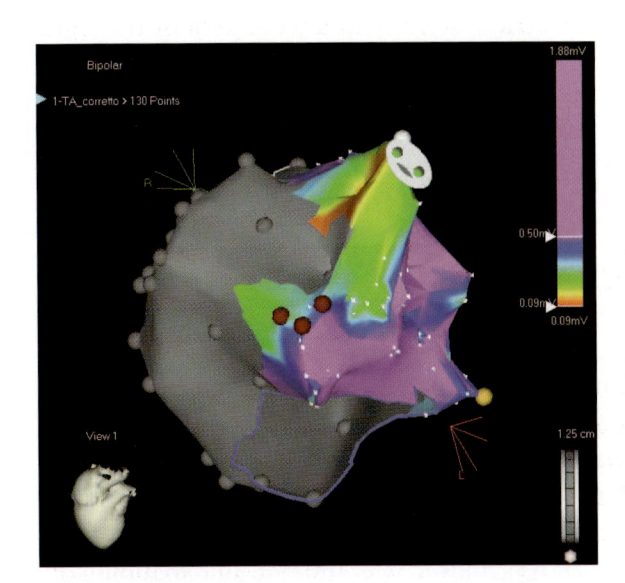

**Fig. 3.** Bipolar voltage mapping of the right atrium during tachycardia in a cranial LAO projection. The lower voltage is 0.09 mV. Areas showing a voltage amplitude >0.5 mV are identified in *purple*

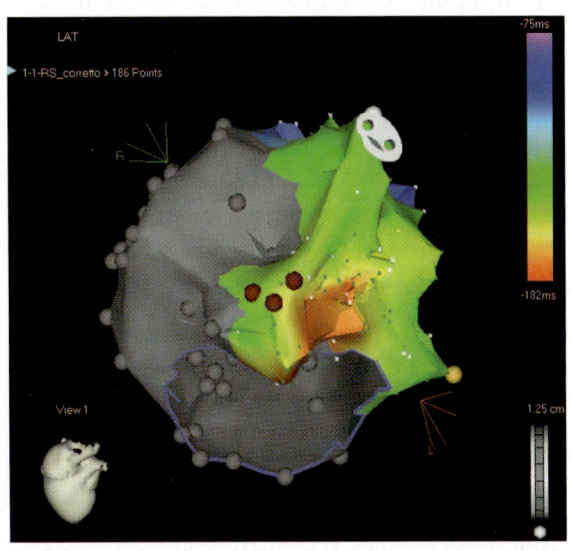

**Fig. 4.** Activation mapping of the right atrium during remapping in sinus rhythm in a cranial LAO projection. Ablation sites have been copied onto this map. The distance between the tachycardia focus and the earliest activated sites in the sinus node area, evident as a relatively large red area, is 16 mm

dia termination, with no sign of damage to sinus-node function. Two other applications, on sinus rhythm, were then delivered just superiorly and inferiorly to the tachycardia focus (Fig. 2a). Afterwards, the tachycardia was no longer inducible even by aggressive programmed electrical stimulation during isoprenaline infusion at the maximal rate, and no other spontaneous ar-

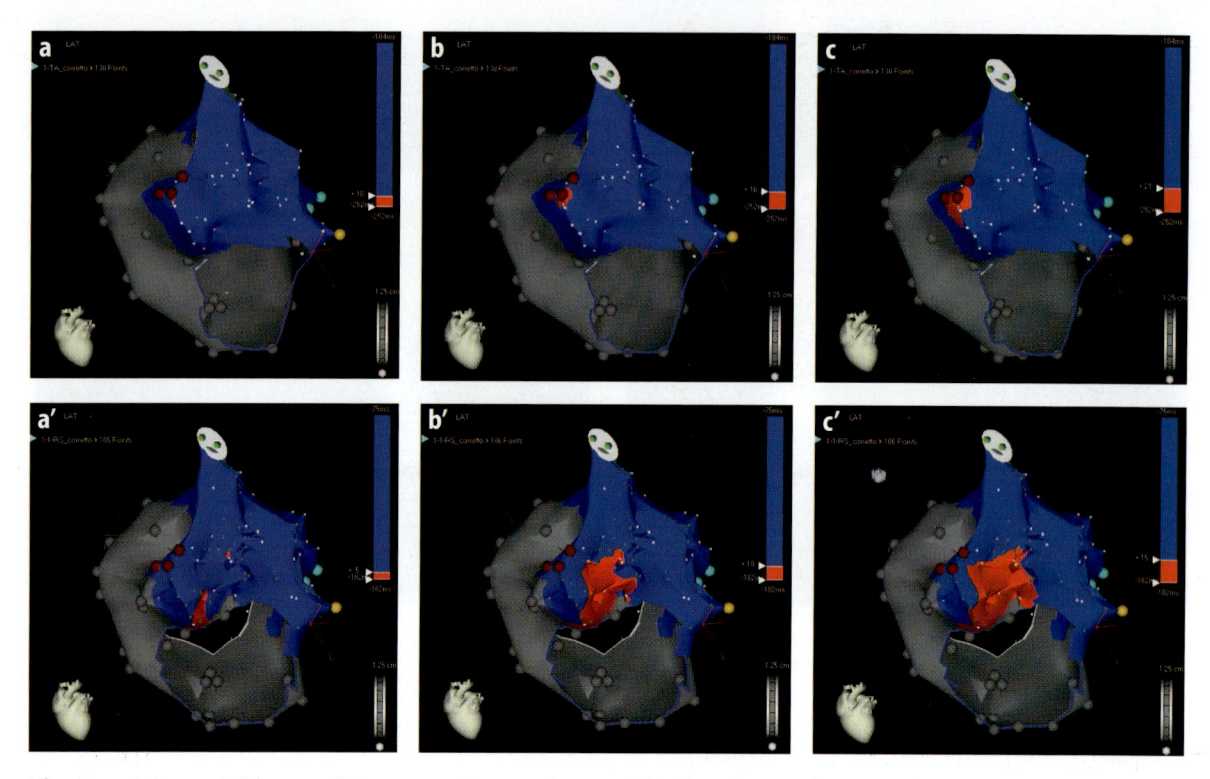

**Fig. 5a–c'.** Sequential frames of the propagation map in a cranial LAO projection during atrial tachycardia (**a–c**) and sinus rhythm (**a'–c'**). The single spot pattern during tachycardia is in contrast to the "multispot" pattern of activation during sinus rhythm; the latter results in activation of a larger area in a shorter time

rhythmia was observed. During a 3-year follow-up, the patient continued the previously ineffective antiarrhythmic agent (low-dose sotalol) and was arrhythmia-free.

## Commentary

Although in patients who have undergone previous cardiac surgery the more frequently expected mechanism of atrial arrhythmias is macroreentry, focal atrial tachycardia in postsurgical patients has been reported [1–8]. In this case, the presence of a focal mechanism could be expected based on iterative presentation of the arrhythmia at baseline and becoming sustained during isoprenaline infusion, without the need for induction by electrical stimulation. As shown in Table 1, focal atrial tachycardia generally accounts for less than 15% of the overall morphologies of atrial tachycardias in series of postsurgical patients. Interestingly, in the majority of these patients the tachycardia focus is located in the anterolateral wall of the right atrium. In such cases, including the present one, it has to be determined whether the finding of a focal atrial tachycardia focus at the border between scar and viable tissue, in an area relatively close to the sinus node and crista terminalis, is casual or due to a cause-effect relationship between degenerative phenomena in this area and tachycardia onset.

The difficulty of this case relies both on the complex anatomy, with wide electrically silent areas requiring precise definition at electroanatomic mapping, and on the absence of information provided by the P wave morphology at preablation evaluation, due to a wide QRS complex, an invariable 1:1 atrioventricular conduction during the arrhythmia and, possibly, the presence of low-voltage P waves related to extensive electrically silent areas in the atrial myocardium. Nev-

Table 1. Overview of focal atrial tachycardias reported in postsurgical patients

| Author | Year | Number of FAT morphologies | Location RA | Location LA | Prevalence of FAT in overall atrial tachycardia morphologies[a] |
|---|---|---|---|---|---|
| Ott [1] | 1995 | 1 | 1 | - | - |
| De Ponti [2] | 1999 | 1 | - | 1 | - |
| Leonelli [3] | 2001 | 11 | 9 | 2 | 35 |
| Shah [4] | 2002 | 1 | 1 | - | 3 |
| Markowitz [5] | 2002 | 3 | 2 | 1 | 27 |
| Zrenner [6] | 2003 | 2 | – | 2 | 13 |
| Nabar [7] | 2005 | 1 | - | 1 | 10 |
| Magnin-Poull [8] | 2005 | 1 | 1 | - | 4 |
| Overall | | 21 | 14 | 7 | 19 |

*FAT* Focal atrial tachycardia, *RA* right atrium, *LA* left atrium
[a] Not available for case reports.

ertheless, the information provided by electroanatomic mapping identified the tachycardia mechanism, excluded involvement of the left atrium, located precisely the arrhythmia focus, and calculated its distance from the sinus node. As a result, the ablation was safe as well as successful.

In this patient, the sinus-node activation pattern was similar to the one observed in normal human subjects [9], but the position of the sinus-node area was downward displaced, as it is commonly located in the high right posterolateral atrium, beneath the superior vena cava os, or in the superior part of the appendage crest, in subjects who had never undergone cardiac surgery. The findings in this case suggested migration of the site of earliest atrial activation during sinus rhythm, as a consequence of either prior surgery or a progressive degenerative process involving the atrial myocardium. The practical implication is that, before approaching right atrial arrhythmias in postsurgical patients, it is mandatory to precisely identify the position of the sinus-node area, which may have an unusual location. In such patients, in whom latent sinus-node dysfunction may be present, this precautionary step prevents inadvertent damage to the sinus node during ablation of focal or macroreentrant atrial tachycardias. Moreover, in our patient, the different propagation patterns of the atrial tachycardia compared to sinus rhythm were peculiar. In fact, in the former, the pattern was consistent with a single and very definite endocardial focus, which should be very sensitive to limited and focal ablation, as occurred in this case. In the latter, the pattern represented an endocardial projection of activation due to a more complex epicardial structure, such as the sinus node.

Finally, the extensive loss of atrial electrical activity seems to be a progressive process, as was concluded from the sequential invasive electrophysiologic evaluation of this patient, with the limitation that only conventional mapping was used in the initial procedure. The possibility of progression of this degenerative phenomenon is intriguing. However, its prevalence is difficult, if not impossible, to determine and its implication on atrial mechanical function remains a topic of further speculation.

# References

1. Ott P, Kelly PA, Mann DE et al. Tachycardia-induced cardiomyopathy in a cardiac transplant recipient: treatment with radiofrequency catheter ablation. J Cardiovasc Electrophysiol 1995; 6: 391-395.

2. De Ponti R, Zardini M, Tritto M et al. Non-fluorscopic system for three-dimensional electroanatomic cardiac mapping (CARTO). Cardiologia 1999; 44 (Suppl. I): 387-390.
3. Leonelli FM, Tomassoni G, Richey M, Natale A. Ablation of incisional atrial tachycardias using a three-dimensional nonfluoroscopic mapping system. Pacing Clin Electrophysiol 2001; 24: 1653-1659.
4. Shah D, Jaïs P, Haïssaguerre M. Electrophysiologic evaluation and ablation of atypical right atrial flutter. Card Electrophysiol Rev 2002; 6: 365-370.
5. Markowitz SM, Brodman RF, Stein KM et al. Lesional tachycardias related to mitral valve surgery. J Am Coll Cardiol 2002; 39: 1973-1983.
6. Zrenner B, Dong J, Schreieck J et al. Delineation of intra-atrial reentrant tachycardia circuits after Mustard operation for transposition of the great arteries using biatrial electroanatomic mapping and entrainment mapping. J Cardiovasc Electrophysiol 2003; 14:1302-1310.
7. Nabar A, Timmermans C, Medeiros A et al. Radiofrequency ablation of atrial arrhythmias after previous open-heart surgery. Europace 2005; 7: 40-49.
8. Magnin-Poull I, De Chillou C, Miljoen H et al. Mechanism of right atrial tachycardia occurring late after surgical closure of atrial septal defects. J Cardiovasc Electrophysiol 2005; 16: 681-687.
9. De Ponti R, Ho SY, Salerno-Uriarte JA et al. Electroanatomic analysis of sinus impulse propagation in normal human atria. J Cardiovasc Electrophysiol 2002; 13: 1-10.

# Case 2
# Focal Atrial Tachycardia in an Enlarged Right Atrium after Rastelli's Operation: Ambiguous Mapping Data in Conflict with the Orthodoxies

## Case Presentation

This is a 39-year-old female patient with transposition of the great vessels and ventricular septal defect. At the age of 5, she underwent Rastelli's operation at the Mayo Clinic. The surgical procedure included an external homograft conduit between the right ventricle and the pulmonary artery. Seven years later, she underwent another operation to replace the conduit. At the age of 35 years, she developed signs and symptoms of congestive heart failure, with enlargement of the right atrium and ventricle. Despite optimal medical therapy, she complained of palpitations due to atrial tachycardia and atrial fibrillation. The concomitant presence of life-threatening ventricular arrhythmias led to the implantation of a dual-chamber ICD. In the months prior to the procedure, despite therapy with amiodarone and beta-blockers, the patient developed atrial tachycardia of 400 ms cycle length with 1:1 atrioventricular conduction and incessant-iterative presentation. This accounted for severe functional limitations and worsening of heart failure. As shown in Fig. 1, two atrial tachycardia morphologies alternated with sinus rhythm/atrial pacing in this patient. The first, more prevalent morphology showed positive P waves in the inferior leads, whereas the second morphology had negative P waves in the same leads. However, the presence of a right bundle branch block and 1:1 atrioventricular conduction greatly complicated analysis of the P wave morphology and onset in all the twelve leads.

## Procedure

At baseline, with the patient under general anaesthesia, stable sinus rhythm was present. Antegrade atrioventricular node conduction properties were normal with right bundle branch block, while ventriculoatrial conduction was absent. During S2S3 programmed atrial stimulation during isoprenaline infusion, the prevalent clinical atrial tachycardia with positive P wave morphology in the inferior leads at a cycle length of 400 ms was reproducibly induced with 1:1 atrioventricular conduction. Electroanatomic mapping of the right atrium was initiated, with a coronary sinus atriogram as reference. A long sheath was used to support the mapping catheter because of the enlarged chamber size. As in the Case 1, the window of interest was set as for focal atrial tachycardia based on presentation of the arrhythmia. The entire mapping procedure was performed during 1:1 tachycardia, since any attempt to change the 1:1 atrioventricular conduction ratio during tachycardia, in order to better evaluate P wave morphology and onset, was unsuccessful or terminated the tachycardia. Despite optimal catheter to tissue contact, atrial

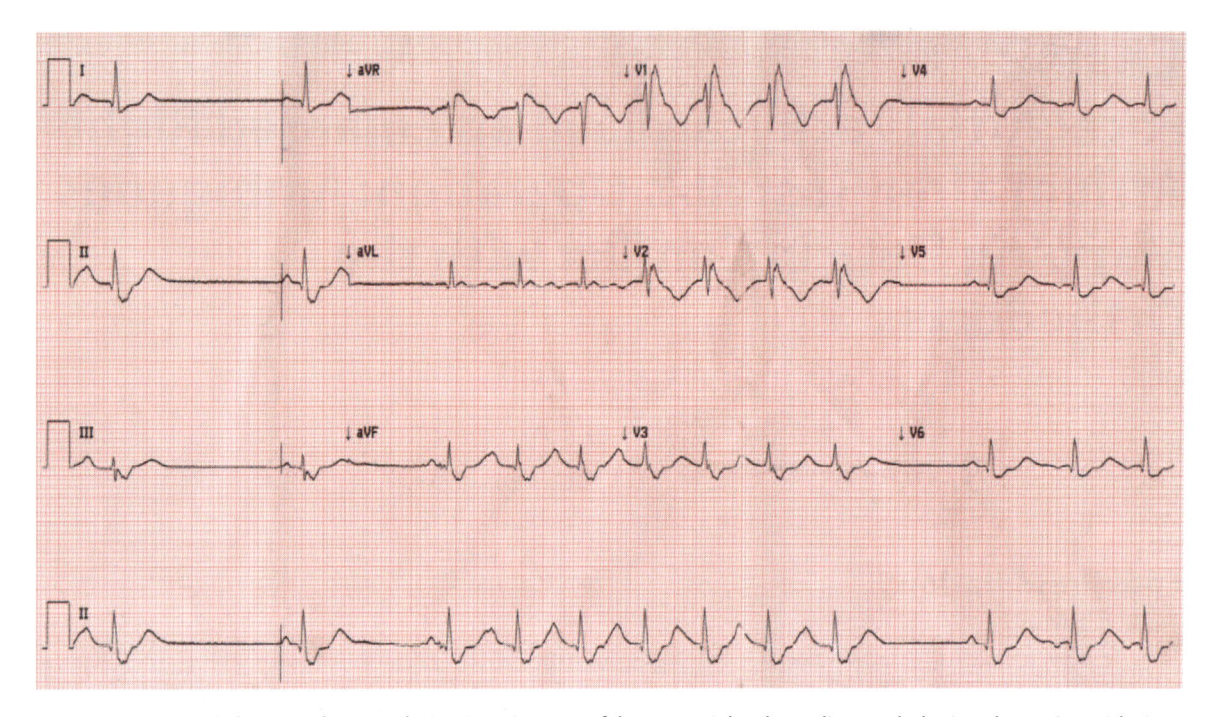

**Fig. 1.** Twelve-lead electrocardiogram during iterative runs of the two atrial tachycardia morphologies, alternating with sinus rhythm. The last tracing is a lead II rhythm strip: after termination of the previous run, an atrial-paced beat and a sinus beat are observed, followed by a 6-beat run of the prevalent tachycardia morphology. Then, after another sinus beat, two beats of the second tachycardia morphology (negative P waves) appear

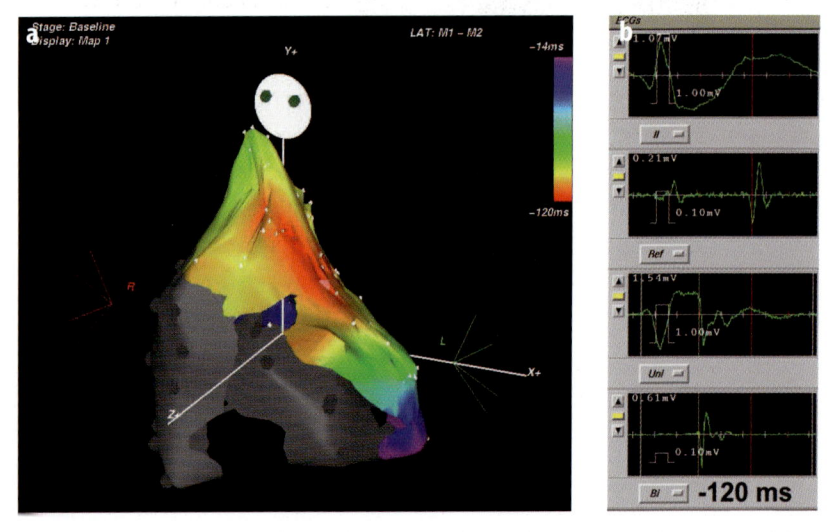

**Fig. 2a, b.** Activation mapping of the right atrium at the first step of mapping of the prevalent morphology of atrial tachycardia in cranial left anterior oblique (LAO) view (**a**) and electrical recordings (**b**) at the site tagged with the *pink dot* on the electroanatomic map. In these, as well as in the next figures, tracings show, from *top* to *bottom*, surface lead II, the coronary sinus signal used as reference, local unipolar and bipolar signals. The number at the bottom of b indicates the local activation time compared to the reference signal. Electrically silent areas are shown in *grey*. Peculiarly, at this phase of mapping, the data were conflicting. In fact, a wide area of earliest activation in the electroanatomic mapping in the medial right atrium could be interpreted as breakthrough from the left atrium, suggesting the presence of a left-sided arrhythmia, while the presence of a completely negative unipolar deflection favoured the hypothesis of a focus located in this site

electrical activity was absent in a vast area of the anterolateral and posterior walls of the right atrium, which, therefore, were tagged by grey dots. At the beginning of mapping (Fig. 2a), the earliest activated site was in the medial upper right atrium, where a bipolar signal with an amplitude of 0.61 mV preceded the reference signal by 120 ms (Fig. 2b). At the same site, a fast neg-

Case 2    23

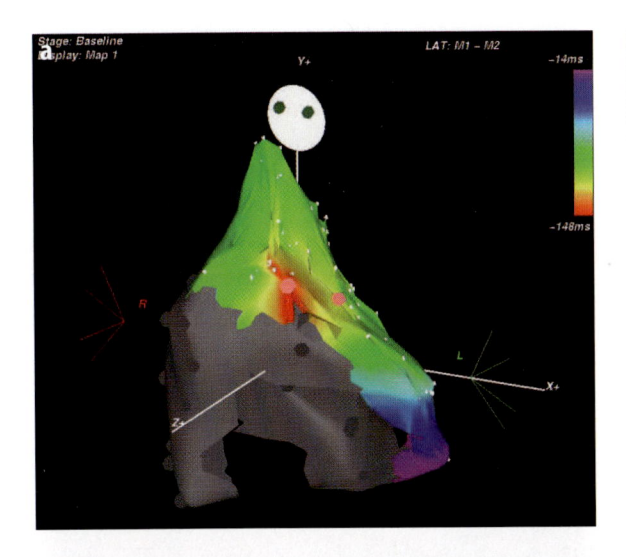

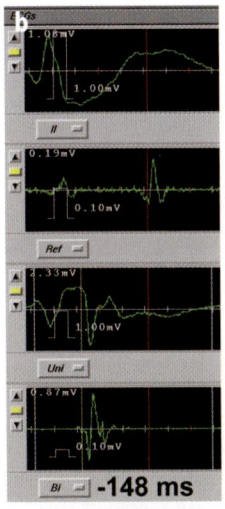

**Fig. 3a, b.** Activation mapping of the right atrium after further mapping of the prevalent morphology of atrial tachycardia in cranial LAO view (**a**) and electrical recordings (**b**) at a more anterior site, marked by the second *pink dot*. The activation map shows a more anterior and more definite area of earliest activation, while the unipolar signal is still negative at this site

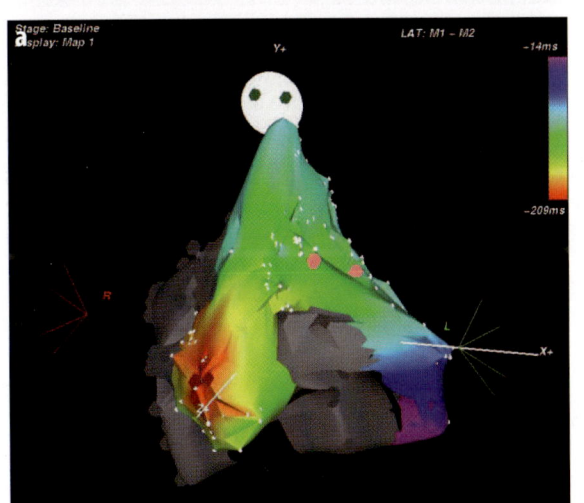

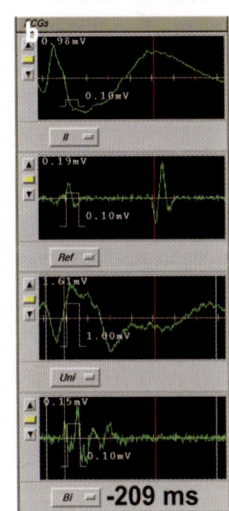

**Fig. 4a, b.** Activation mapping after almost complete reconstruction of the right atrium during the same morphology of atrial tachycardia, in cranial LAO view (**a**) and electrical recordings (**b**) at the site of successful ablation, identified by the red dots at the end of the channel of viable tissue between two electrically silent areas

ative initial unipolar deflection was recorded and a centrifugally spreading propagation pattern from this area was evident. At this point, these mapping data were ambiguous. On the one hand, completely negative unipolar deflection suggested that the distal electrode of the mapping catheter was positioned at the site of origin of a right-sided focal atrial tachycardia. On the other hand, a larger area of earliest activation in the upper medial right atrium may have been the result of left-to-right propagation of a left-sided arrhythmia. Since the geometry of the chamber appeared incomplete, especially in its anterosuperior area, mapping was continued. This revealed a more anterior site (Fig. 3a) that showed an earlier activation (-28 ms compared to the previous site) with a similar unipolar pattern and a bipolar amplitude of 0.87 mV (Fig. 3b). Mapping was continued from that site in an anterolateral direction, and a channel of very-low-amplitude bipolar signals between two areas of scar tissue (Fig. 4a) was thus identified. This led to the earliest activated site, which preceded the reference signal by 209 ms (Fig. 4b). At this site, the first component of unipolar deflection could not be accurately evaluated, since it was superimposed on the one from the previous ventricular beat. Although the bipolar signal at this site was inscribed in the previous QRS complex, its atrial nature was confirmed by a single ventricular extra-stimulus that anticipated the ventricular activity and dissociated the local atrial potential. Interestingly, analysis of the voltage map (Fig. 5) showed extremely low voltage (0.07–0.15 mV) along the channel leading to the tachycardia focus, located at the border zone between viable

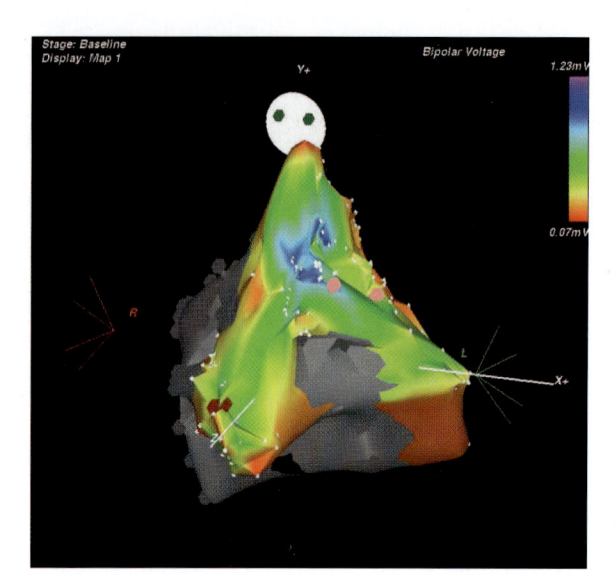

**Fig. 5.** Bipolar voltage mapping of the right atrium in the same view and rhythm as in Fig. 4a

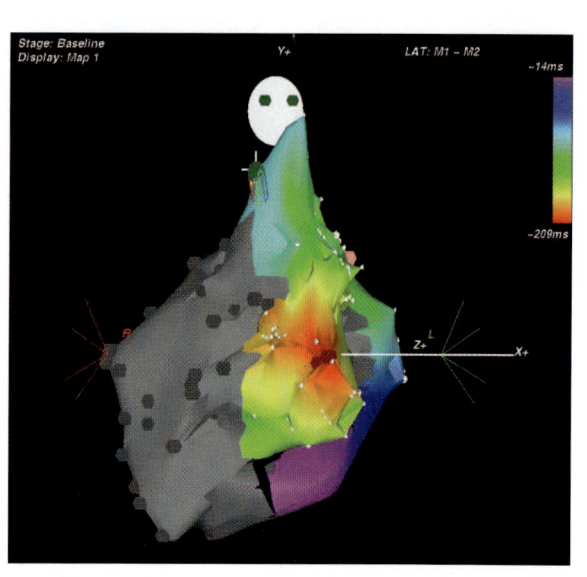

**Fig. 6.** Activation mapping of the right atrium during the prevalent morphology of atrial tachycardia in right anterior oblique (RAO) view. The relative position of the earliest activated site during sinus rhythm, identified by the catheter icon in a preacquired site, is compared to the tachycardia focus

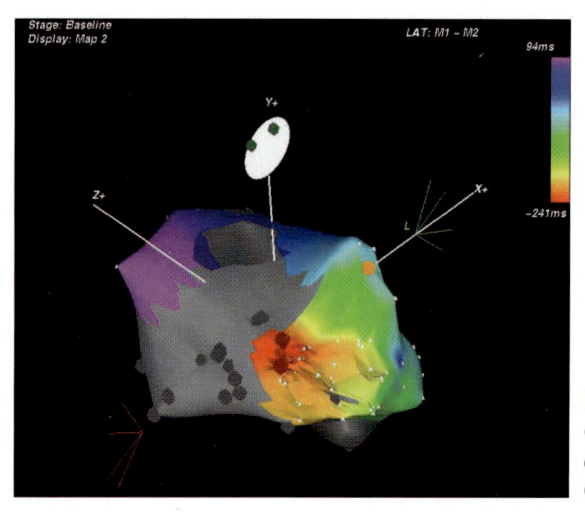

**Fig. 7.** Activation mapping of the right atrium during the second tachycardia morphology in a caudal LAO view. The *orange dot* identifies the His-bundle area. *Red dots* show sites of successful ablation

and scar tissue, whereas a preserved bipolar voltage (>0.5 mV) was observed at the channel exit. Based on the evidence obtained up to that point and the remote position of the sinus node, as previously assessed (Fig. 6), radiofrequency energy was delivered by cool-tip catheter (maximum power 30 W, cut-off temperature 45°C, duration 60 s). This produced early termination and complete suppression of the tachycardia. Subsequently, atrial tachycardia with a 500 ms cycle length and negative P wave in the inferior lead was reproducibly inducible. Accordingly, the tachycardia was mapped and the site of earliest activation was identified in the central part of the cavotricuspid isthmus (Fig. 7). Although a prolonged right atrial activation on tachycardia (335 ms, equal to 67% of the tachycardia cycle length) was present, also this tachycardia had a focal origin. In this morphology, the usual centrifugally spreading activation pattern from the earliest activated site was modified by the presence of a wide electrically silent area just lateral to the tachycardia focus. This prolonged the right atrial activation time and simulated a counter-clockwise loop around the tricuspid annulus. However, macroreentry was excluded by the lack of electrical activity in the area between the earliest and the latest activated sites. Limited radiofrequency energy delivery in the area of earliest activation with the same parameters as before resulted in persistent suppression of the tachycardia. During follow-up, the patient showed relevant clinical improvement, with persistent suppression of the treated forms and only rare non-sustained runs of slow well-tolerated atrial tachycardia.

## Commentary

Similar to the previous case, this is a postsurgical patient with focal tachycardia–here, with two morphologies and foci–in the absence of macroreentrant atrial tachycardia. As in Case 1, the dominant focus was located in the upper right atrium and this corroborates the considerations made for the previous case (see Commentary and Table 1 of Case 1).

The main difficulty of the present case was the diffuse presence of very-low-amplitude bipolar potentials, especially in the area close to the prevalent tachycardia focus. In fact, at an early stage of mapping, the tachycardia origin was missed and a left atrial origin was suspected. Especially in cases involving an enlarged atrial chamber and multiple previous interventions, reconstruction of as much of the atrial endocardial surface as possible is of vital importance for correct diagnosis and successful ablation. Since the atrial tachycardia focus in this setting is usually located at the border zone between the scar and the viable tissue, and frequently exhibits very-low-amplitude potentials, discrimination between an electrically silent site and a site with a minimal (0.06–0.07 mV) signal amplitude is very important. Furthermore, adequate increase of the gain setting of the bipolar signal from the mapping catheter is mandatory.

This case is also paradigmatic in its contradictions of the general rules of focal atrial tachycardia. In fact, general rules may not apply to this particular subset of patients. It was reported [1, 2] that at the site of the tachycardia focus a rapid downstroke is observed in minimally filtered unipolar signals. In the present case, the unipolar signal showed a completely negative initial deflection at sites remote from the tachycardia focus. The most likely explanation is that activation of the very-low-voltage channel where the tachycardia originated was not detectable by unipolar recording. Therefore, at the exit of this channel, where the highest voltage amplitude (0.8–1.2 mV) was observed, the wavefront propagating from this site to the atria generated a negative unipolar deflection, albeit remote from the site of tachycardia origin. Moreover, in focal atrial tachycardias, intracardiac mapping has been reported to generally show a significant portion of the cycle length without recorded activity, even when recordings from the entire right atrium, left atrium and/or coronary sinus are considered [2]. In this case (first morphology) and in the previous one, the earliest activated site preceded the reference coronary sinus signal by 209 and 252 ms, respectively. Therefore, electrical activity spanned at least 52 and 87% of the tachycardia cycle, combining both right atrial activation and activation at the reference signal in the coronary sinus. Certainly, this was due to major conduction disturbances in these two patients. However, even in the presence of these "extreme" features, the activation map showed an unambiguous, centrifugally spreading activation pattern, which allowed correct diagnosis and focus localisation.

The second morphology of this case is a good example of how a wide electrically silent area close to the tachycardia focus is able to greatly modify the usual activation pattern of a focal atrial tachycardia, prolonging the activation time and potentially simulating a macroreentrant loop. High-density mapping assessed the lack of electrical activity in the area between the earliest and the latest activated sites in the right atrium and, hence, ruled out a macroreeentrant loop around the tricuspid annulus.

The effect of general anesthesia on focal atrial tachycardia, i.e. complete suppression, as observed in this patient, must also be considered. Fortunately, in this patient, stimulation combined with isoprenaline infusion induced the clinical tachycardia and allowed the procedure to continue.

**Acknowledgement.** *The images for this case were provided by Antonio Dello Russo, MD, and Gemma Pelargonio, MD, Institute of Cardiology, Department of Cardiovascular Medicine, Catholic University of the Sacred Heart, Rome, Italy.*

## References

1. Delacretaz E, Soejima K, Gottipaty VK et al. Single catheter determinants of local electrogram prematurity using simultaneous unipolar and bipolar recordings to replace the surface ECG as a timing reference. Pacing Clinc Electrophysiol 2001; 24: 441-449.
2. Saoudi N, Cosio F, Waldo A et al. Classification of atrial flutter and regular atrial tachycardia according to electrophysiologic mechanism and anatomic bases: a statement from the Joint Expert Group from the Working Group of Arrhythmias of the European Society of Cardiology and the North American Society of Pacing and Electrophysiology. J Cardiovascular Electrophysiol 2001; 12: 852-866.

# Case 3
# Focal Atrial Tachycardia Associated with a Macroreentrant Tachycardia: Two Arrhythmias with Different Mechanisms and Similar Morphologies in a Non-surgical Left Atrium with Electrically Silent Areas

## Case Presentation

This 67-year-old female patient was referred for recurrent episodes of atrial tachycardia. She was repeatedly hospitalised for these episodes in order to undergo pharmacologic or electrical cardioversion. The patient was known to have mitral valve disease with moderate stenosis and regurgitation; left ventricular function was mildly impaired. Since prior oral antiarrhythmic drugs failed to prevent arrhythmia recurrences, an electrophysiologic procedure was planned. On admittance, the patient presented with a tachycardia recurrence. The surface electrocardiogram (Fig. 1) showed atrial tachycardia at a cycle length of 330 ms with a variable atrioventric-

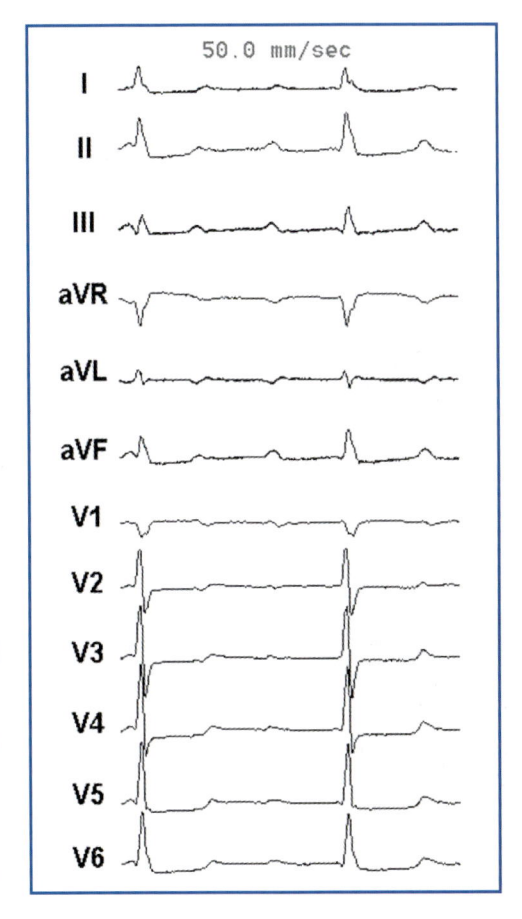

**Fig. 1.** Twelve-lead electrocardiogram of the clinical atrial tachycardia at 330 ms cycle length

ular conduction and positive P waves in lead I, inferior and left precordial leads, biphasic (negative/positive) in aVL, biphasic (positive/negative) in V1, and flat in V2, V3.

## Procedure

At the beginning of the electrophysiologic procedure, the patient was still in the same tachycardia with a stable cycle length of 330 ms. A multipolar catheter was placed in the coronary sinus and an atriogram from the mid-coronary sinus was used as reference. Electroanatomic mapping of the right atrium was initiated, setting the window of interest as for reentry. As shown in Fig. 2a, the right atrium was activated for only 29% (96/330 ms) of the tachycardia cycle length, with a wide area of early activation in the medial right atrium, corresponding to the right insertion of Bachmann's bundle and to the fossa ovalis. The bipolar signal recorded in the earliest activated area (Fig. 2b), which preceded the reference signal by 87 ms, had a presystolic chronology, while the unipolar signal showed a clearly positive initial deflection. The location and the extension of the earliest activated area, together with the characteristics of the signal in the early activated area, strongly favoured the hypothesis of a left atrial substrate. Interestingly, although the right atrium showed a mild dilation (volume of 96 ml), no region of low-amplitude bipolar signal was present (Fig. 3a, b), with the exception of small areas close to the superior and inferior venae cavae. After transseptal catheterisation was accomplished, mapping was continued in the left atrium. Early during mapping, two small electrically silent areas in the anterior and posterior walls (Fig. 4a, b) were identified. After roughly 100 sites had been acquired, 99% of the tachycardia circuit was reconstructed. A macroreentrant circuit and a mid-diastolic isthmus, between the electrically silent area in the anterior wall and the anterior mitral annulus (Fig. 4a), were clearly identified. In fact, using the specific setting of the window of interest (see pp. 2 and 3), the mid-diastolic isthmus is identified by the area where the red colour encounters the purple. The left atrial volume was 150 ml. Analysis of the colour distribution in the activation map and of the sequential frames of the propagation map (Fig. 5) showed that the arrhythmia had a double-loop reentry mechanism, with one loop rotating clockwise around the anterior scar area

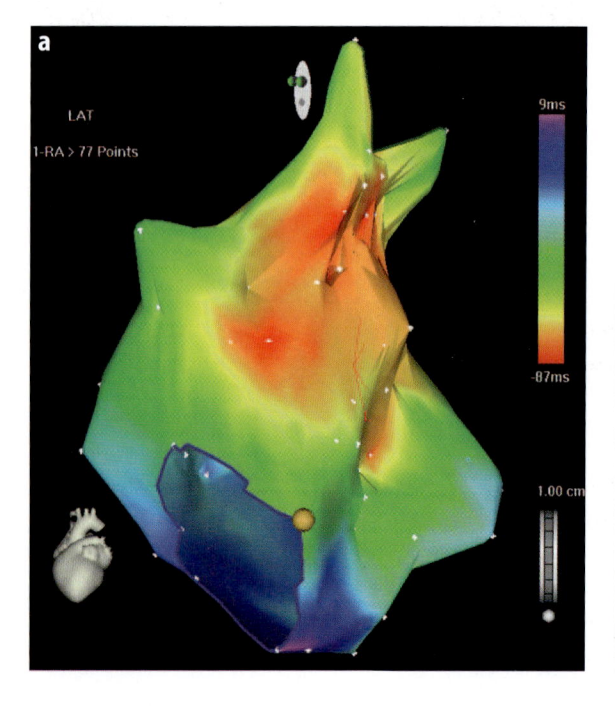

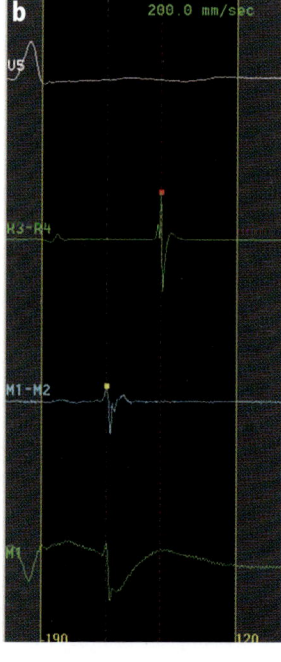

**Fig. 2a, b.** Activation map of the right atrium in a left anterior oblique (LAO) view during clinical tachycardia (**a**) and intracavitary signals at the earliest activated site in the right atrium (**b**). The wide earliest activated area in the activation map corresponds to Bachmann's bundle insertion in the right atrium. The area of the His-bundle recording is marked by the *orange dot*. In **b**, from *top* to *bottom*, a surface lead (V5), coronary sinus bipolar signal (R3–R4), bipolar (M1–M2) and unipolar (M1) signals from the earliest activated site in the right atrium are displayed

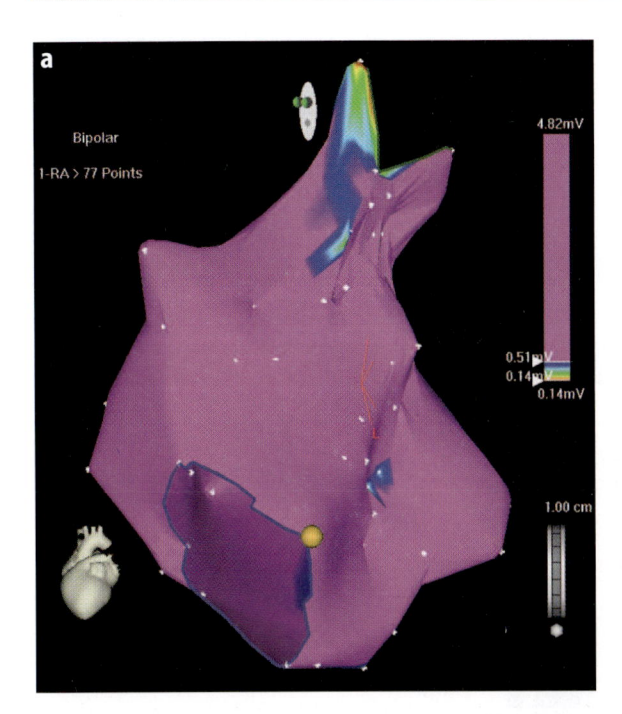

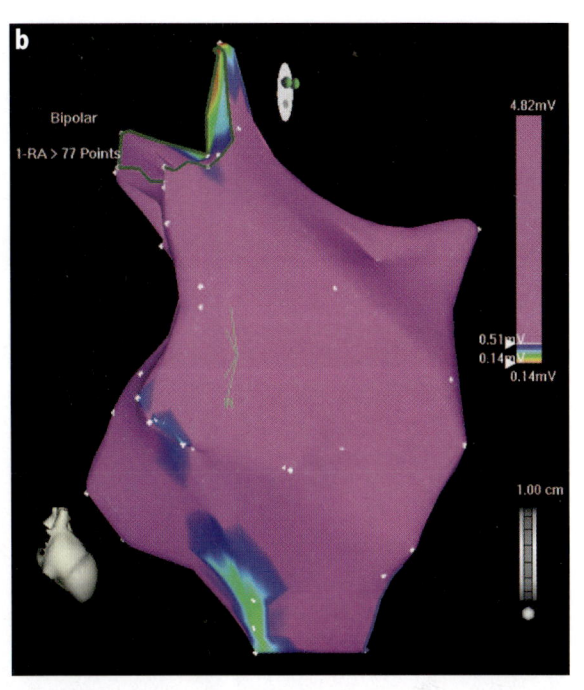

**Fig. 3a, b.** Bipolar voltage map of the right atrium in LAO (**a**) and RAO (**b**) views during clinical tachycardia. According to the setting of the colour-coded scale, areas with preserved voltage are shown in *purple*

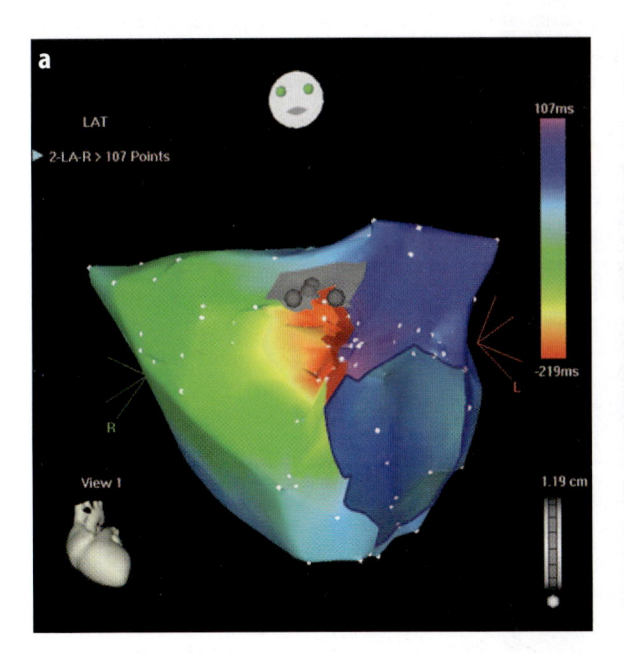

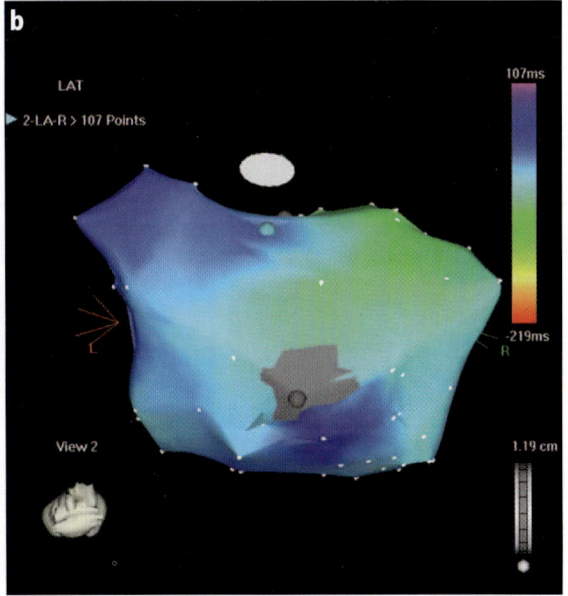

**Fig. 4a, b.** Activation map of the left atrium in anteroposterior (AP) (**a**) and cranial posteroanterior (PA) (**b**) views during clinical tachycardia. As indicated by the limits of the colour-coded scale, the reconstructed activation accounts for 99% of the tachycardia cycle length. *Grey* areas are electrically silent

and the second loop rotating counter-clockwise around the mitral annulus. The two loops shared the mid-diastolic isthmus, whose vertical extension was 17 mm. As shown in Fig. 5c' and 5d', the scar area in the posterior wall was responsible for the delayed propagation of the first loop to the posterior left atrium. Interestingly, as a consequence of the counter-clockwise rotation of the second loop around the mitral annulus, the posterolateral wall close to the mitral annulus was activated from medial to lateral, consistent with the sequence of activation recorded

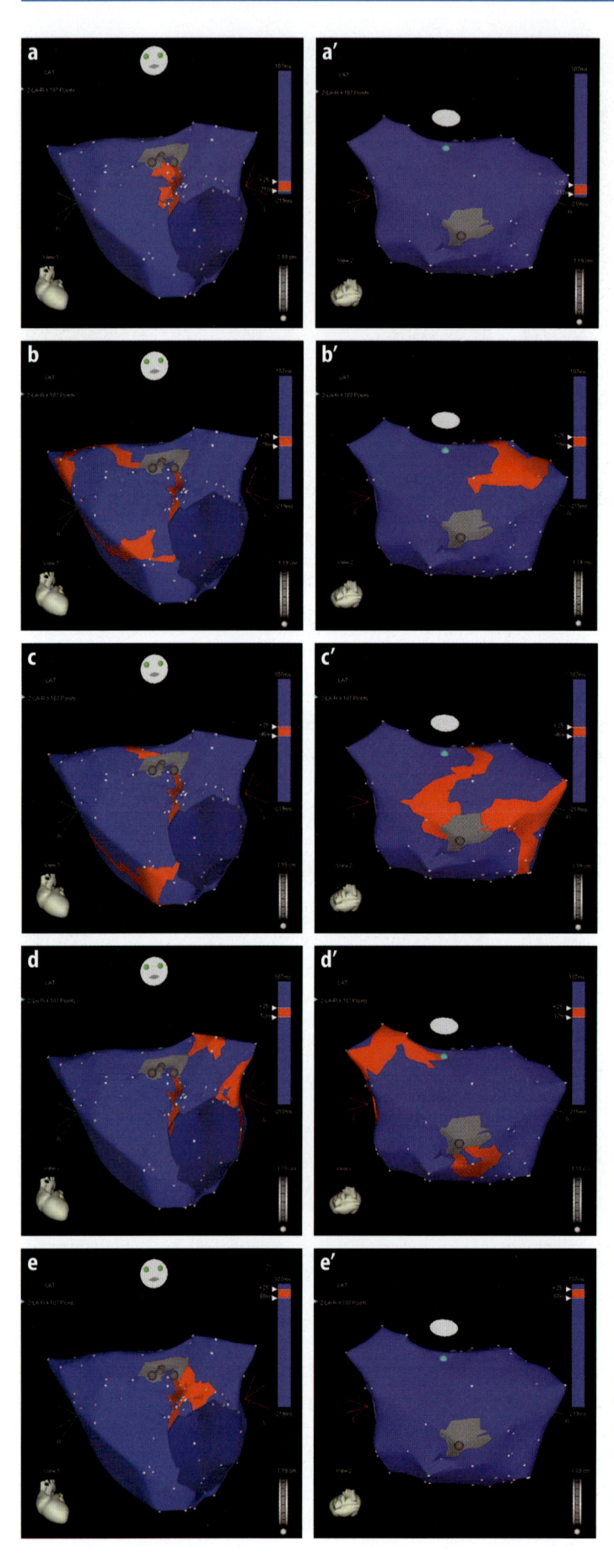

**Fig. 5a-e'.** Sequential frames of the propagation map of the left atrium in AP (**a–e**) and cranial PA (**a'–e'**) views during clinical tachycardia. The two loops separate upon exiting the mid-diastolic isthmus (**a**); the first proceeds clockwise around the electrically silent area at the roof, whereas the second rotates counterclockwise around the mitral annulus (**b**, **c**). The two loops rejoin just before entering the mid-diastolic isthmus (**d**, **e**). The area close to the os of the right superior pulmonary vein shows dead-end activation (**b**). The posterior electrically silent area modifies propagation in the posterior wall, by splitting the propagation wavefront (**c'**) and delaying activation of the posteromedial left atrium (**d'**)

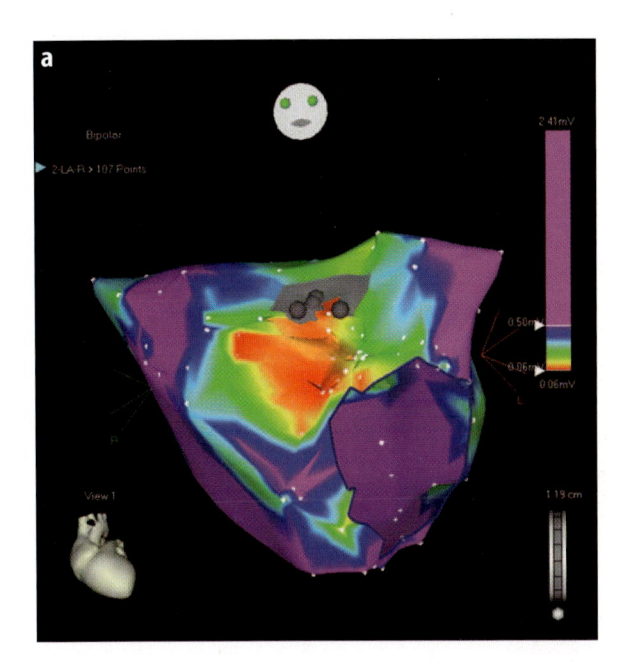

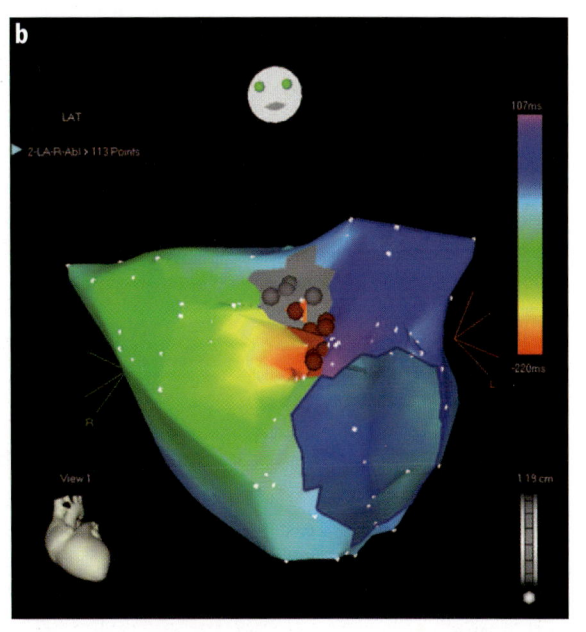

**Fig. 6a, b.** Bipolar voltage map of the left atrium in the AP view during clinical tachycardia (**a**) and activation map in the same view and rhythm (**b**), showing ablation tags (*red dots*). In **a**, the voltage threshold on the colour-coded scale is as in Fig. 3. In **b**, the lesion was deployed linearly from the electrically silent area and the mitral annulus

conventionally in the coronary sinus. The bipolar voltage map of the left atrium (Fig. 6a) showed a low-voltage amplitude in the anterior wall around the electrically silent area, with the lowest voltage in the mid-diastolically activated area. Ablation was targeted to the mid-diastolic isthmus (Fig. 6b) by delivering radiofrequency energy with an irrigated-tip catheter (maximum power 30W, cut-off temperature 43°C, duration 60 s). After two 60-s applications, the tachycardia terminated and sinus rhythm was restored. Four more sequential applications, from the upper to the lower part of the mid-diastolic isthmus up to the mitral annulus, produced complete disappearance of the intracavitary signals in this area. Subsequently, S1S2 programmed atrial stimulation reproducibly induced a second sustained tachycardia with a cycle length of 420 ms and a P wave morphology not very dissimilar (especially in the limb leads) to the index one (Fig. 7). This new morphology could have been the same arrhythmia but modified by the previous ablation, which might have prolonged the cycle length and slightly modified the surface P wave morphology, related to modification of the exit site from the mid-diastolic isthmus. Hypothetically, this scenario was possible, since the effect of ablation was assessed only by the disappearance of local signals, and a conduction block in the ablated isthmus was not demonstrated by pacing due to the absence of a second catheter in the left atrium and the poor discrimination provided by pacing from the coronary sinus. Therefore, the left atrium was remapped and, since another macroreentrant arrhythmia was expected, the window of interest was set accordingly. During mapping it soon became clear that the previously ablated area was now electrically silent and thus did not participate in this second arrhythmia. After the left atrium had been remapped, including the acquisition of 56 new mapping sites (Fig. 8a, b), it was evident that it was activated for 30% of the tachycardia cycle length, with an activation pattern suggesting a focal origin from the left atrial roof. In fact, the earliest activated area was located in the anterior wall, superior to the electrically silent area already identified in the first mapping (Fig. 8a), whereas the latest activated area was identified in the posteromedial left atrium (Fig. 8b), in an area almost diametrically opposite to the earliest one, as usually observed in focal tachycardias. Although the centrifugally spreading pattern from the early activated site, typical of focal arrhythmias, was preserved, it was clearly affected by the presence of the electrically silent areas,

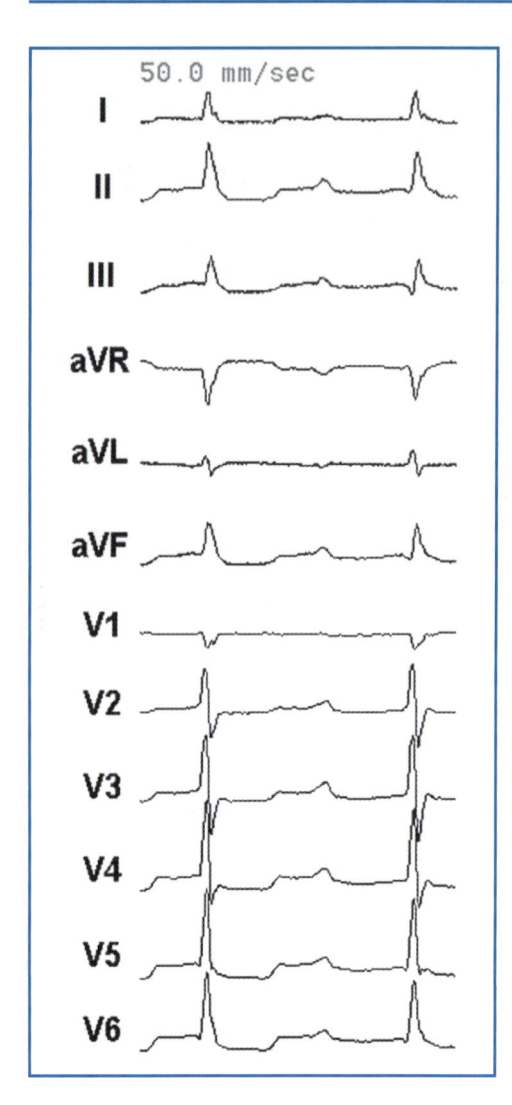

**Fig. 7.** Twelve-lead electrocardiogram of the second tachycardia, induced after ablation of the clinical arrhythmia

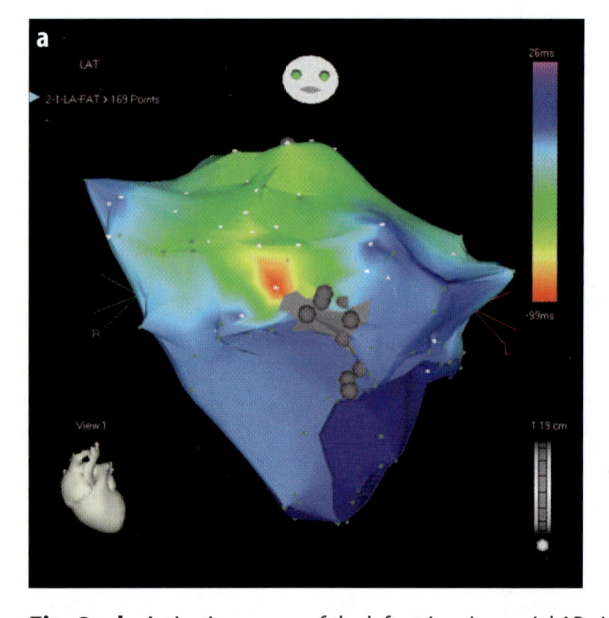

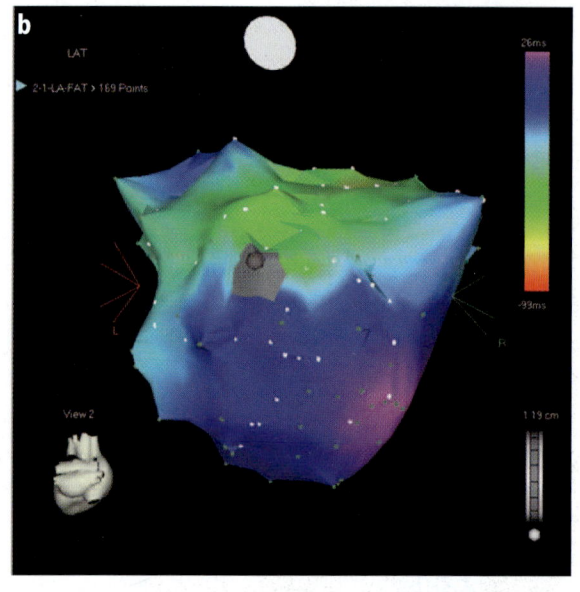

**Fig. 8a, b.** Activation remap of the left atrium in cranial AP view (**a**) and caudal PA view (**b**) during the second tachycardia, induced after ablation of the clinical arrhythmia. Spreading of activation from the earliest site, located posteriorly to the electrically silent area at the left atrial roof, is observed

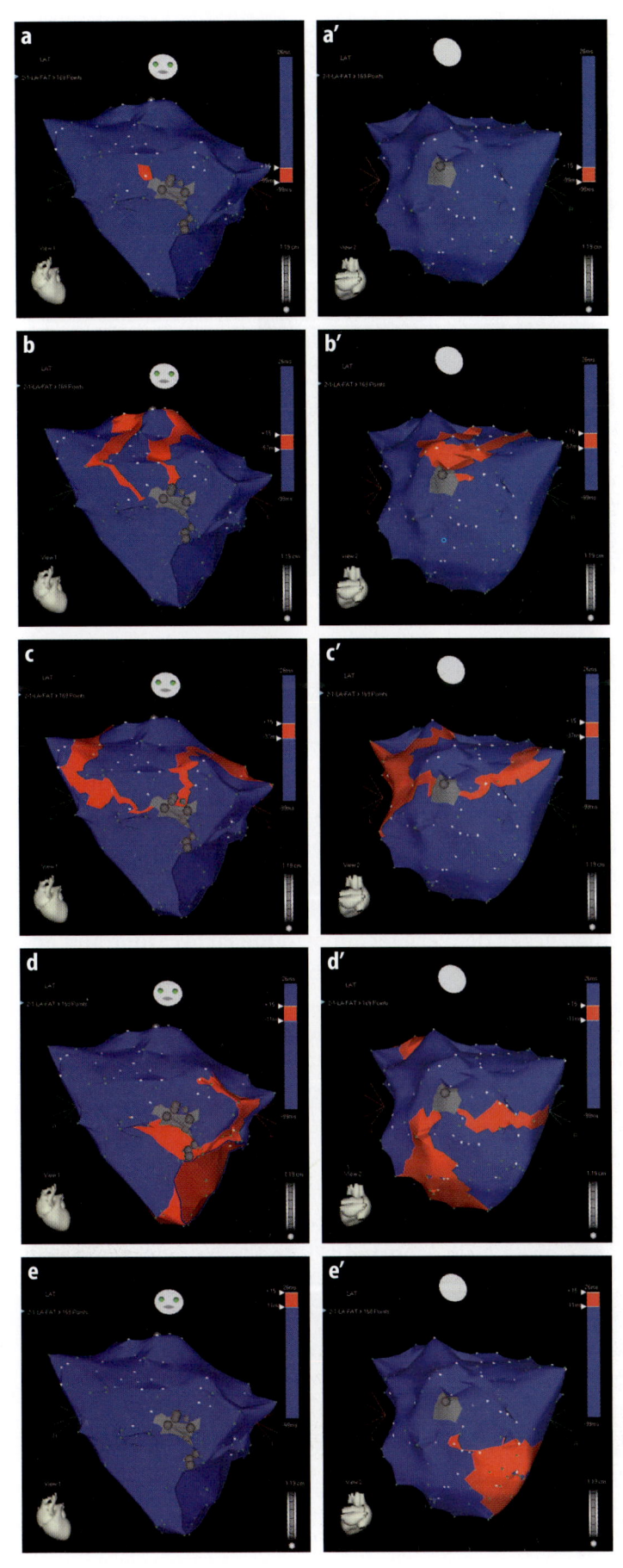

**Fig. 9a-e′.** Sequential frames of the propagation map of the left atrium in cranial AP (**a–e**) and caudal PA (**a′-e′**) views during the focal tachycardia, induced after ablation of the index tachycardia

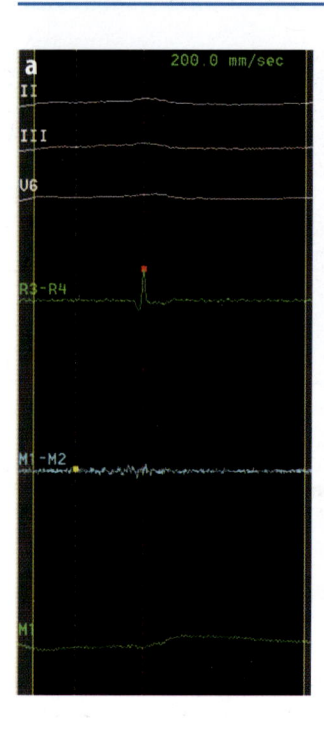

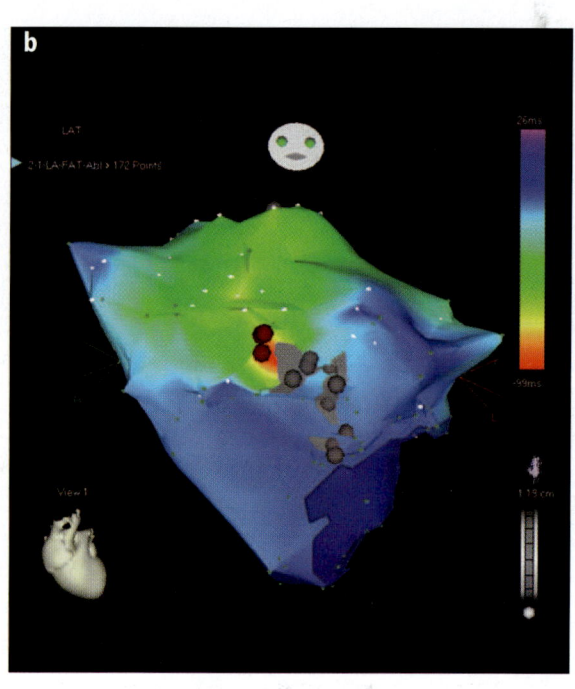

**Fig. 10a, b.** Intracavitary signals at the site of successful ablation (**a**) and activation map of the left atrium in the same view and rhythm as in Fig. 8a, with the ablation tags of both the successful application and the insurance applications delivered immediately thereafter in sinus rhythm (**b**). In **a**, from *top* to *bottom*, the surface leads II, III and V6, reference signal (R3–R4), bipolar (M1–M2) and unipolar (M1) signals from the earliest activated site are shown

previous ablation and, possibly, the fibre orientation, as shown in the sequential frames of the propagation map in Fig. 9. Particularly, collision of medial and lateral wavefronts at the site acting as the mid-diastolic isthmus in the previous tachycardia (Fig. 9d) further ruled out reentry and confirmed the conduction block along the previous ablation line. Analysis of the bipolar signals in the earliest activated area was unusually difficult due to the very low amplitude of these signals. In fact, the earliest activated site (Fig. 10a) exhibited a very low voltage (0.08 mV), fragmentation and a long-lasting bipolar signal, which preceded by 49 ms the P wave onset and was automatically annotated by the system on its first positive sharp deflection. The unipolar signal from this site was flat. The first radiofrequency energy application, using the same parameters as before (Fig. 10b), early during energy delivery terminated the tachycardia, and another two applications were delivered in the same area in sinus rhythm. Afterwards, since no other tachycardia was inducible by S2S3 programmed atrial stimulation, the procedure was terminated. During a 2-year follow-up, the patient was free from arrhythmia recurrences without antiarrhythmic therapy.

## Commentary

The coexistence in a nonsurgical patient of macroreentrant and focal tachycardias in a right atrium showing spontaneous scarring was previously reported [1]. In the patient considered here, definitive clinical evidence of the focal tachycardia was lacking prior to ablation of the macroreentrant one; however, clinical occurrence of the focal tachycardia could not be excluded, since not all palpitation episodes were systematically and extensively documented by electrocardiogram recordings. Nonetheless, the fact that the focal tachycardia was easily and reproducibly inducible in a sustained form suggested that it would pose a clinical problem during follow-up if left untreated. It is likely that the macroreentrant tachycardia initially prevailed, since its cycle length was 90 ms shorter, whereas it is quite unlikely that the focal tachycardia was in some way elicited by the previous ablation.

As in Case 2, in the present case involving the left atrium, the focus was located adjacent to scar tissue, and very low voltage was recorded at the earliest activated area. This certainly represents an adjunctive difficulty, since discrimination between electrically silent and electrically active areas is not trivial. Moreover, unipolar recordings may be of no help in defining the earliest activated site. In fact, the unipolar signal at the tachycardia focus did not show, as expected, a downstroke, but instead was flat, likely due to the very-low-voltage amplitude of this area so that it scarcely contributed to the unipolar signal.

This case is also paradigmatic of how, in an enlarged left atrium with electrically silent areas and a previous ablation line, the centrifugally spreading pattern, characteristic of a focal arrhythmia, may be less typical than expected.

Since the second arrhythmia was initially assumed to be macroreentrant, the window of interest was set accordingly. This was not misleading and did not affect correct annotation of all acquired sites. In our experience, the window of interest can be set as for macroreentry if, at the beginning of the procedure, the tachycardia mechanism is unclear.

## References

1. Stevenson IH, Kistler PM, Spence SJ et al. Scar-related right atrial macroreentrant tachycardia in patients without prior atrial surgery: electroanatomic characterization and ablation outcome. Heart Rhythm 2005; 2: 594-601.

# Case 4
# Focal Atrial Tachycardia From the Right Superior Pulmonary Vein with Irregular Cycle and P Wave Morphology: the Missing Link in the Chain Connecting Organized and Disorganized Atrial Arrhythmias?

## Case Presentation

This 38-year-old female patient had mild hypertension with a 2-year history of poorly tolerated irregular palpitations. During symptoms, the surface electrocardiogram showed short runs of atrial arrhythmia (Fig. 1), with irregular cycle length (between 275 and 340 ms) and beat-to-beat variations of the P wave morphology although its polarity was constantly negative in aVL and aVR and positive in the other leads. The variations of the P wave morphology were more evident in leads $V_1$-$V_2$. During prolonged electrocardiographic monitoring, longer salvos of atrial tachycardia were observed. These were characterised by a more constant P wave morphology and shorter cycle-length variations, between 270 and 310 ms, with 2:1 atrioventricular conduction (Fig. 2). Degeneration into atrial fibrillation was never observed, even at prolonged monitoring. The findings suggested the presence of a multifocal automatic atrial tachycardia, likely originating from the left atrium. Symptoms worsened over the six months before the procedure, and at the time of the procedure the patient complained of iterative palpitation with dizziness, especially during daily activities. Therapy with IC antiarrhythmic drugs and beta-blockers, even

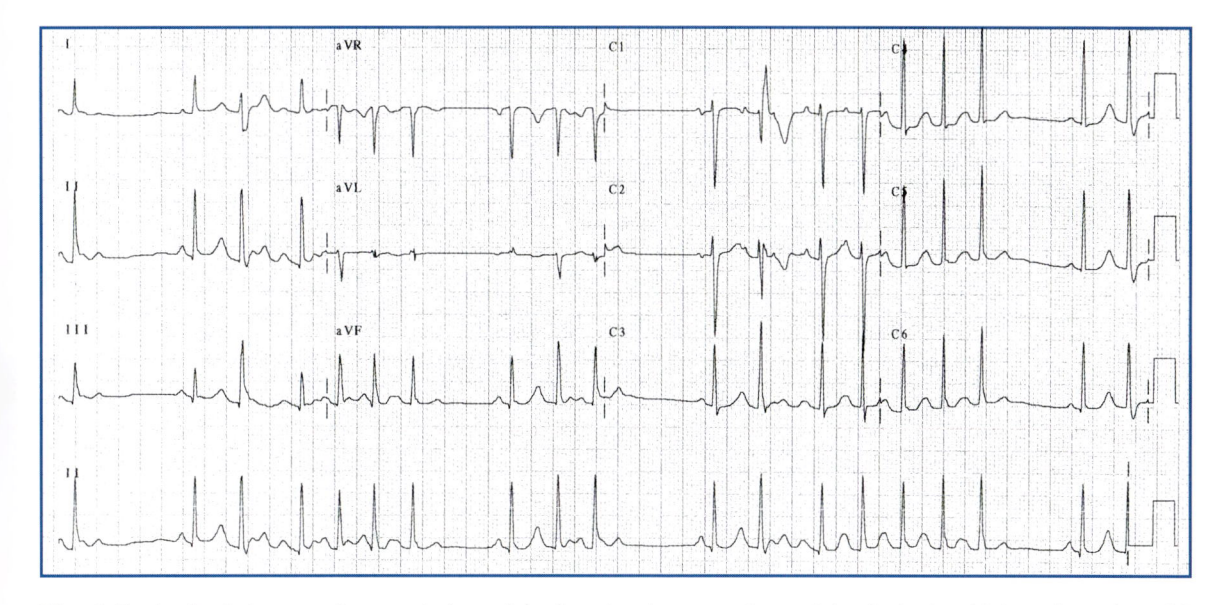

**Fig. 1.** Twelve-lead electrocardiogram during palpitation, showing runs of an atrial arrhythmia with irregular cycle and P wave morphology

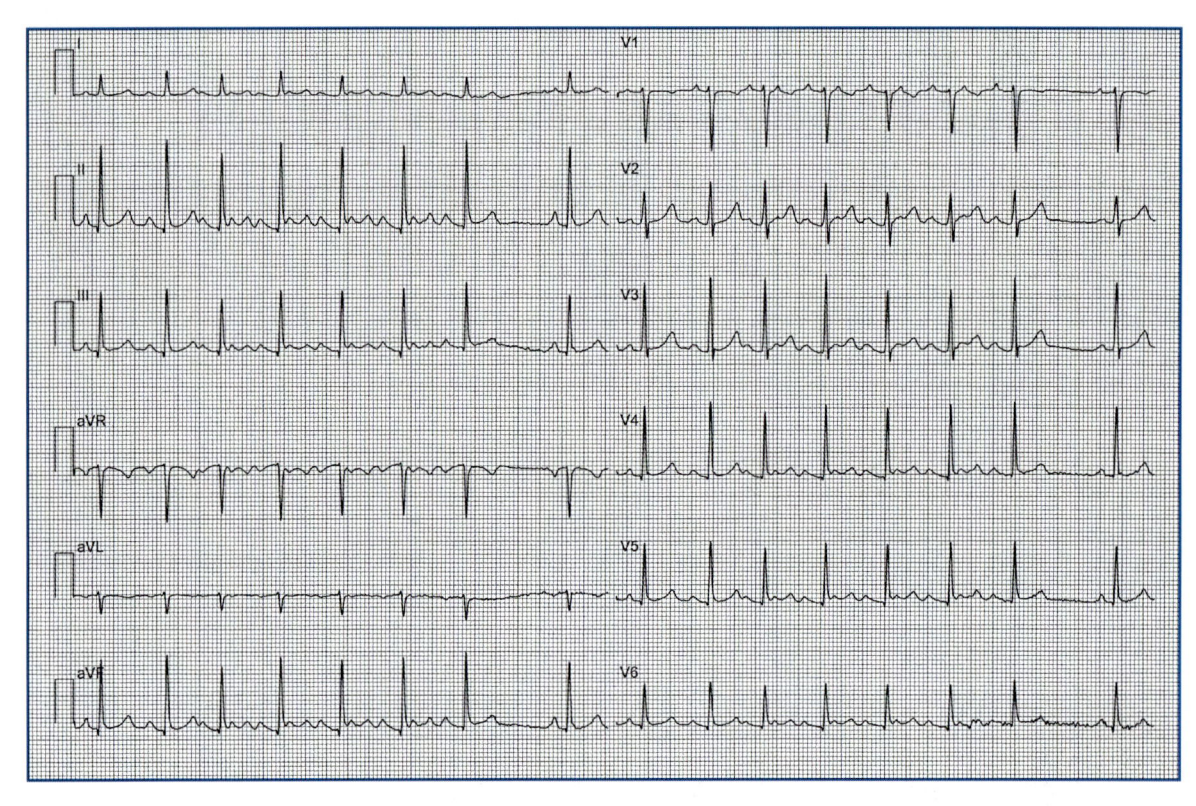

**Fig. 2.** Twelve-lead electrocardiogram during monitoring, showing a prolonged run of atrial tachycardia with more constant cycle and P wave morphology

in combination, was only minimally effective. Blood pressure values were constantly within the normal range with the administration of ACE inhibitors. Transthoracic and transesophageal echocardiograms showed normal findings. Thyroid function was also normal.

## Procedure

The procedure was performed after withdrawal of any antiarrhythmic drugs and with the patient in a non-sedated state. Iterative runs of the arrhythmia were constantly present during isoprenaline infusion. Electroanatomic mapping of the right atrium was initiated, with an atriogram in the mid-coronary sinus as reference. For each mapping site, using the 10-beat buffer option, annotation was made on the first tachycardia beat, which showed a rather constant coupling interval (330–350 ms) with the previous sinus beat. After acquisition of about fifty points, the activation map (Fig. 3a, b) showed a larger (1 × 1 cm) area of earliest activation in the high medial right atrium. As expected, the site of latest activation was diametrically opposite, in the low lateral right atrium. At the site of earliest activation, a double-component bipolar signal was recorded (Fig. 3c), with a maximum amplitude of 1.21 mV and the first low-amplitude component synchronous with the P wave onset in lead II and preceding the reference signal by 59 ms. The corresponding unipolar signal showed a small initial positive deflection followed by a slow negative deflection. The characteristics of the local signals and the extension and location of the earliest activated area strongly suggested a left-sided arrhythmia. Accordingly, transseptal catheterisation was accomplished. Electroanatomic reconstruction of the left atrium very soon showed that the area of early activation was located around the os of the right superior pulmonary vein (Fig. 4a), which activated 43 ms earlier than the corresponding area in the right

Case 4    39

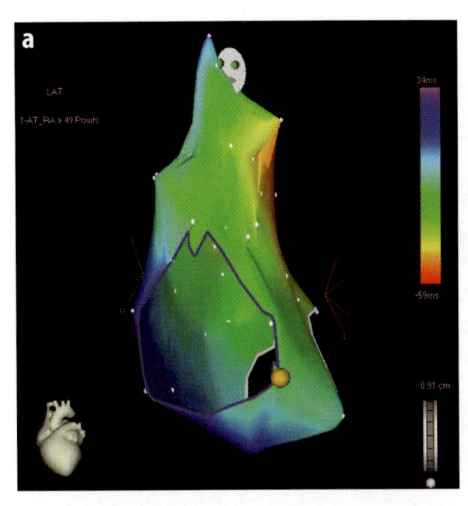

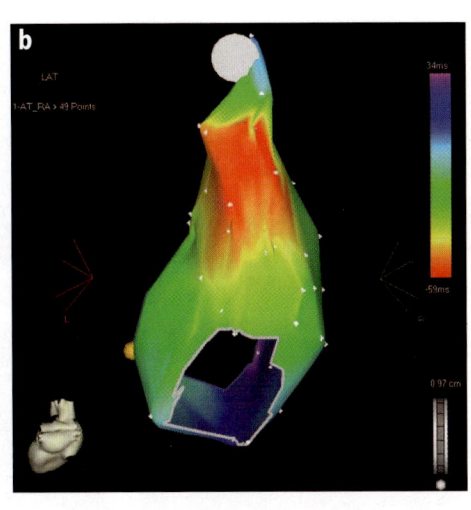

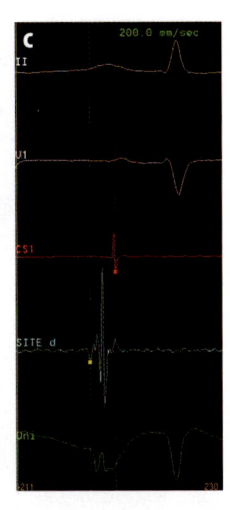

**Fig. 3a-c.** Activation map of the right atrium during the first tachycardia beat in the left anterior oblique (LAO) (**a**) and PA (**b**) views, and display of the intracavitary signals at the site of earliest activation in the right atrium during the first tachycardia beat (**c**). The *orange dot* identifies the His-bundle area. In **c**, from *top* to *bottom*, surface leads II and V1, bipolar reference signal (CS1) and bipolar (Sited) and unipolar (Uni) signals at the earliest activated site are shown

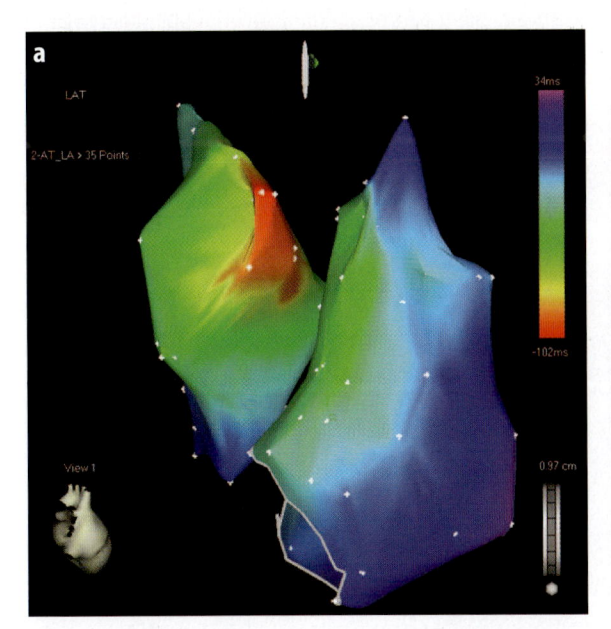

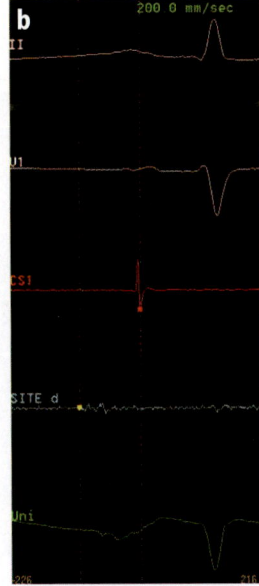

**Fig. 4a, b.** Activation map of the right and left atria during the first tachycardia beat in right lateral view (**a**) and display of the intracavitary signal at the earliest activated site in the left atrium (**b**). In **b**, signals are shown as in Fig. 3c

atrium. Here, as shown in Fig. 4b, a low-amplitude (0.08 mV) fragmented bipolar signal preceded a completely negative unipolar signal by 17 ms and the P wave onset by 43 ms. To better characterise the area of earliest activation, mapping was continued in the right superior pulmonary vein, which was electroanatomically reconstructed (Fig. 5a, b). After this further mapping, the site of earliest activation during the first atrial tachycardia beat was identified in the anterior wall of the vein, 8 mm from the ostium. In this site, bipolar activation preceded activation at the ostium by 71 ms, in the absence of a discernible unipolar signal coincident with the earliest bipolar potential. To better record this focal activity, a 20-pole circular mapping catheter (Lasso Variable 2515, Biosense-Webster, USA) was inserted distally in the vein. The recordings are displayed in Fig. 6. Interestingly, multipolar simultaneous recordings inside the vein showed that most of the focal activity remained concealed inside it. Moreover, the sequence of vein activation during focal activity showed beat-to-beat variations, suggesting different activation sources and courses inside the vein, although the vein activity that generated the first tachycardia beat

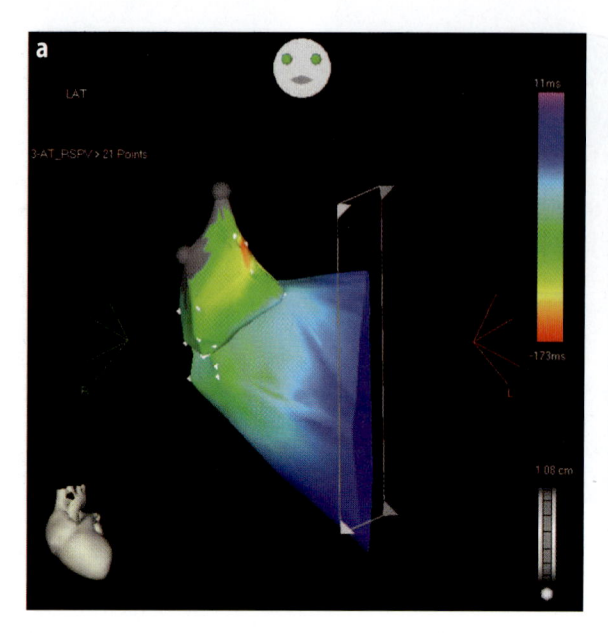

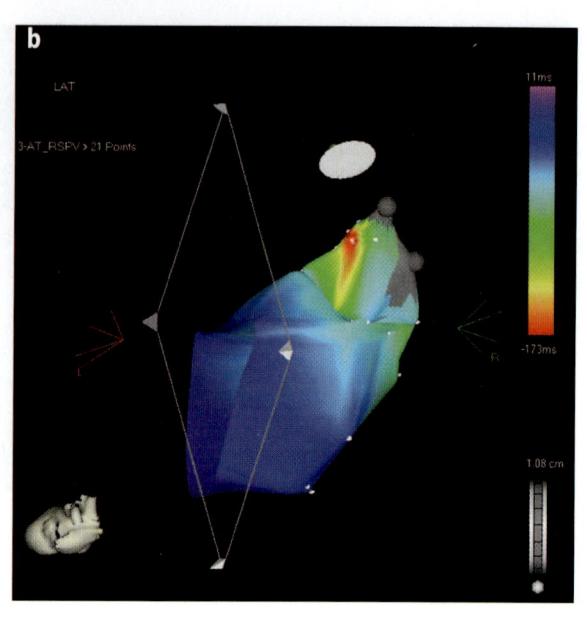

**Fig. 5a, b.** Activation map of the medial part of the left atrium and of the right superior pulmonary vein during the first tachycardia beat in AP (**a**) and cranial PA (**b**) views. The distal, electrically silent part of the right superior pulmonary vein is tagged with *grey dots*

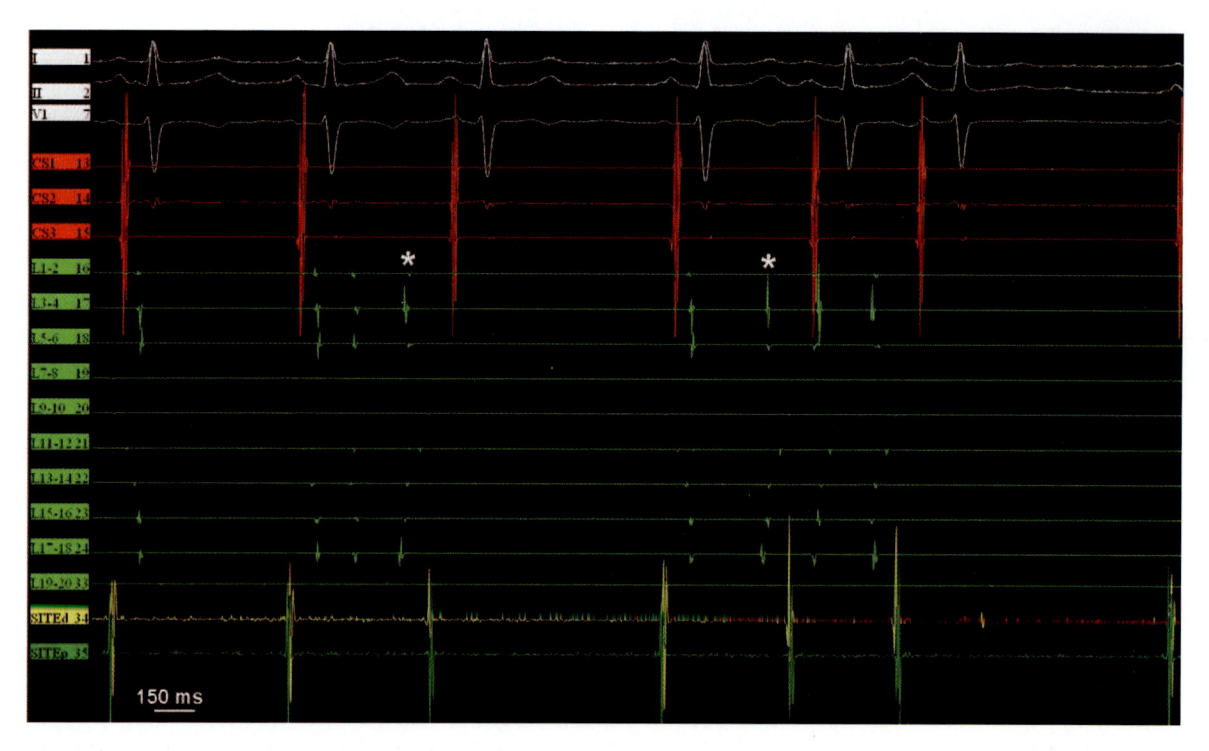

**Fig. 6.** Surface and intracavitary signals during iterative runs of tachycardia. From *top to bottom*, surface leads I, II, V1, bipolar signals of the coronary-sinus catheter, from *distal to proximal* (CS1–CS3), bipolar signals from the 20-pole circular mapping catheter inserted in the right superior pulmonary vein (L1-2 to L19-20) and bipolar signals from the distal (SITEd) and proximal (SITEp) electrode pairs of the mapping catheter. Focal activity from the pulmonary vein is only partially conducted to the left atrium and shows an irregular activation sequence. Only the first conducted beat during each run, marked by the *asterisk*, shows a constant activation pattern

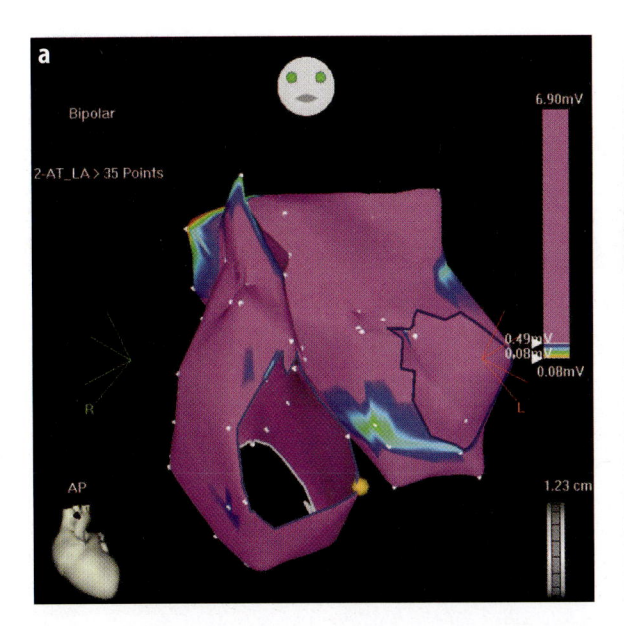

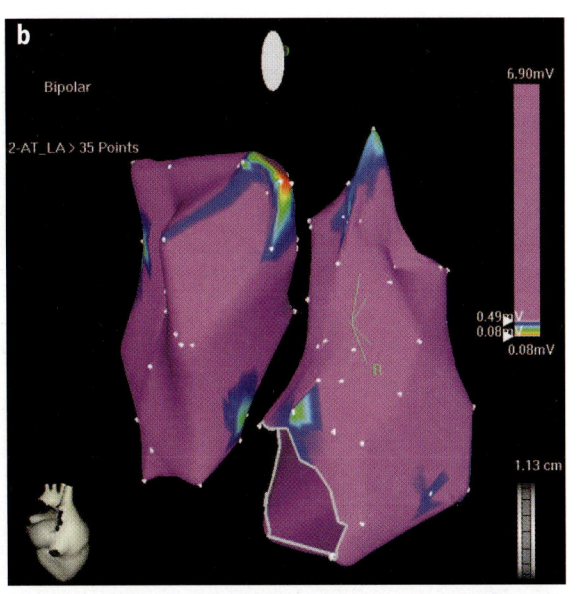

**Fig. 7a, b.** Bipolar voltage map of both atria in AP (**a**) and right lateral (**b**) views. According to the setting of the colour-coded scale, *purple* indicates preserved voltage. Other than at the os of the right superior pulmonary vein, low voltage is observed only in very limited areas close to the superior and inferior venae cavae orifices and in the proximity of the medial and lateral mitral annulus

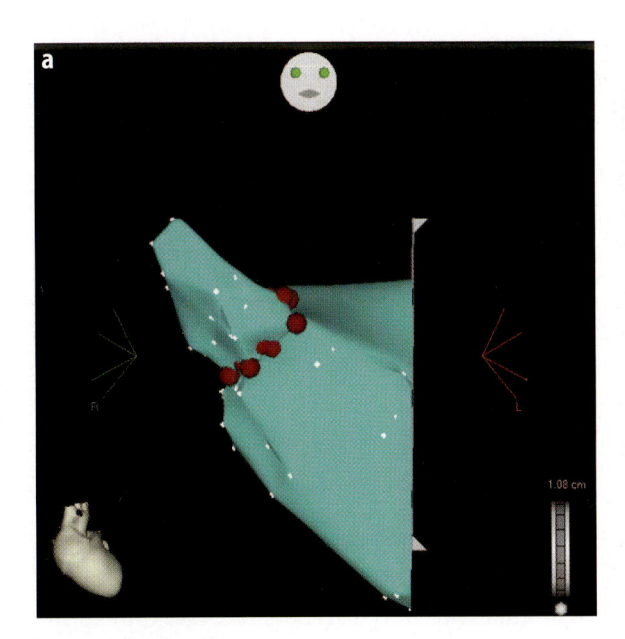

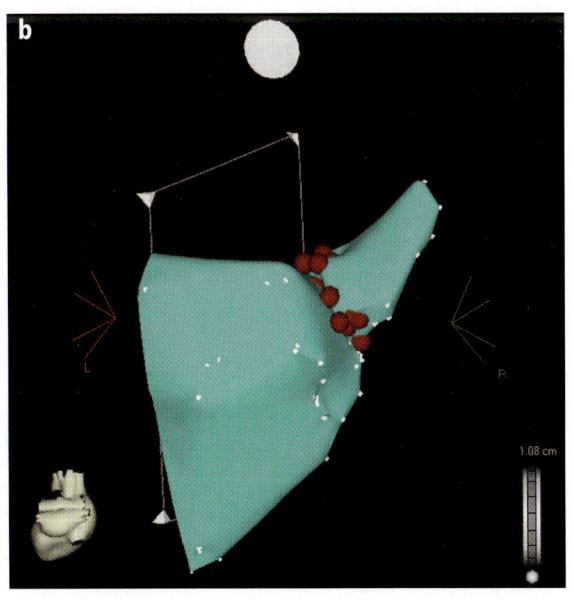

**Fig. 8.** Anatomic map of the medial left atrium and of the right superior pulmonary vein in AP (**a**) and PA (**b**) views, showing the ablation tags, which were deployed circularly to obtain vein electrical disconnection

conducted to the atrium (asterisks in Fig. 6) had a constant activation sequence. An analysis of the bipolar voltage map (Fig. 7a, b) showed substantially normal values, both in the right and in the left atrium, and low-amplitude potentials (0.08–0.16 mV) confined at the os and inside the right superior pulmonary vein. It was then decided to proceed to electrical isolation of the pulmonary vein rather than to focal ablation inside the vein due to the high risk of pulmonary-vein stenosis and the likely presence of multiple foci in the vein. Radiofrequency energy was delivered with an irrigated-tip catheter (maximum power 30 W, cut-off temperature of 43°C, duration 60 s) at the venoatrial junction, thus achieving pulmonary-vein electrical disconnection (Fig. 8a, b). Afterwards, during maximal isoprenaline infusion, dissociated pulmonary vein ac-

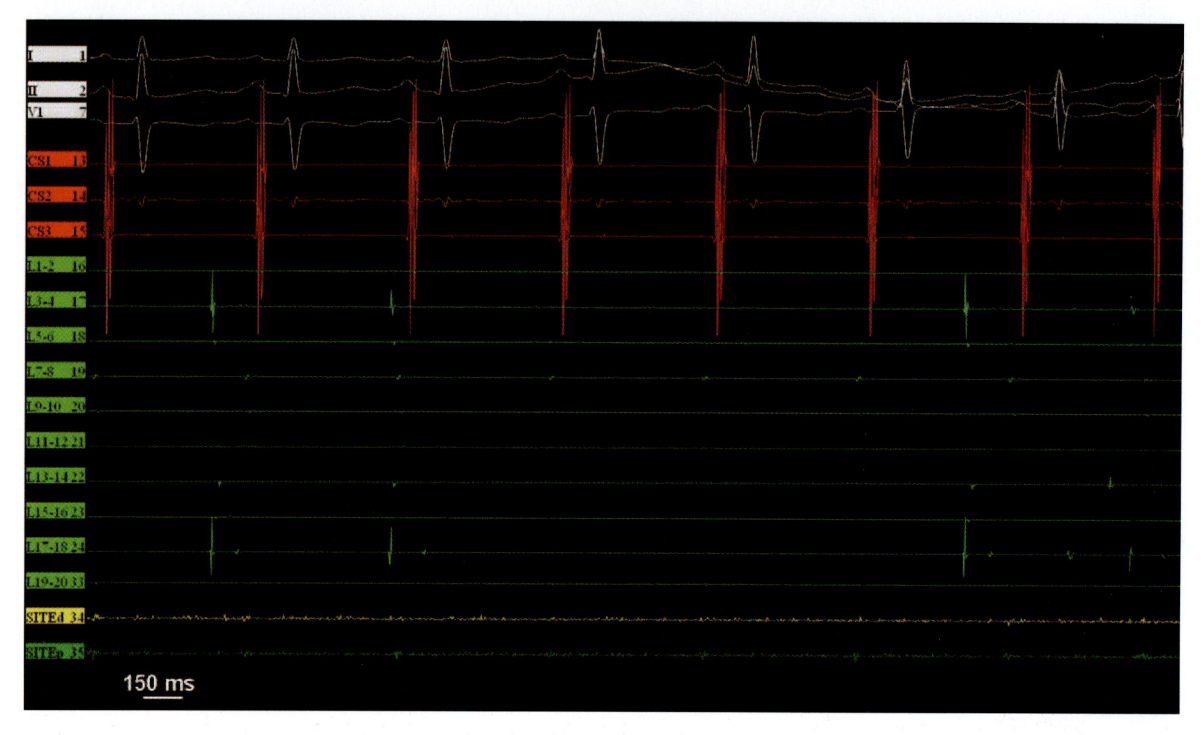

**Fig. 9.** Display of the signal from the 20-pole circular mapping catheter inserted in the right superior pulmonary vein after pulmonary-vein electrical disconnection during maximal isoprenaline infusion. Signals are displayed as in Fig. 6. A low-rate dissociated electrical activity was still present in the vein, with irregular beat-to-beat variations of the activation sequence

tivity was still present while the patient was in sinus rhythm (Fig. 9). Electrical disconnection of the vein persisted after a 12 mg intravenous adenosine bolus. During a 1-year follow-up, the patient remained asymptomatic and in sinus rhythm, as assessed by repeated Holter monitoring, without antiarrhythmic drugs.

## Commentary

The pulmonary veins are well-recognised sources of the focal activity responsible for atrial fibrillation, especially in paroxysmal forms. They are also the main sources of left focal atrial tachycardia with a stable cycle length and P wave morphology [1, 2]. According to these studies, in the majority of cases (74%) the focus of tachycardias originating from the pulmonary veins is located at the vein os and can be abolished by focal ablation; only rarely is it located deep inside the vein, as assessed by accurate electroanatomic mapping [2].

This peculiar case could be paradigmatic of those forms of arrhythmias representing the missing link in the chain joining atrial fibrillation and atrial tachycardias with regular activation pattern. In this patient, disorganised activity with multiple activation patterns in the right superior pulmonary vein originated a self-limiting atrial tachycardia in which the electrical activity in the atria remains organised, although beat-to-beat variations of the cycle length and P wave morphology are present. Modification of the surface P wave morphology in an arrhythmia originating from the same vein can be explained by the fact that irregular and multifocal vein activity may find a different venoatrial pathways with different exits to the atrium. Especially for the right superior pulmonary vein (very close to the septum on one side and to the left atrial roof and Bachmann's bundle on the other), this may result in minimal but appreciable beat-to-beat variations of the surface P wave, as observed in lead V1 in Fig. 1.

The difficulty of mapping an irregular tachycardia was overcome in this case by considering only the first tachycardia beat, which showed a relatively stable coupling interval with the previous sinus beat. Systematic analysis and annotation of only the first tachycardia beat, using the 10-beat buffer option, allowed reconstruction of a consistent activation map, although it obviously prolonged the mapping time. Eventually, when the multipolar circular mapping catheter was inserted in the vein, it turned out that only the first beat conducted to the atrium during each run of pulmonary vein activity showed a constant activation pattern, thus representing the expression of a contant phoenomenon. Whether the stratey of mapping the first tachycardia beat in irregular atrial tachycardia could be in other patients as successful as it was here remains to be assessed.

The unipolar deflection was undetectable at the site of tachycardia origin inside the vein and showed a negative deflection at the vein os, remote from the tachycardia focus. Similar to the observations in Cases 2 and 3, areas of low-amplitude potentials inside the vein were unable to generate a unipolar deflection, which, nonetheless, could be recorded as a negative deflection only at the site of exit to the atrial myocardium, where preserved voltage was present.

A multifocal activation pattern in a pulmonary vein was recorded by simultaneous high-density mapping upon arrhythmia initiation in patients suffering from paroxysmal, frequently recurrent atrial fibrillation [3]. It is hard to assess why our patient had a relatively organised and self-limiting arrhythmia rather than sustained atrial fibrillation, although he had the same kind of "trigger". The finding of preserved voltage in both atria might support the hypothesis of a very limited atrial electrical disease in this patient. This may have prevented degeneration of the arrhythmia into atrial fibrillation, even in the presence of a very active pulmonary-vein focus with disorganised electrical activity inside the vein.

## References

1. Kistler PM, Sanders P, Fynn SP et al. Electrophysiological and electrocardiographic characteristics of focal atrial tachycardia originating from the pulmonary veins; acute and long-term outcomes of radiofrequency ablation. Circulation 2003; 108: 1968-1975.
2. Dong J, Zrenner B, Schreieck J et al. Catheter ablation of left atrial focal tachycardia guided by electroanatomic mapping and new insights into interatrial electrical conduction. Heart Rhythm 2005; 2: 578-591.
3. De Ponti R, Tritto M, Lanzotti M et al. Computerized high-density mapping of the pulmonary veins: new insights into their electrical activation in patients with atrial fibrillation. Europace 2004; 6: 97-108.

# Case 5
# Focal Atrial Tachycardia from the Right Superior Pulmonary Vein with Stable P Wave Morphology and Cycle Length: the Problem of Discriminating between a Right and Left Origin

## Case Presentation

This is a 62-year-old female patient with a long history of arrhythmia. Eleven years earlier, in our centre, she underwent ablation of a slow atrioventricular node pathway for a frequently recurrent and drug-refractory common atrioventricular nodal reentrant tachycardia. The procedure was successful and follow-up was initially uneventful. Six years later, her complaints of palpitations resumed and were electrocardiographically documented as atrial tachycardia. The palpitations worsened during the following three years and the patient was referred to another centre for an electrophysiology procedure. There, a focal atrial tachycardia was diagnosed and the patient underwent two unsuccessful ablation procedures in the posterior right atrium. In the following 24 months, antiarrhythmic drug therapy with flecainide, sotalol and then with amiodarone did not prevent recurrences and the arrhythmia worsened, becoming in some cases iterative-incessant. Surface electrocardiograms showed the same tachycardia morphology (Figs. 1, 2) with flat P waves in leads I and aVL, negative in aVR and positive in all the other leads, not very dissimilar from the sinus morphology (Fig. 1a). In different recordings, the arrhythmia showed a variable presentation and cycle length, i.e. sustained with 2:1 atrioventricular conduction and a regular atrial cycle of 300 ms (Fig. 1b), or iterative with short tachycardia runs (Fig. 1c) or, on occasion, sustained with a beat-to-beat variation of the cycle length from a minimum of 280 ms to a maximum of 460 ms (Fig. 2). Finally, the patient was referred to our institution for further evaluation. An echocardiogram showed no dilatation of the heart chambers and ventricular function was preserved. This suggested that the ventricular repolarization abnormality observed on surface electrocardiogram should have been interpreted as tachycardia-related rather than an expression of the presence of structural heart disease or tachycardiomyopathy. Systemic hypertension was also present, but blood pressure values were controlled with ACE-inhibitor therapy.

## Procedure

The procedure was performed after withdrawal of any anti-arrhythmic drugs and with the patient in a non-sedated state. At the beginning of the procedure, sinus rhythm was present. A decapolar catheter was positioned into the coronary sinus and two tetrapolar catheters in the His-bundle area and high right atrium, respectively. Baseline conduction intervals were normal. At baseline electrophysiologic study, atrioventricular conduction was normal with no sign of dual

46   Focal Atrial Arrhythmias

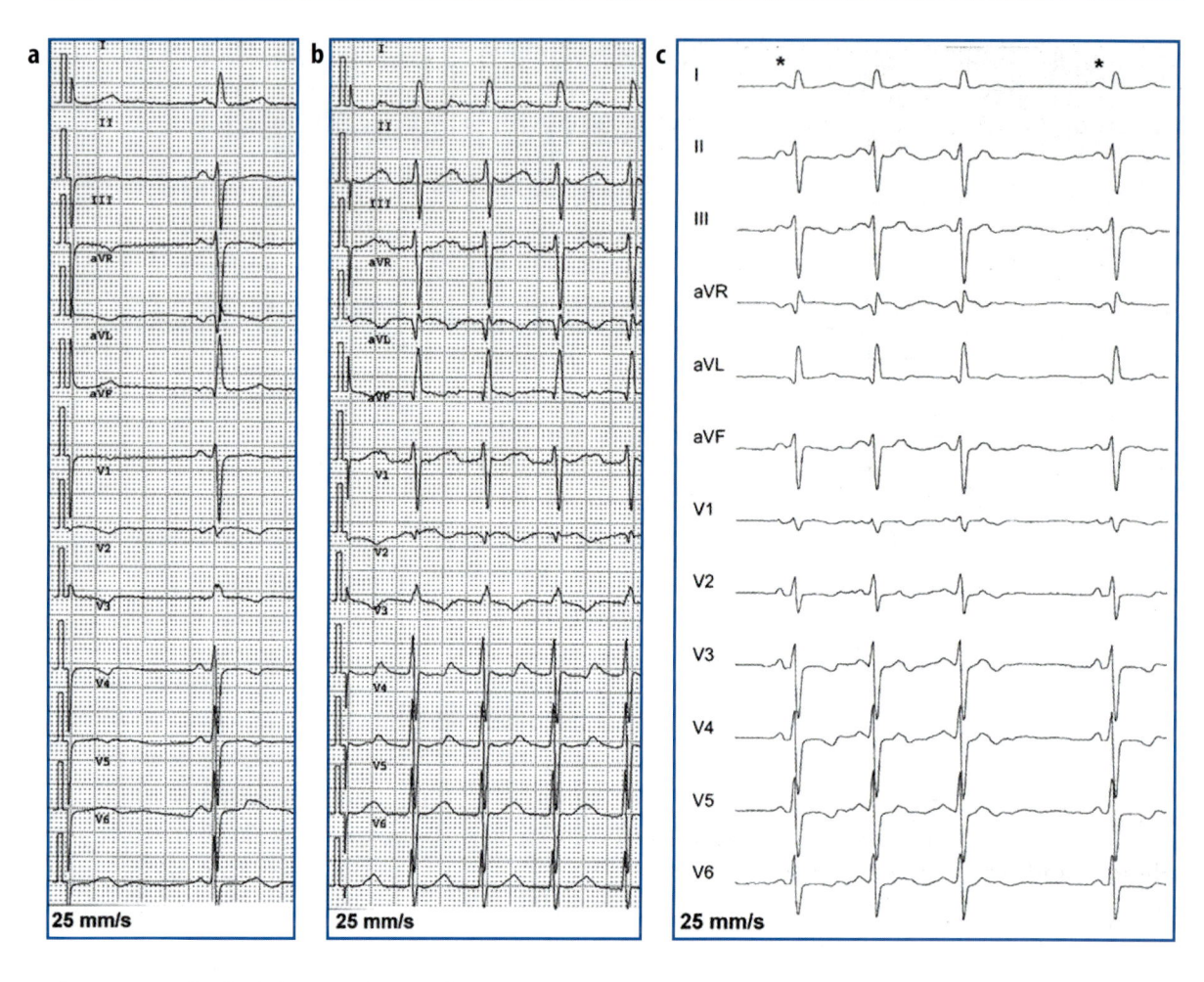

**Fig. 1a-c.** Twelve-lead electrocardiogram during sinus rhythm (**a**), sustained focal atrial tachycardia with 2:1 atrioventricular conduction (**b**) and a non-sustained run of focal atrial tachycardia (**c**). In **c**, sinus beats are marked by an *asterisk*

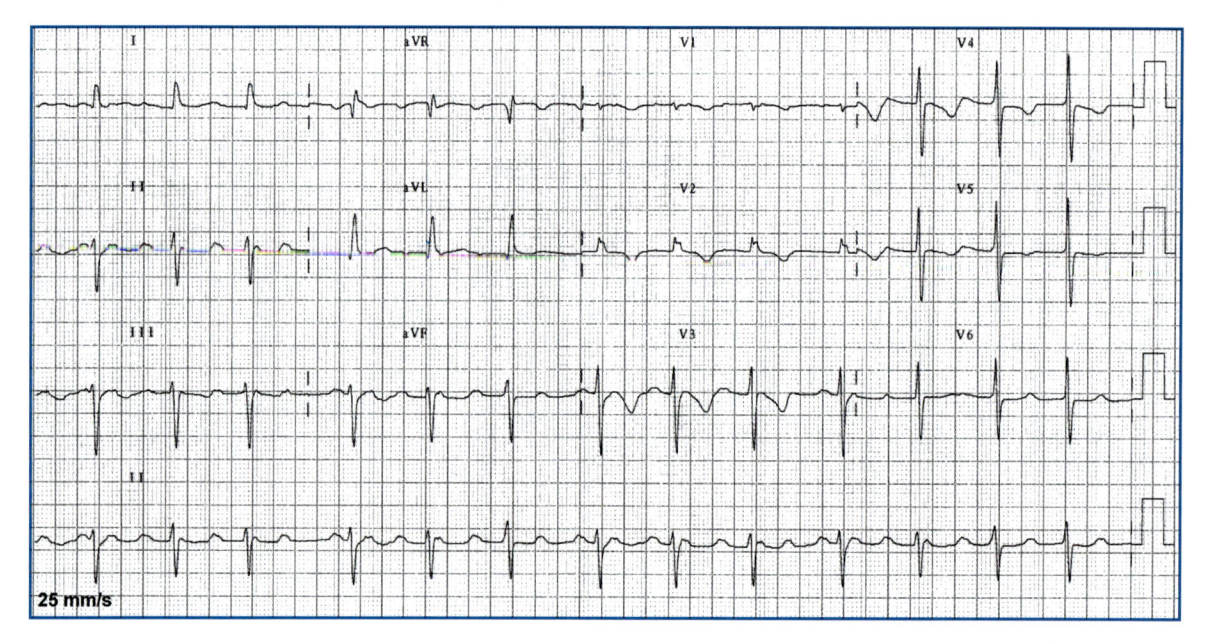

**Fig. 2.** Another twelve-lead electrocardiogram during focal atrial tachycardia. The *bottom line* is a lead II rhythm strip that shows beat-to-beat variations of the tachycardia cycle with no change in P wave morphology

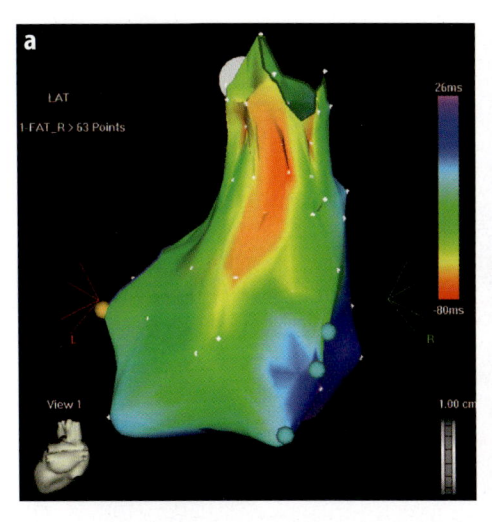

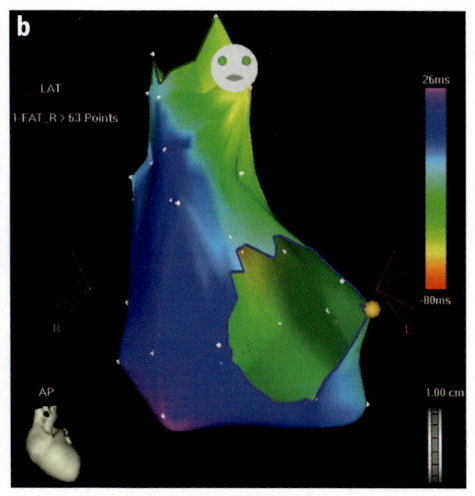

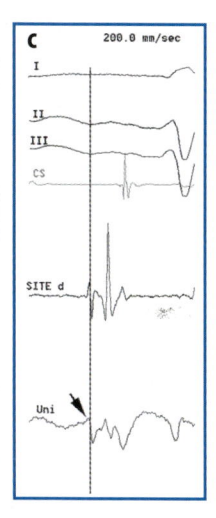

**Fig. 3a-c.** Activation map of the right atrium during focal atrial tachycardia in PA (**a**) and AP (**b**) views, and display of the intracavitary signal at the site of earliest activation in the right atrium (**c**). In the electroanatomic map, the *orange dot* marks the His-bundle area and the *blue dots* indicate a line of double potentials in the lower part of the posteromedial right atrium. In **c**, from *top to bottom*, leads I, II, III, reference coronary sinus signal (CS), bipolar (Sited) and unipolar (Uni) signals from the mapping catheter are shown

atrioventricular node conduction; no arrhythmia was inducible. During isoprenaline infusion, clinical tachycardia appeared in an iterative non-sustained form. Incremental atrial pacing during isoprenaline infusion reproducibly induced a sustained form of the clinical tachycardia with a fast and stable cycle length (240 ms), 2:1 atrioventricular conduction and fixed P ware morphology and intracavitary activation sequence. An atriogram from the coronary sinus catheter was used as the reference signal and electroanatomic mapping commenced in the right atrium with a window-of-interest setting as for focal tachycardia. After the right atrial chamber had been reconstructed, mapping focused on the medial part of the upper right atrium, where a larger area of earliest activation was identified (Fig. 3a). A centrifugally spreading activation pattern was present that resulted in the low lateral right atrium, diametrically opposite the earliest activated site, being activated late, as expected in a focal activation pattern (Fig. 3b). Thus, the crucial issue became discrimination of a left from a right origin of the tachycardia; in other words, did the tachycardia originated from a wider area in the medial upper right atrium, incompletely treated during the previous unsuccessful procedures because of focus extension? Or was the activation pattern observed in the right atrium simply the result of left-to-right propagation from a medial left atrial focus, thus explaining why the previous procedures, limited to the right atrium, were unsuccessfu? After further analysis, all the evidence favoured a left atrial origin, although a proximal to distal activation of the coronary sinus was present. Several observations supported this conclusion: (1) the bipolar signal at the site of earliest right atrial activation (Fig. 3c) preceded the reference signal by 80 ms, but was only simultaneous with the surface P wave onset. (2) The corresponding unipolar signal at this site showed a minimal, but still evident, initial positive upstroke (arrow in Fig. 3c), inconsistent with the site of origin of a focal atrial tachycardia. (3) The finding of three separate spots of earliest activation, evident in the first 15 s of the propagation map (Fig. 4a), is unusual for a focal tachycardia and is more consistent with an activation breakthrough in the right atrium from a left-sided arrhythmia. (4) Although this last finding could be interpreted as the presence of a multifocal atrial tachycardia possibly originating from the myocardial sleeves at the os or inside the superior vena cava, and thus requiring isolation of the latter, it was clear from the bipolar voltage map (Fig. 4b) that the area of earliest activation was in the right atrium, where a preserved bipolar voltage was present. The muscular sleeves penetrating the superior vena cava, identified by voltages < 0.5 mV, were

**48** Focal Atrial Arrhythmias

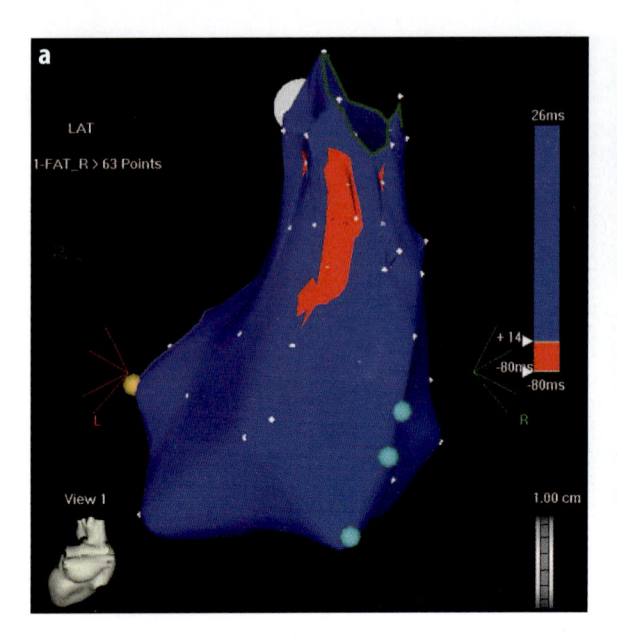

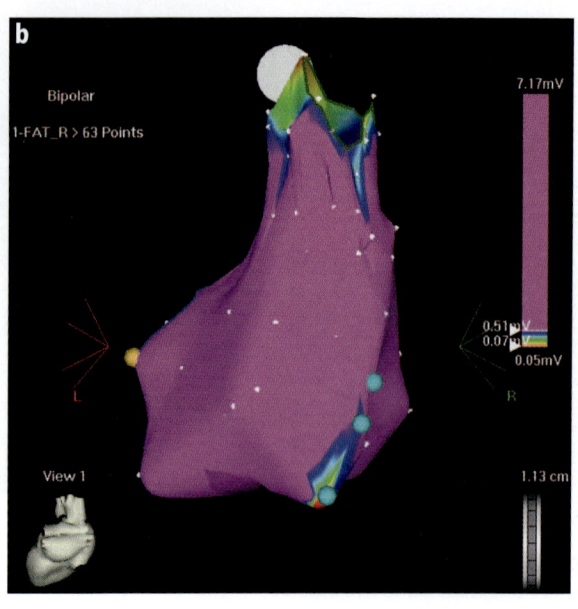

**Fig. 4a, b.** Propagation map of the right atrium of the first 15 ms of activation during tachycardia (**a**) and bipolar voltage map of the right atrium during tachycardia (**b**) in PA view. In **a**, three different spots (two small ones and a wider one in between) of early activation are evident in the upper posteromedial right atrium. In **b**, according to the setting of the colour-coded scale, areas of preserved voltage are shown in *purple*

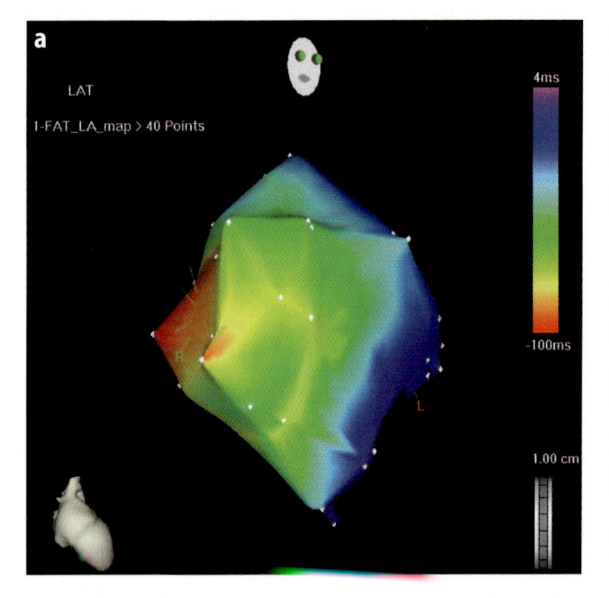

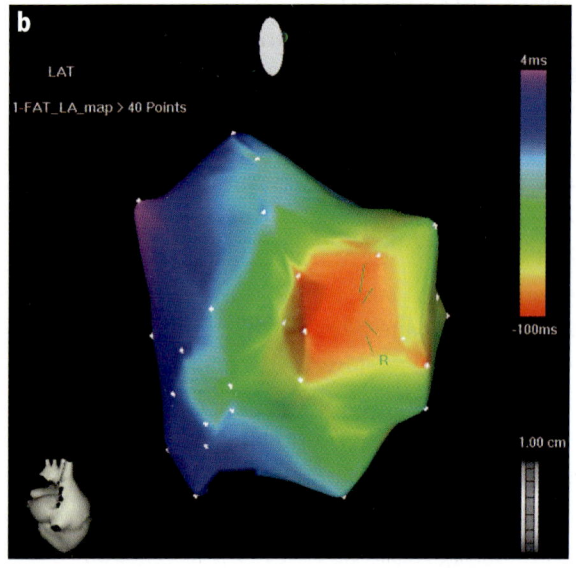

**Fig. 5a, b.** Activation map of the left atrium during tachycardia in RAO (**a**) and posteriorly tilted right lateral (**b**) views

located in a more medial and more superior area. (5) The site of the earliest activated area corresponded to the insertion in the right atrium of the posteromedial accessory interatrial connections, whose role in interatrial propagation becomes relevant when a rhythm originating from the medial left atrium is present. For these reasons, transseptal catheterization was performed and mapping was continued in the left atrium. This confirmed expectations that the upper medial left atrium around the os of the right pulmonary veins was the earliest activated area, with a centrifugal propagation pattern resulting in the posterolateral wall being activated last (Fig. 5a, b). In the area of early activation, the earliest activated site (-100 ms with respect to

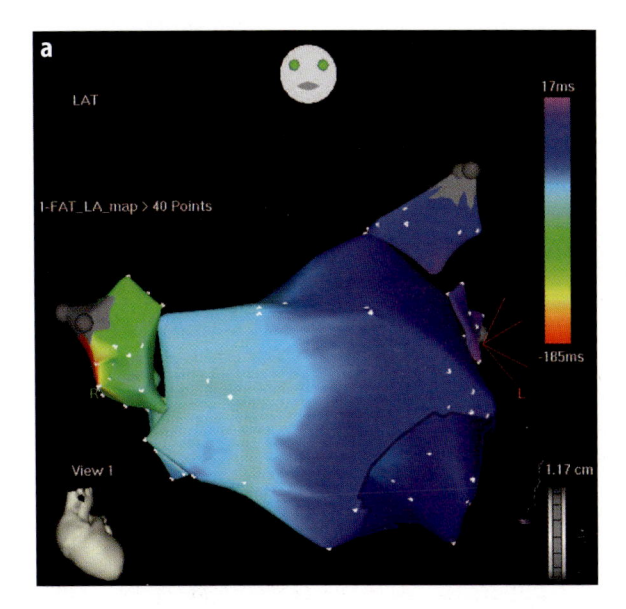

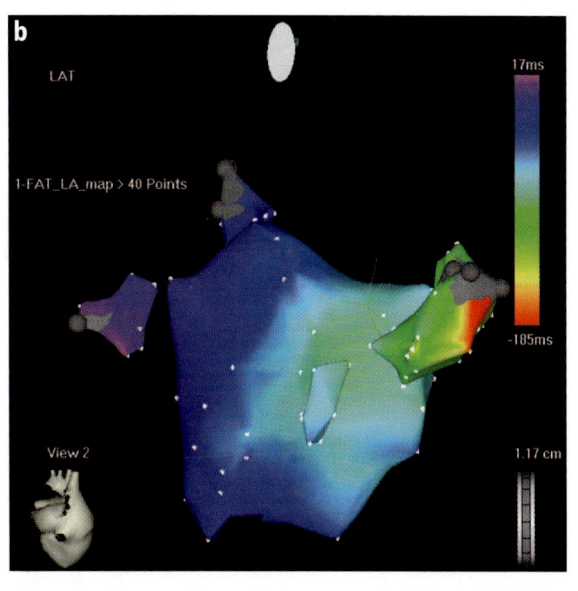

**Fig. 6a, b.** Activation map of the left atrium and pulmonary veins during tachycardia in AP (**a**) and posteriorly tilted right lateral (**b**) views. The four pulmonary veins are electroanatomically reconstructed as separate chambers. The electrically silent, distal part of the pulmonary veins is tagged with *grey dots*

the reference signal, 20 ms earlier than the right atrium) was relatively posterior, while the anterior part of the atriovenous junction of the right superior pulmonary vein activated 10–15 ms later and preceded activation of the corresponding area in the right atrium by a few ms. This led to doubt as to whether the arrhythmia focus was located in the right inferior and not in the right superior pulmonary vein. Mapping was then continued by reconstructing the electrically active areas of the four pulmonary veins as separate chambers (Fig. 6a, b). This further mapping showed that there was a regular activation sequence inside the right superior pulmonary vein, with the earliest activated area being the posteroinferior one. The right inferior pulmonary vein was activated later than the os of the right superior vein, while the left pulmonary veins were activated last, with an activation time similar to the latest activated area in the right atrium. Activation of the site of tachycardia origin preceded left atrial activation by 85 ms, suggesting prolonged propagation inside the vein before exiting to the left atrium. The unipolar potential at the site of tachycardia origin was difficult to evaluate, partly because it was superimposed onto the electrical activity of the previous beat and partly because of the low amplitude of the potential, likely related, as in the previous case, to the minimal myocardial mass present in the pulmonary vein. Figure 7 shows the stable cycle length present at the site of tachycardia origin and the time interval between the pulmonary-vein potential and the far-field potential of the left atrium, during tachycardia (Fig. 7a) and during sinus rhythm (Fig. 7b). It should be noted that this interval was maximal during the 240 ms cycle-length tachycardia, while it decreased to 67 ms during temporary restoration of sinus rhythm, suggesting the presence of rate-dependent decremental conduction in the vein. Figure 7a as well as Figs. 5 and 6 provide evidence of how a rhythm emerging from the right superior pulmonary vein results in proximal to distal activation of the coronary sinus. The CARTO_Merge software was then used to superimpose a pre-acquired and pre-segmented three-dimensional 64-slice computed tomography scan image of the left atrium and pulmonary veins onto electroanatomic mapping. Figure 8 shows the location of the tachycardia focus in the posteroinferior area of the right superior vein, between the origins of two sub-branches. The sequential frames of the propagation map (Fig. 9a–f) show the delayed propagation inside the right superior vein, from the focus to the left atrium following a preferential posterior route (Fig. 9a–c), resulting in earliest activation of the posterior area of the vein os

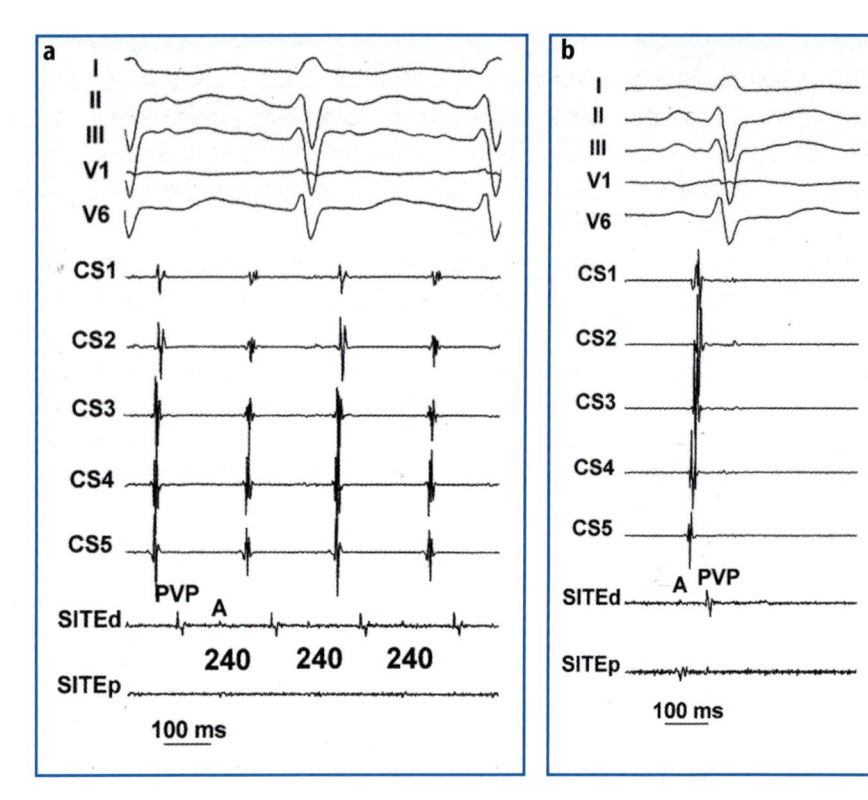

**Fig. 7a, b.** Surface and intracavitary signals during tachycardia (**a**) and sinus rhythm (**b**). From *top to bottom*, surface leads I, II, III, V1 and V6, bipolar recording of the coronary sinus catheter, from distal to proximal (CS1–5), bipolar signals from distal (SITEd) and proximal (SITEp) electrode pairs from the mapping catheter positioned in the right superior pulmonary vein are shown. The time interval between the pulmonary vein potential (*PVP*) and the left atrial deflection (*A*) is longer (85 vs. 67 ms) during tachycardia than during sinus rhythm, when the potential sequence in reversed. Note the proximal to distal activation sequence of the coronary sinus during tachycardia. Numbers are in milliseconds and refer to the tachycardia cycle

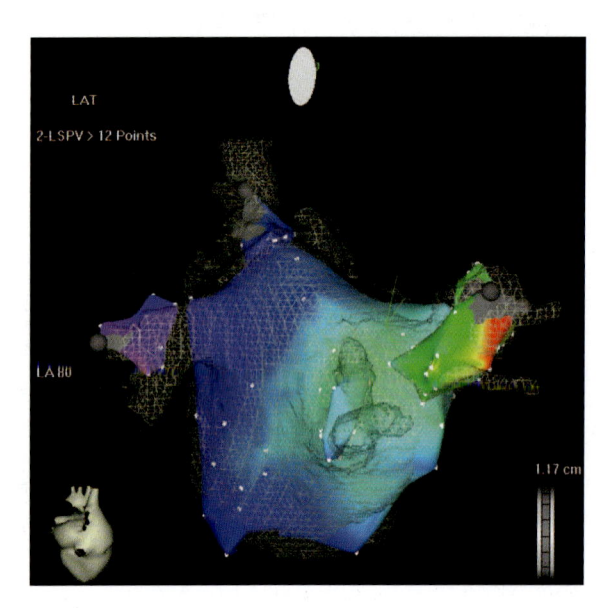

**Fig. 8.** Activation map of the left atrium and pulmonary veins during tachycardia in a posteriorly tilted right lateral view. The three-dimensional reconstruction of the computed tomography scan image of the left atrium and pulmonary vein (displayed as a mesh) is superimposed on the electroanatomic reconstruction. The image has been registered using a single left-atrial roof site and visual alignment with surface registration options

(Fig. 9d) and passive activation of the right inferior pulmonary vein from the left atrium, with a proximal to distal sequence (Fig. 9e–f). Voltage mapping of the left atrium and the pulmonary veins (Fig. 10a, b) diffusely showed preserved bipolar voltage, with the exception of the myocardial sleeves in the pulmonary veins, particularly at the sites of tachycardia origin in the right su-

Case 5 51

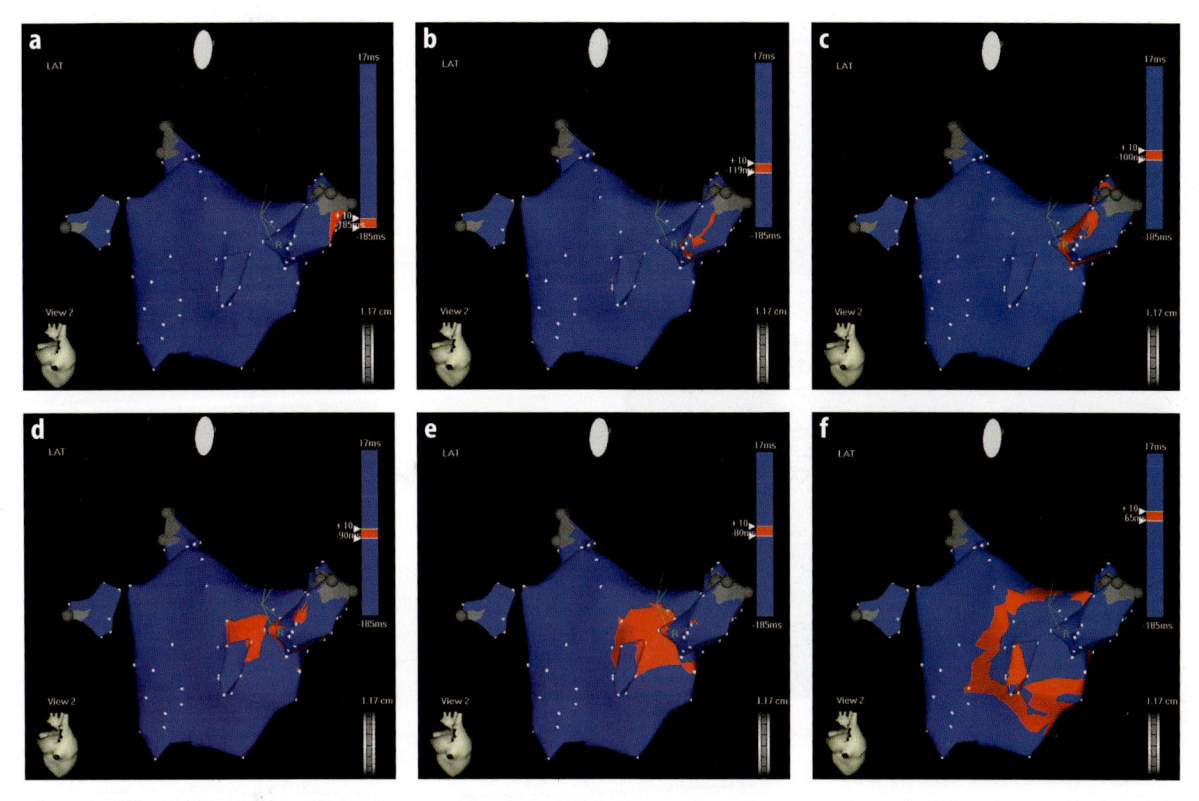

**Fig. 9a-f.** Sequential frames of initial propagation from the right superior pulmonary vein to the left atrium and right inferior pulmonary vein during tachycardia in a posteriorly tilted right lateral view

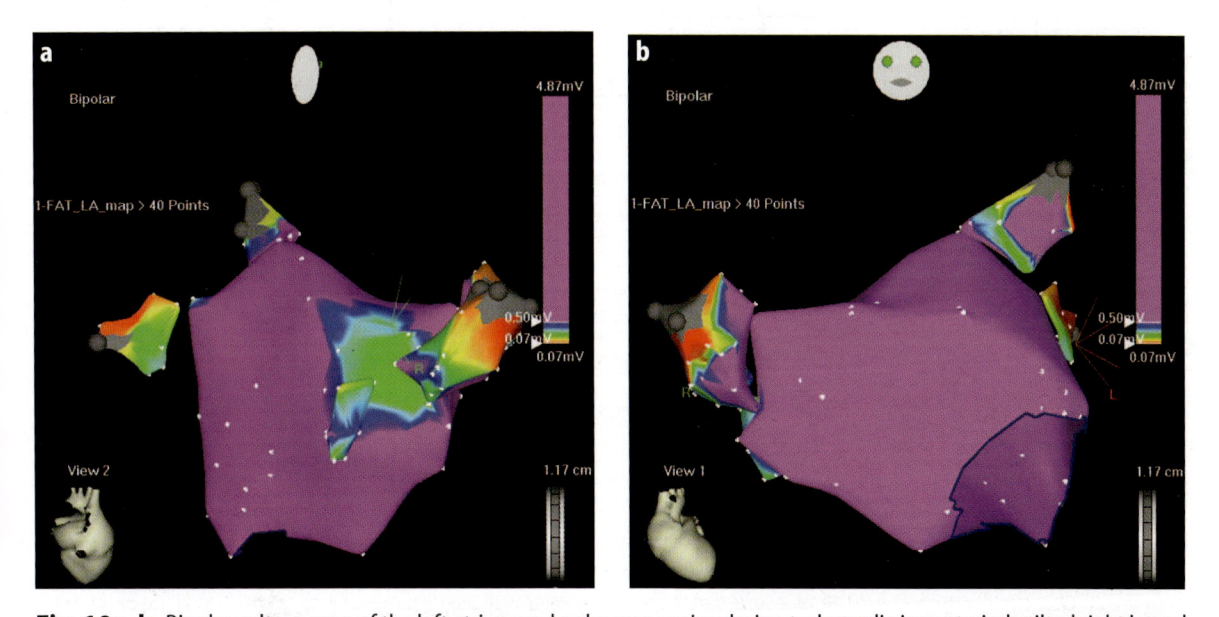

**Fig. 10a, b.** Bipolar voltage map of the left atrium and pulmonary veins during tachycardia in posteriorly tilted right lateral (**a**) and AP (**b**) views. According to the setting of the colour-coded scale, areas of preserved voltage are shown in *purple*. Low voltage is observed not only in the culprit vein, but also in wide areas of the other pulmonary veins

perior vein (where voltage was 0.07–0.09 mV) and of the antrum of the right veins (where the voltage was 0.3 mV). After isoprenaline withdrawal, the right superior pulmonary vein was electrically isolated, mainly in sinus rhythm, by sequential radiofrequency energy applications using an irrigated-tip catheter (maximum power 30 W, cut-off temperature 43°C, duration 60 s), as

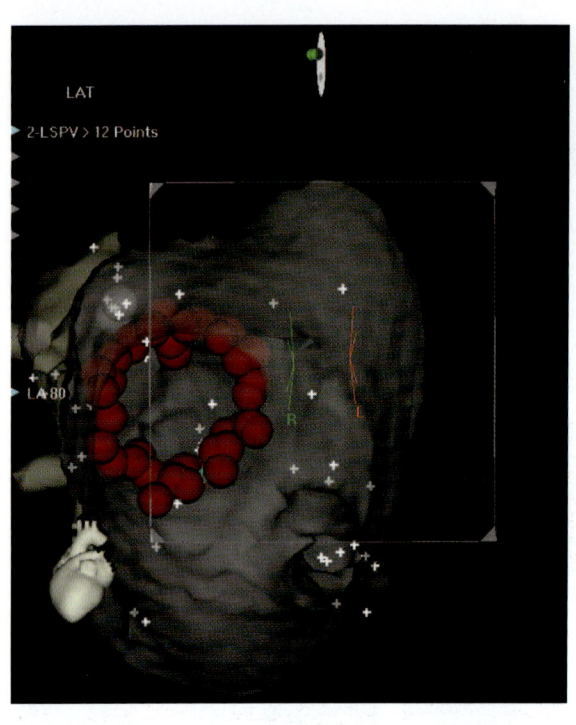

**Fig. 11.** Three-dimensional rendering of the computed tomography scan image of the medial right atrium and pulmonary veins, in a left lateral endocardial view with a sagittal clipping plane. *Red dots* indicate the site of circular ablation around the os of the right superior pulmonary vein

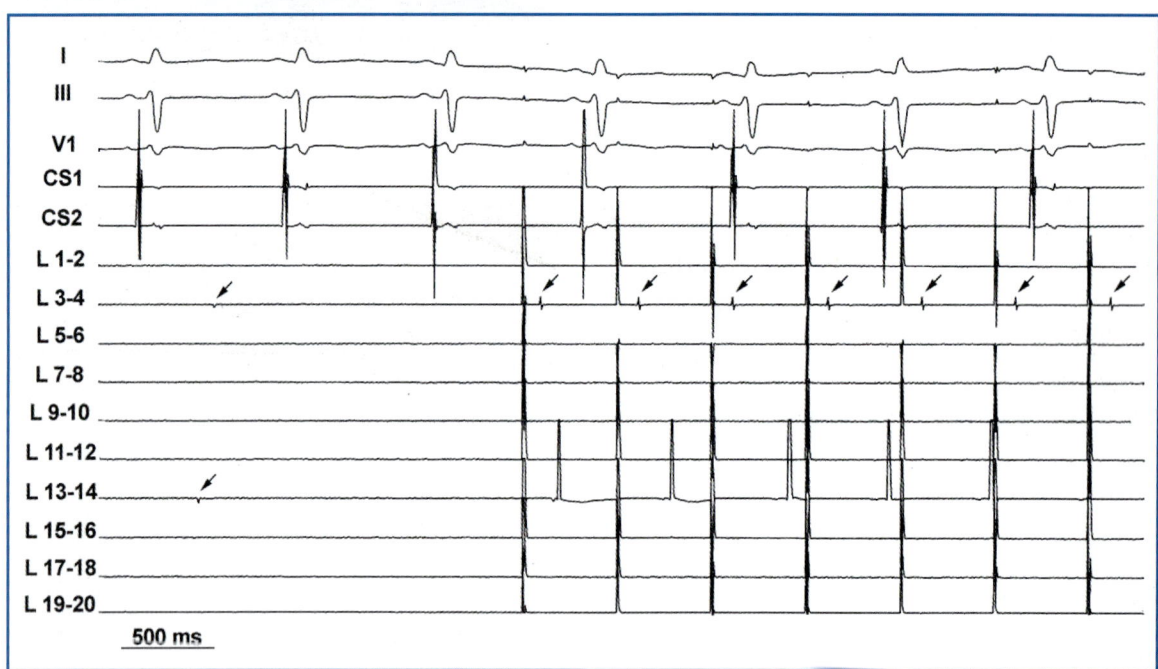

**Fig. 12.** Surface and intracavitary signals after electrical disconnection of the right superior pulmonary vein. From *top to bottom*, surface leads I, III, V1, bipolar recordings from the coronary sinus, from distal to proximal (CS1–2) and bipolar recordings from the 20-pole circular mapping catheter inserted in the right superior vein are displayed. On the right hand side of the tracings, two *arrows* indicate a spontaneous residual electrical activity still present in the pulmonary vein. Pacing artefacts are due to stimulation from poles 13 and 14 of the circular mapping catheter. Stimulation from this site captures the vein potential (*arrows* in L3–4 after the pacing artefact) and demonstrates the exit block to the atrium, which is still in sinus rhythm

shown in Fig. 11. After achievement of complete pulmonary-vein electrical isolation, sinus rhythm was stably restored. A 20-pole circular mapping catheter (Lasso Variable 2515, Biosense-Webster, USA) was then inserted into the vein to verify residual activity. As shown in Fig. 12, a dissociated low-rate electrical activity was still spontaneously present in the vein. Electrical

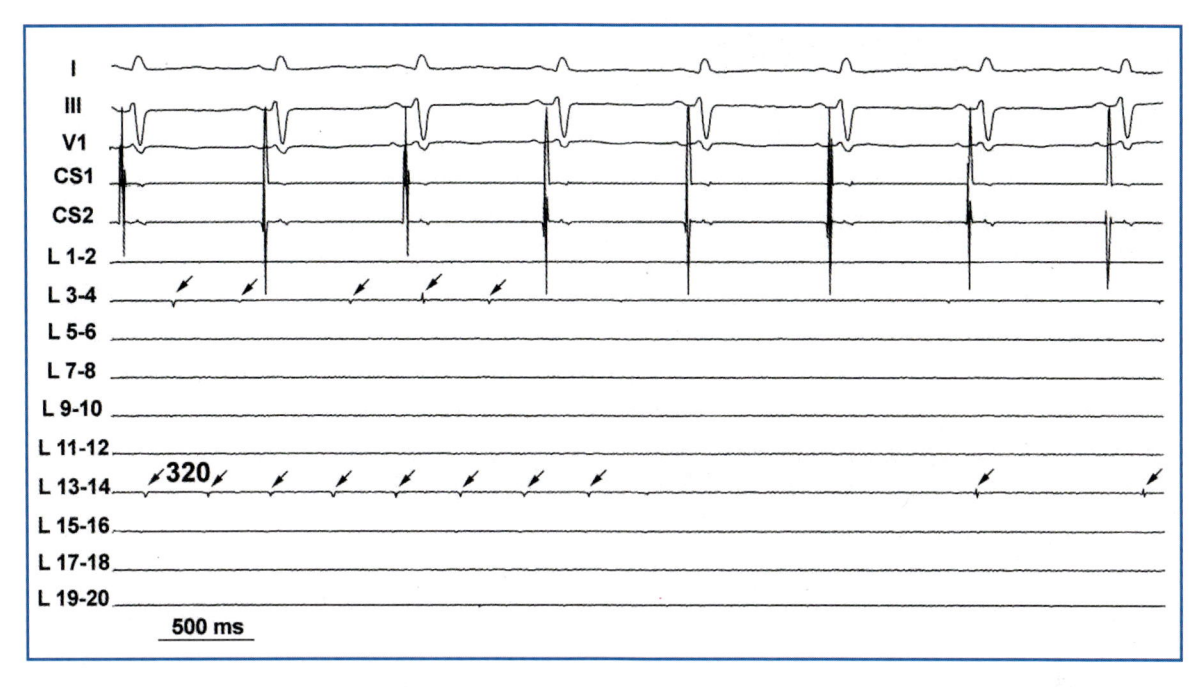

**Fig. 13.** Surface and intracavitary signals after electrical disconnection of the right superior pulmonary vein during isoprenaline infusion. Tracings are displayed as in the Fig. 12. A fast, although irregular, vein electrical activity is still recorded in L3–4 and L13–14 and is completely dissociated from sinus rhythm, further confirming exit conduction block from the vein

stimulation from the poles of the circular mapping catheter resulted in local capture of pulmonary-vein potentials with demonstration of exit block from the isolated pulmonary vein. Interestingly, during maximal isoprenaline infusion, it was still possible to observe (Fig. 13) a non-sustained dissociated tachycardia at 320 ms cycle length present in a localized area inside the vein, while nearby areas in the vein were irregularly activated by the residual focus with a variable degree of conduction block. After a 30-min verification of a persisting bidirectional atrio-venous conduction block, the procedure was terminated. At 8 months follow-up, the patient was arrhythmia free without antiarrhythmic drug therapy.

## Commentary

Unlike the previous case, electrical activity in the right superior pulmonary vein was quite regular and stable during isoprenaline administration in this patient. In the surface electrocardiogram, a tachycardia with stable P wave morphology and cycle length was detected. Variations of the tachycardia cycle length observed clinically could be explained by decremental conduction inside the vein, more evident at higher heart rates (85 ms during tachycardia and 67 ms during sinus rhythm) and probably influenced by adrenergic tone. The conduction time in the culprit pulmonary vein was relatively longer even in sinus rhythm. A previous study showed that, in patients with atrial fibrillation, the average conduction time from the proximal to the distal right superior pulmonary vein, assessed in sinus rhythm by high-density mapping, is 36±19 ms [1]. Significant conduction delay during arrhythmia has been reported in some patients with focal atrial tachycardia originating from the pulmonary vein [2]. Decremental conduction in pulmonary veins was previously demonstrated in patients with atrial fibrillation. The increment in conduction time from the pulmonary vein to the left atrium was significantly higher in these patients than in controls [3]. In the present case, delayed conduction from the pulmonary vein to the left atrium during tachycardia, corresponding to 35% of the tachycardia cycle, was mainly responsible for the fact that electrical activity was recorded for 88% of the tachycardia cycle: if activation times of both atria and of the right superior pulmonary vein were combined, then they accounted for a total of 211 ms. Therefore, other than inter- or intra-atrial conduction disturbances, such as observed in Cases 1 and 2, a pulmonary-vein conduction delay during focal atrial tachycardia originating inside the vein may represent another exception to the general rule that during focal atrial tachycardia a significant portion of the cycle length lacks recorded activity even when recordings from multiple chambers are considered [4]. However, the presence of a macroreentrant circuit in the atria was clearly excluded by electroanatomic mapping. Evidence of a macroreentrant circuit could also be excluded in the right superior pulmonary vein, where a centrifugal, although delayed, propagation pattern was present with activation of the entire vein spanning a reduced portion of the tachycardia cycle.

The main difficulty in this case centred on the discrimination between a right and left atrial origin. Nonetheless, all the considerations made during the procedure, based on an analysis of conventional signals and electroanatomic mapping, clearly indicated the presence of a breakthrough in the right atrium from a left-sided focus. Under such conditions, ablation attempts in the right atrium should be avoided, since there is no evidence that they will be effective. During tachycardia, propagation from the left to the right atrium, which was particularly fast in this case, occurs over posteromedial accessory connections, originating from the left atrium around the right pulmonary vein oses and inserting in the medial upper right atrium [5]. As already reported, although these accessory connections contribute minimally to interatrial propagation during sinus rhythm [6], they become crucially important during focal atrial tachycardias originating from the pulmonary veins [2], resulting in an area of relatively early activation in the posteromedial right atrium (as observed here and in Case 4) that is different from the Bachmann's-bundle insertion in the right atrium. In this case and in the previous one, there was no evidence of a direct connection between the muscular sleeves of the pulmonary veins and the right atrium, by-passing propagation to the left atrium. This rendered ostial isolation of the vein a safe and effective ablation strategy in these patients. Minimal and individual variants of breakthrough in the right atrium are observed; they may be of limited extension and "multifocal", such as in this case, or larger and "single spot", as in the previous case. These variants are likely related to individual anatomic variants of the posteromedial connections and the location of earliest activation in the left atrium.

In this as in other cases (Cases 24 and 25), the complex and variable anatomy of the pulmonary vein can be better approached by extensive electroanatomic mapping and imaging integration after electroanatomic reconstruction of the left atrium and pulmonary veins.

## References

1. De Ponti R, Tritto M, Lanzotti M et al. Computerized high-density mapping of the pulmonary veins: new insights into their electrical activation in patients with atrial fibrillation. Europace 2004; 6: 97-108.
2. Dong J, Zrenner B, Schreieck J et al. Catheter ablation of left atrial focal tachycardia guided by electroanatomic mapping and new insights into interatrial electrical conduction. Heart Rhythm 2005; 2: 578-591.
3. Jaïs P, Hocini M, Macle L et al. Distinctive electrophysiological properties of pulmonary veins in patients with atrial fibrillation. Circulation 2002; 106: 2479-2485.
4. Saoudi N, Cosio F, Waldo A et al. Classification of atrial flutter and regular atrial tachycardia according to electrophysiologic mechanism and anatomic bases: a statement from the Joint Expert Group from the Working Group of Arrhythmias of the European Society of Cardiology and the North American Society of Pacing and Electrophysiology. J Cardiovascular Electrophysiol 2001; 12: 852-886.

5. Ho SY, Sanchez-Quintana D, Cabrera JA et al. Anatomy of the left atrium: implications for radiofrequency ablation of atrial fibrillation. J Cardiovasc Electrophysiol 1999; 10:1525-1533.
6. De Ponti R, Ho SY, Salerno-Uriarte JA et al. Electroanatomic analysis of sinus impulse propagation in normal human atria. J Cardiovasc Electrophysiol 2002; 13: 1-10.

# Part II

# Macroreentrant Atrial Tachycardia/Flutter

# Case 6
## Counter-clockwise Atrial Flutter in the Donor's Right Atrium After Heart Transplantation: a Peculiar Example of Single-Loop Right Atrial Reentry

## Case Presentation

This is a 75-year-old male patient who, 17 years earlier, underwent an orthotopic heart transplantation for idiopathic dilated cardiomyopathy, carried out according to the Lower and Shumway technique. In this technique, large portions of the recipient's right and left atria are kept in place and an atrio-atrial anastomosis is performed with the donor's atria. Before transplantation, the patient was in sinus rhythm with complete left bundle branch block. Early after transplantation, the patient exhibited sinus-node dysfunction with the appearance of junctional rhythm; for this reason, a VVI pacemaker was eventually implanted. Over the 3 months prior to examination in our centre, the patient had suffered recurrent episodes of persistent palpitations. An electrocardiogram during palpitations documented atrial flutter with a P wave morphology resembling that of typical atrial flutter (Fig. 1), although the classical "sawtooth" morphology was not present. The arrhythmia had predominantly a 2:1 atrioventricular conduction. After two episodes terminated by electrical cardioversion, the arrhythmia recurred; for this reason, the patient was admitted for an electrophysiologic procedure.

## Procedure

At the beginning of the procedure, the clinical arrhythmia was present at a cycle length of 265 ms. A decapolar catheter was positioned in the lateral right atrium and a second multipolar catheter was positioned in the coronary sinus. An atriogram from the coronary sinus was used as reference signal and the window of interest was set as for macroreentry (see pp. 1-3). A long sheath was introduced to stabilise the roving catheter during mapping, since the right atrium appeared enlarged. At the end of electroanatomic mapping, its volume was determined to be 184 ml. During mapping, areas corresponding to the recipient's right atrium were electrically silent or showed a fast and very irregular rhythm (Figs. 2, 3). Circular mapping around the site of anastomosis showed that there was a complete electrical dissociation, with no conducting gap, between the recipient's and donor's right atria. The latter showed a stable cycle length of 265 ms, with beat-to-beat variations of less than 10 ms. Therefore, even the electrically active sites of the recipient's right atrium were not annotated and were uniformly tagged in grey, since they were of no interest for electroanatomic reconstruction of the arrhythmia. Mapping was then continued until the duration of the reconstructed right atrial activation equalled the tachycardia cycle length (Fig. 4a–c). It was clear that: (1) the recipient's right atrium represented a relevant volume

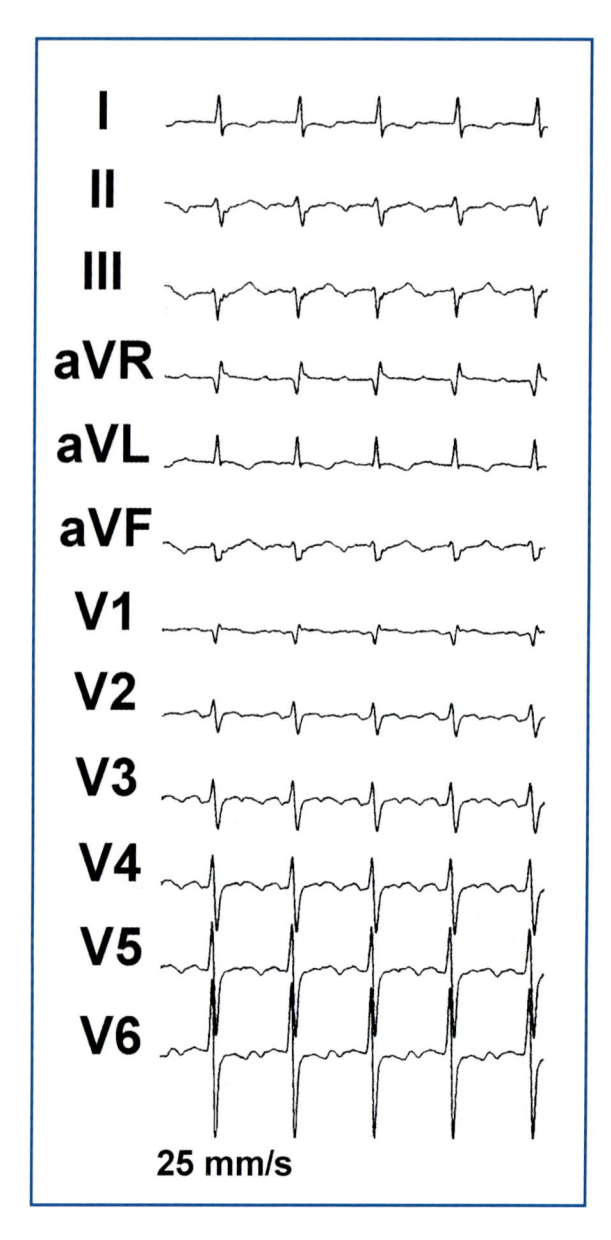

Fig. 1. Twelve-lead electrocardiogram of clinical flutter with 2:1 atrioventricular conduction

of the "new" right atrium, including the region of the right atrial appendage, while the donor's right atrium was limited to a relatively narrow band of atrial myocardium around the tricuspid annulus; (2) the "new" right atrium showed a marked clockwise rotation with the tricuspid valve orifice oriented leftward; (3) the donor's right atrial activation spanned the entire tachycardia cycle length; (4) the arrhythmia was sustained by single-loop counter-clockwise reentry in the donor's right atrium; (5) the mid-diastolically activated area was located in the lateral cavo-tricuspid isthmus, where the red colour encountered the purple one (Fig. 4a). The course of reentry was particularly evident during analysis of the propagation map (Fig. 5a–f): upon exiting from the mid-diastolic area, the reentrant wavefront travelled in the cavotricuspid isthmus from lateral to medial (Fig. 5a–c), then moved to the medial right atrium and upwards in the atrial septum (Fig. 5d, e). Finally, the propagation wavefront returned to the anterolateral right atrium (Fig. 5f) before reentering the mid-diastolic area. The anatomic irregularity of this area combined with the presence of preserved voltage (Fig. 6) led us to argue that this was the area of the donor's lower crista terminalis and not the result of poor catheter contact. The ablation

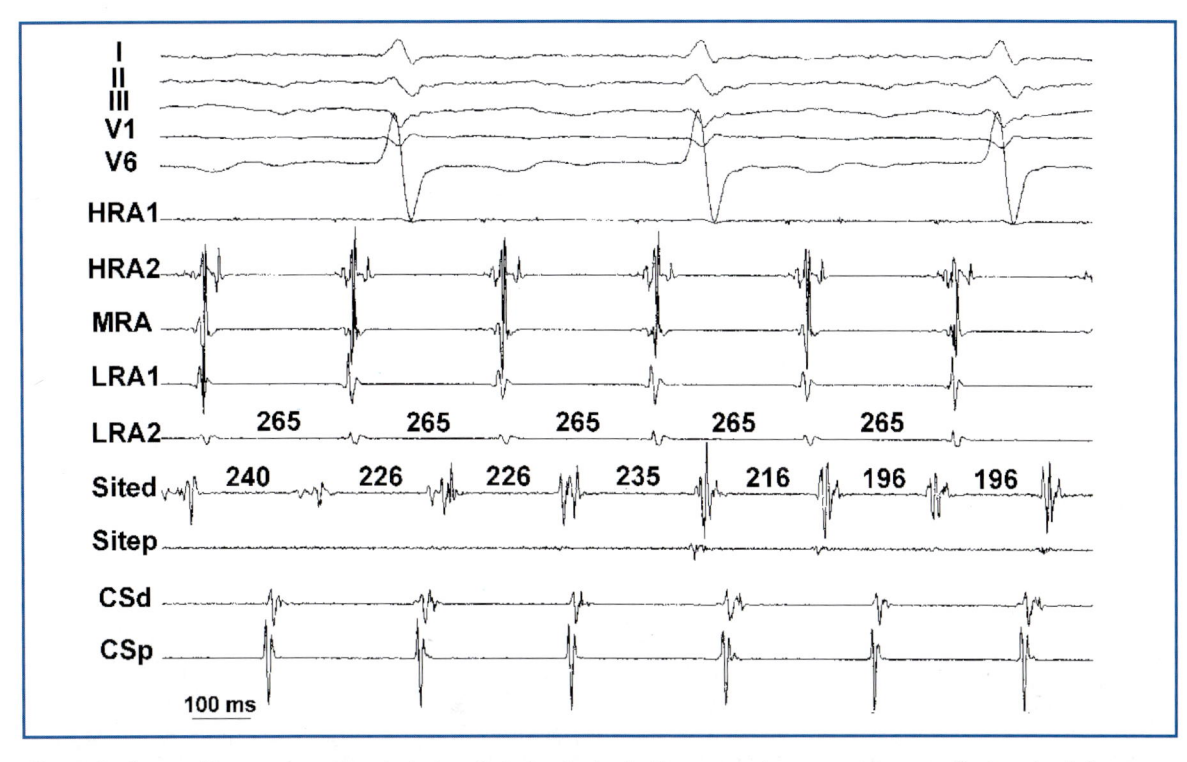

**Fig. 2.** Surface and intracavitary signals during clinical arrhythmia. From *top to bottom*, tracings are displayed as follows: surface leads I, II, III, V1, V6, bipolar signals from proximal (HRA1) to distal (LRA2) electrode pairs of the decapolar catheter placed in the lateral wall of the donor's right atrium, bipolar signals from the distal (Sited) and proximal (Sitep) electrode pair of the mapping catheter and bipolar signals from the distal (CSd) and proximal (CSp) electrode pairs of the coronary-sinus catheter. The mapping catheter was positioned in the recipient's right atrium, where an irregular dissociated electrical activity was recorded. Numbers are in milliseconds and indicate the cycle length of the tachycardia in the donor's lower right atrium (LRA2) and of the irregular activity in the recipient's right atrium (Sited)

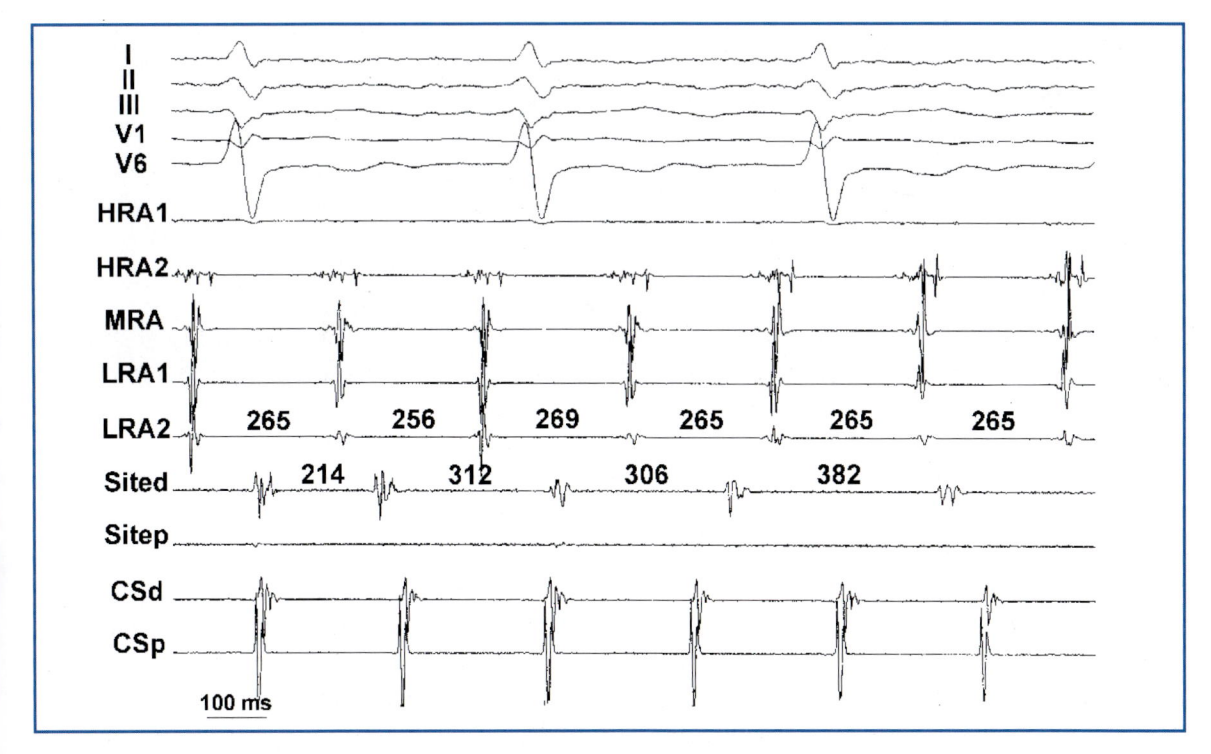

**Fig. 3.** Surface and intracavitary signals during clinical arrhythmia; same catheter positioning and tracing display as in Fig. 2. As shown in tracing Sited, in some areas of the recipient's atrium the cycle length of the electrical activity spontaneously prolongs before the site becomes temporarily silent.

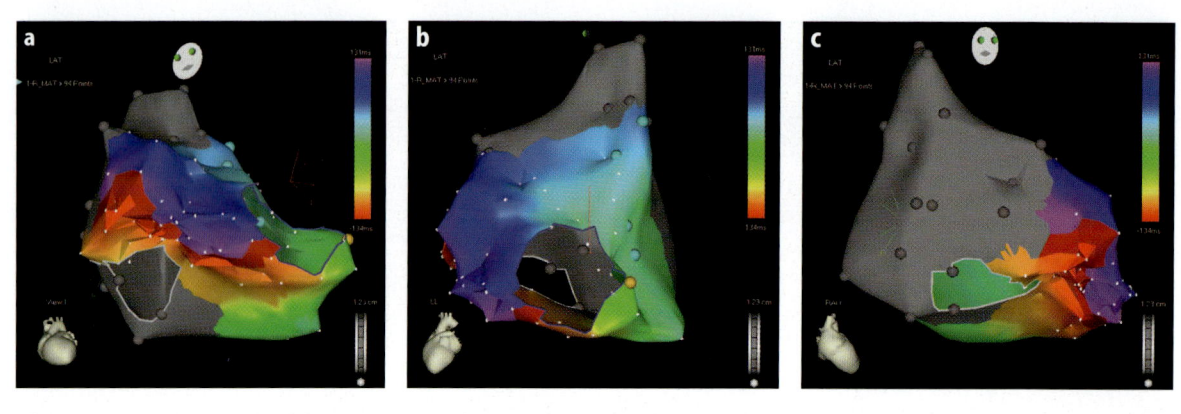

**Fig. 4a–c.** Activation map of the right atrium during atrial flutter in caudal left anterior oblique (LAO) (**a**), left lateral (**b**) and RAO (**c**) views. The *orange dot* indicates the position of the His-bundle area, while *blue dots* indicate the site of double potentials. The recipient's right atrium, electrically silent or with an irregular and dissociated electrical activity, is tagged with *grey dots*. Clockwise rotation of the donor's right atrium with the tricuspid valve orifice oriented leftward is evident

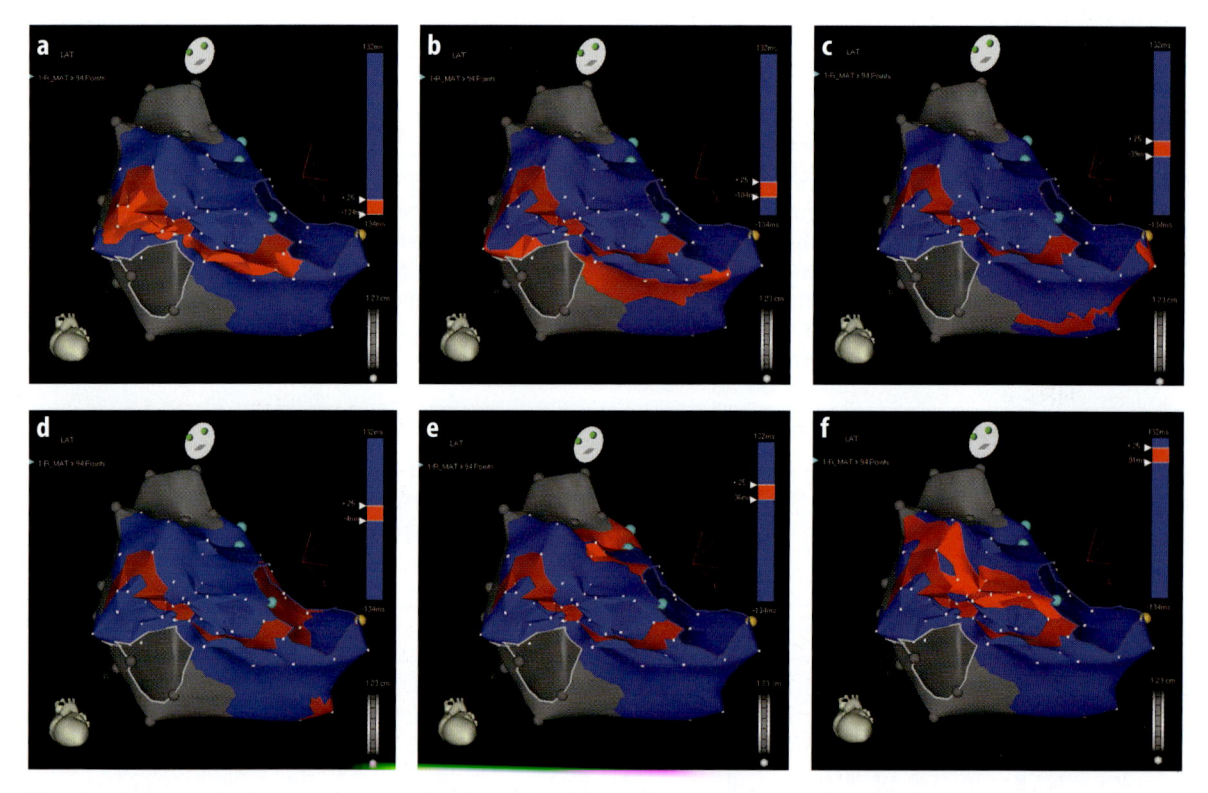

**Fig. 5a–f.** Sequential frames of the propagation map of the right atrium during clinical arrhythmia in caudal LAO view. Counter-clockwise single-loop reentry around the tricuspid annulus is evident. In **b**, the wavefront exiting from the posterior part of the mid-diastolic area (*fixed dark red band*) does not participate in the reentrant circuit and terminates as a dead-end pathway against the inferior vena cava os

strategy was aimed at the mid-diastolic isthmus, but, since its posterior part led to a dead-end pathway against the inferior vena cava os, the ablation line was limited to the anterior part of the mid-diastolic area, which corresponded to the narrowest anatomic isthmus between the tricuspid annulus and the inferior vena cava (Fig. 7). Sequential radiofrequency energy applications using an irrigated-tip catheter (maximum power 40 W, cut-off temperature 43°C, duration 45 s) first prolonged the tachycardia cycle length by 30 ms, then interrupted the arrhythmia, and eventually blocked conduction over the cavotricuspid isthmus, as assessed during coronary-si-

**Fig. 6.** Bipolar voltage map of the right atrium during clinical arrhythmia in caudal LAO view. According to the setting of the colour-coded scale, areas with preserved voltage are shown in *purple*

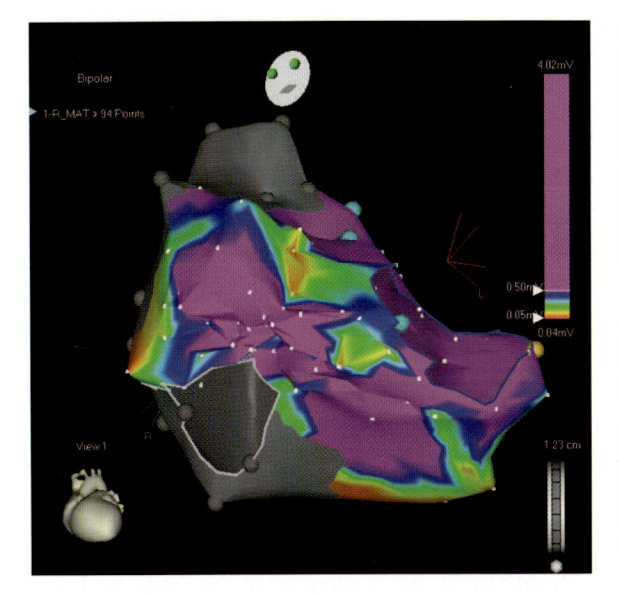

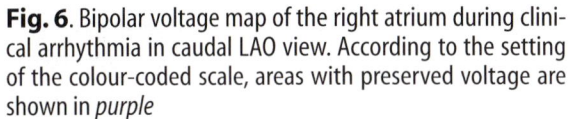

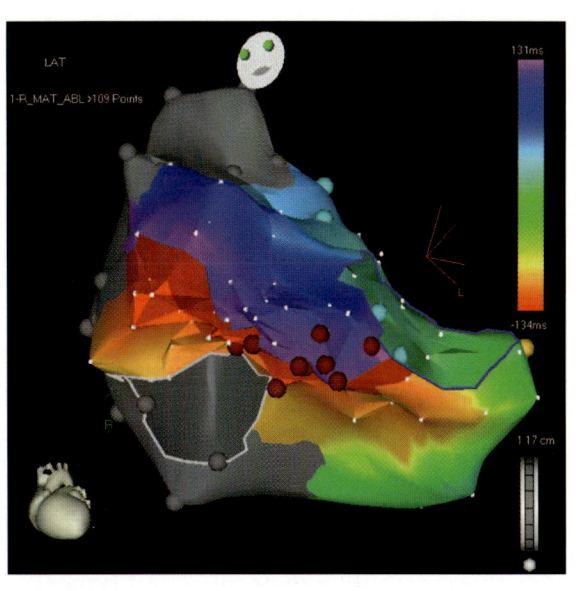

**Fig. 7.** Activation map of the right atrium in the same rhythm and view as in Fig. 4a, with the ablation tags (*red dots*) along the part of the mid-diastolic area involved in the reentrant circuit

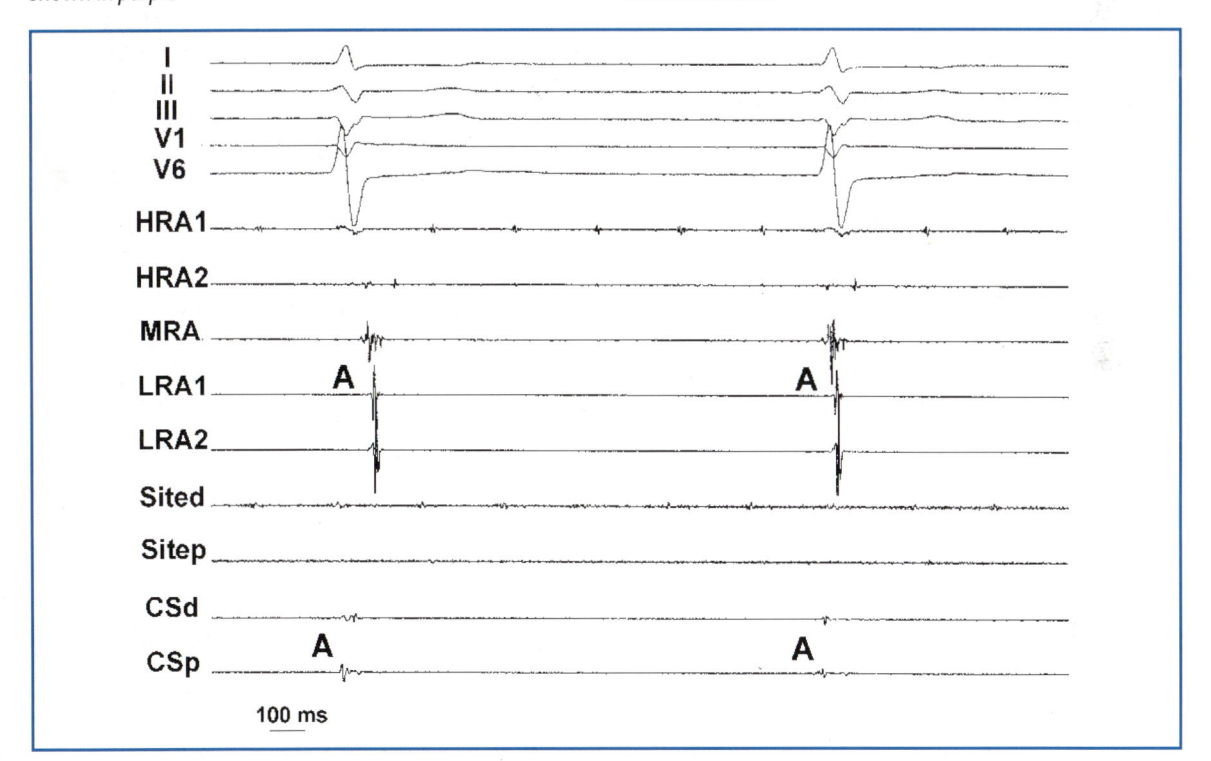

**Fig. 8.** Spontaneous rhythm after termination of atrial flutter by ablation of the cavotricuspid isthmus conduction. Same catheter positioning and tracing display as in Figs. 2 and 3 with the difference that now HRA1 is in the recipient's right atrium. The donor's atrium now has a slow junctional rhythm, with retrograde activation (*A*) to the lower part of the crista terminalis (MRA, LRA1 and LRA2) and to the coronary sinus (CSd and CSp), while the recipient's atrium is now in a dissociated fast atrial tachycardia (HRA1 and Sited)

nus pacing. After the arrhythmia had been terminated, a junctional rhythm with retrograde activation to the donor's right atrium and coronary sinus became apparent, while fast, irregular and dissociated electrical activity was still present in some areas of the recipient's right atrium (Fig. 8). No arrhythmia was inducible and the bidirectional block of the cavotricuspid isthmus conduction persisted after 30 min; accordingly, the procedure was terminated. The patient was arrhythmia free after a 2-year follow-up.

## Commentary

Counter-clockwise isthmus-dependent atrial flutter confined in the donor's right atrium is the most common form of atrial flutter in transplanted hearts with atrio-atrial anastomosis; the approximate prevalence is 4–5% in patients undergoing heart transplantation [1, 2]. Only rarely, the arrhythmia in the donor's heart originates from the development of a neo-atrioatrial electrical connection, and thus requires limited ablation aimed at the site of electrical continuity between the recipient's atrium and that of the donor [3].

The complexity of this case can mainly be ascribed to the distorted anatomy of the enlarged right atrium and to the need for careful mapping to assess electrical isolation between the two portions of the right atrium, since the recipient's right atrium was still electrically active. However, this case, although peculiar, is a typical example of single-loop reentry in the right atrium, which is observed in a minority of postsurgical macroreentrant tachycardia morphologies. In fact, in our experience (see Case 8) as well as in that of others [4], right atrial double-loop reentry may account for up to 65% of the morphologies in postsurgical patients with macroreentrant tachycardias. Moreover, even typical atrial flutter in a structurally normal heart may be sustained in half of the cases by double-loop reentry around the tricuspid annulus and the inferior vena cava [5]. In the present case, the limited portion of the donor's right atrium allowed only single-loop reentry around the tricuspid annulus.

This case represents an exception to the general rule of ablating the entire extension of the mid-diastolic isthmus [6]. In fact, in this patient only the anterior part of the mid-diastolically activated area in the lateral cavotricuspid isthmus was crucial for reentry, while the posterior one caused dead-end activation of the lateral wall and, obviously, did not require ablation. This underlines the need for careful, individual evaluation to define a tailored ablation strategy for each patient.

## References

1. Heist EK, Doshi SK, Singh JP et al. Catheter ablation of atrial flutter after orthotopic heart transplantation. J Cardiovasc Electrophysiol 2004; 15: 1366-1370
2. Marine JE, Schuger CD, Bogun F et al. Mechanism of atrial flutter occurring late after orthotopic heart transplantation with atrio-atrial anastomosis. Pacing Clin Electrophysiol 2005; 28: 412-420.
3. Marine JE, Bogun F, Krishnan SC, Schuger CD. Supraventricular tachycardia in a heart transplant recipent: what is the mechanism? Heart Rhythm 2004; 1: 632-633
4. Magnin-Poull I, De Chillou C, Miljoen H et al. Mechanism of right atrial tachycardia occurring late after surgical closure of atrial septal defects. J Cardiovasc Electrophysiol 2005; 16: 681-687
5. Fujiki A, Nishida K, Sakabe M et al. Entrainment mapping of dual-loop macroreentry in common atrial flutter: new insights into the atrial flutter circuit. J Cardiovasc Electrophysiol 2004; 15: 679-685
6. De Ponti R, Verlato R, Bertaglia E et al. Treatment of macroreentrant atrial tachycardia based on electroanatomic mapping: identification and ablation of the mid-diastolic isthmus. Europace 2007; 9: 449-457

# Case 7
## Single-loop Macroreentry in the Left Atrium in an "Atrial Cardiomyopathy": Discrimination between Right and Left Circuits and the Paradox of Proximal-to-distal Coronary Sinus Activation in a Left-sided Arrhythmia

## Case Presentation

This is a 44-year-old female patient with an initial form of familiar cardiomyopathy characterised by impairment of left ventricular function and sudden death. In sinus rhythm, a very low voltage surface P wave associated with a right bundle branch block and left axis deviation was present. The patient's sister, who showed the same electrocardiographic pattern, had previously died suddenly. The patient's echocardiogram showed enlarged right and left atria, mild mitral valve regurgitation and normal-sized left ventricle with ejection fraction just below the normal range (50%). Over the last 6 months, the patient complained of recurrent episodes of persistent atrial tachycardia with an almost undetectable surface P wave morphology (Fig. 1); the only lead with a discernible positive P wave was V1. The tachycardia cycle length was 310 ms with a prevalent 2:1 atrioventricular conduction, although not infrequently a 1:1 conduction was observed. During sinus rhythm and tachycardia, frequent monomorphic ventricular ectopies were recorded (Fig. 1). Since the arrhythmia recurred early after cardioversion, the patient was highly symptomatic and oral amiodarone was considered a second-choice option, an ablation procedure was planned.

## Procedure

At baseline, the patient was in sinus rhythm. One tetrapolar catheter was positioned into the coronary sinus and a second catheter for electroanatomic mapping was advanced into the right atrium. The H-V interval and atrioventricular nodal conduction were normal, with a normal Wenckebach point. Clinical tachycardia at a stable cycle length of 310 ms could be reproducibly induced by S2S3 coronary-sinus stimulation. The window of interest was set as for macroreentrant tachycardias, calculating the P wave duration only in lead V1, during a transient modification of the 2:1 atrioventricular conduction due to the occurrence of a spontaneous ventricular ectopy. Right atrial mapping was then started and a large, uniform electrically silent area extending from the superior to the inferior venae cavae along the posterolateral wall was evident early during mapping (Fig. 2a). Right atrial activation lasted 192 ms, corresponding to 62% of the tachycardia cycle length. Earliest right atrial activation was simultaneously observed in the upper medial region and in the area of the fossa ovalis (Fig. 2b), whereas the latest activated area, with a mid-diastolic chronology, was in a diametrically opposite site, in what was defined by detailed mapping as a dead-end pathway adjacent to the electrically silent area in the posterolateral wall (Fig. 2a). The right atrial volume was 238 ml. This activation pattern was highly

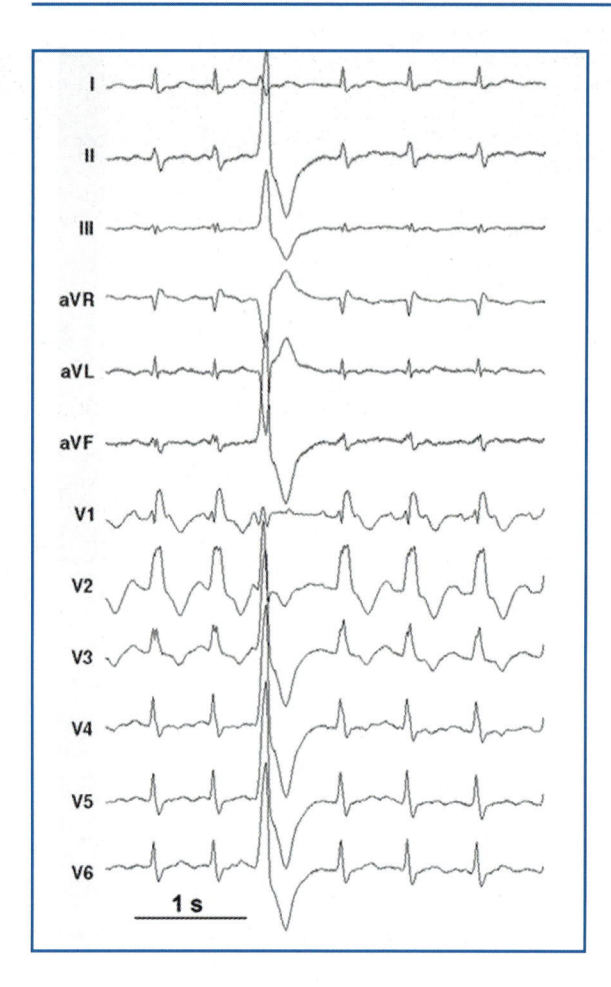

**Fig. 1.** Twelve-lead electrocardiogram of clinical tachycardia with a 2:1 atrioventricular conduction and right bundle branch block. The P wave morphology is not clearly discernible; however, after the ventricular ectopy, two positive P waves are evident in lead V1

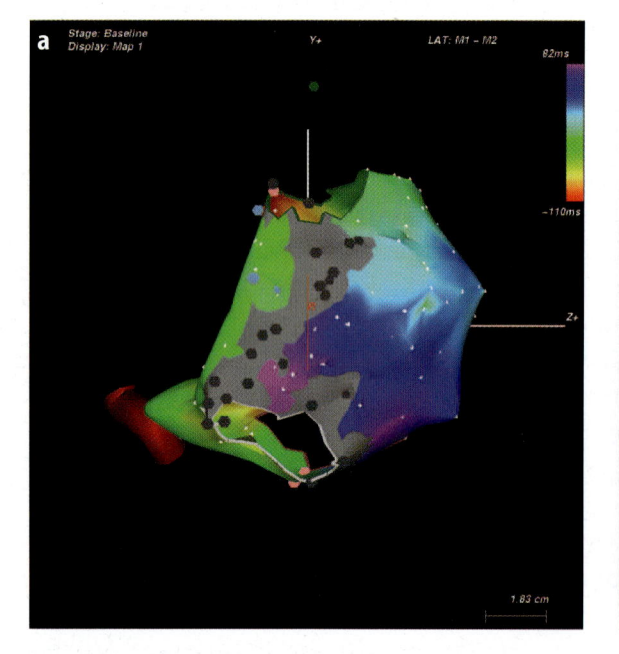

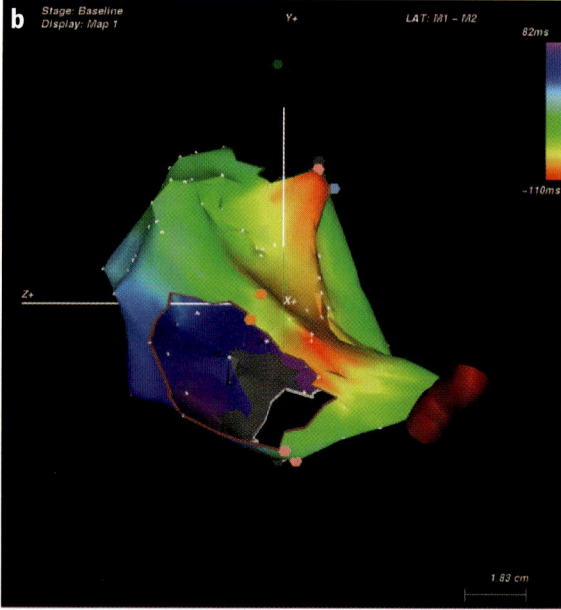

**Fig. 2a,b.** Activation map of the right atrium during tachycardia in right lateral (**a**) and left lateral (**b**) views. Electrically silent areas are tagged in *grey* and sites of double potentials are tagged in *blue*. The two *orange dots* indicate the positions of the proximal and distal His bundle. The proximal coronary sinus is tagged by a tubular icon

**Fig. 3.** Activation map of the left atrium during tachycardia in left anterior oblique (LAO) view. The electrically silent areas are tagged in *grey*; *blue dots* indicate the line of double potentials extending from the posterior part of the electrically silent area to the left superior pulmonary vein os

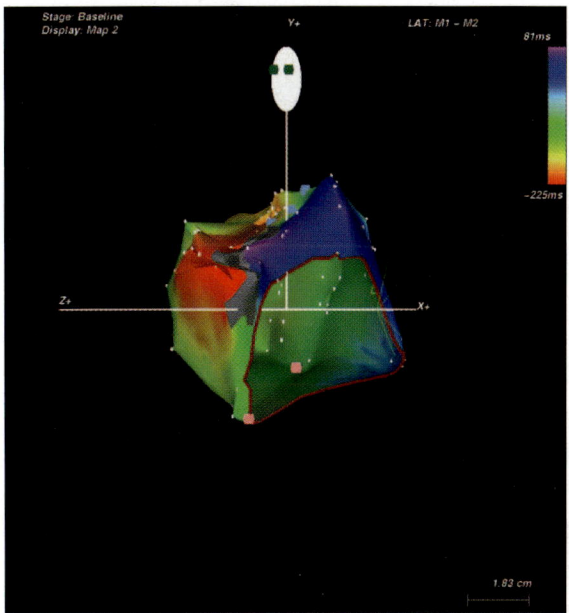

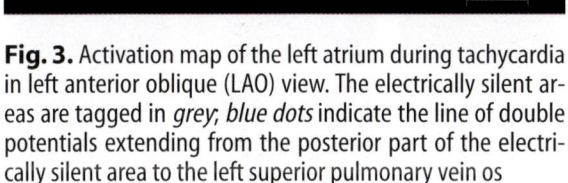

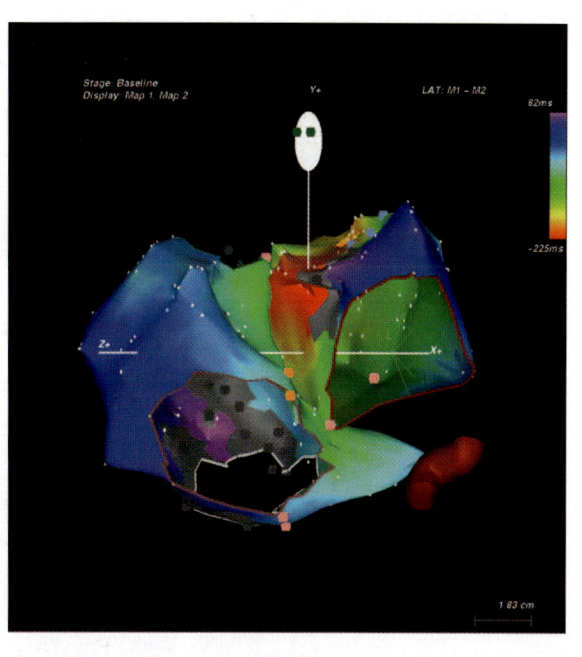

**Fig. 4.** Activation map of both atria during tachycardia in a LAO view

suggestive of a left atrial origin of the arrhythmia despite the fact that: (1) the low-voltage surface P wave morphology was of no use in discriminating a right vs. left origin; (2) the activation sequence of the coronary-sinus catheter was from proximal to distal; and (3) right atrial activation spanned > 50% of the tachycardia cycle length. Therefore, mapping was continued in the left atrium, after transseptal catheterisation was accomplished. The left atrium was then reconstructed until its activation corresponded to 99% of the tachycardia cycle length. A single-loop counter-clockwise reentry was identified (Fig. 3), with a narrow mid-diastolically activated isthmus at the roof. In fact, the mid-diastolic isthmus was represented by a small channel of conducting tissue extending from lateral to medial within an electrically silent area, which anteriorly was adjacent to the mitral annulus and posteriorly was in continuity with an uninterrupted line of double potentials extending up to the left superior pulmonary vein. This line of double potentials, separated by >50–70 ms, was indicative of conduction block in this area. The left atrial volume was 131 ml. Analysis of the biatrial activation map (Fig. 4) identified the presence of two areas of equally late activation (shown in purple in Fig. 4): the first was located, as expected, at the entrance of the mid-diastolic isthmus in the left atrium and was involved in the reentry circuit, whereas the second was in the inferior part of the posterolateral wall in the right atrium and was the result of delayed propagation in this dead-end channel, boundered anteriorly and posteriorly by two electrically silent areas. Analysis of the biatrial propagation map (Fig. 5 a–h) showed diffuse delayed propagation. In fact, the 20-ms red wavefront rotated counter-clockwise and very slowly in the left atrium with a dead-end propagation to the right superior pulmonary vein os (Fig. 5c). Occurrence of a second loop in the left atrium was prevented in this case by the extension of the electrically silent areas and the line of double potentials extending up to the left superior pulmonary vein (Fig. 5b–d). Delayed interatrial propagation was also evident, with earliest activation occurring almost simultaneously in the right atrium at the site of Bachmann's bundle insertion and fossa ovalis (Fig. 5d). The delayed right atrial propaga-

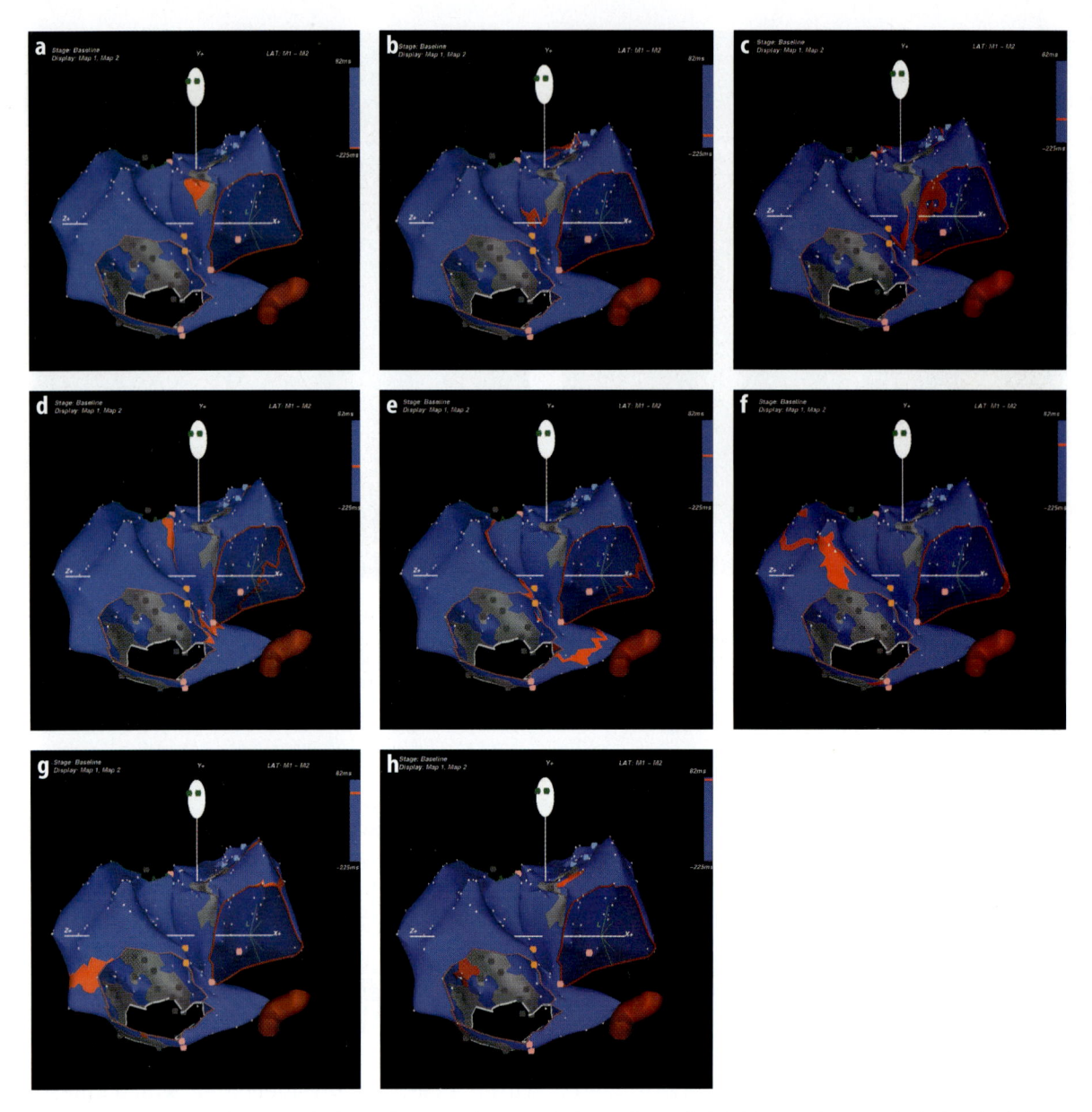

**Fig. 5a-h.** Sequential frames of the biatrial propagation map during tachycardia in LAO view. Counter-clockwise single-loop reentry in the left atrium with by-stander activation of the right atrium is evident. Also note the medial to lateral activation (**c–g**) of the left atrial wall adjacent to the coronary sinus

tion, responsible for its activation spanning 62% of the tachycardia cycle length, was due both to global delayed propagation in this enlarged heart chamber and to dead-end activation in the posterolateral channel (Fig. 5e–h). The finding of delayed propagation was complemented by the evidence of diffuse low-amplitude potentials, as shown by bipolar voltage mapping of both atria (Fig. 6). The extension of the mid-diastolic isthmus was 13 mm and the voltage in this site ranged from 0.07 to 0.1 mV. This area was then targeted for ablation (Fig. 7). Here, stimulation attempts before ablation for entrainment validation resulted in no capture. The first radiofrequency energy application by an irrigated-tip catheter (maximum power 35 W, cut-off temperature 43°C, duration 60 s) prolonged the tachycardia cycle length by 40 ms, resulting temporarily in 1:1 atrioventricular conduction; the second interrupted the arrhythmia (Fig. 8). Another three applications were delivered in the same area to complete the ablation line and this pro-

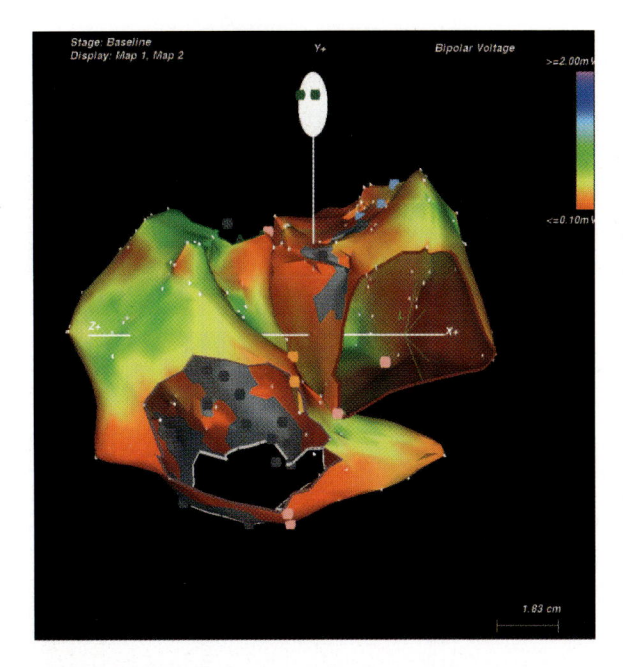

**Fig. 6.** Bipolar voltage map of both atria in LAO view. According to the setting of the colour-coded scale, areas with voltage amplitude < 0.5 mV are shown in *red/yellow*

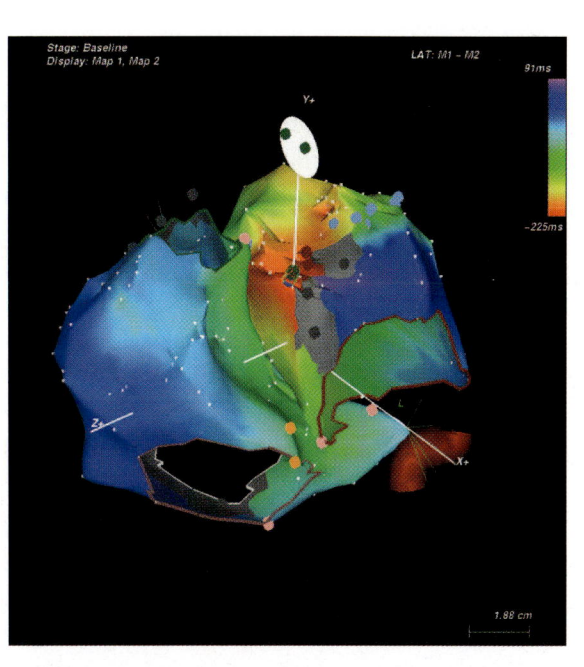

**Fig. 7.** Activation map of both atria during tachycardia in cranial LAO view. The catheter icon is positioned at the narrow mid-diastolic isthmus. The ablation sites are tagged in *red*

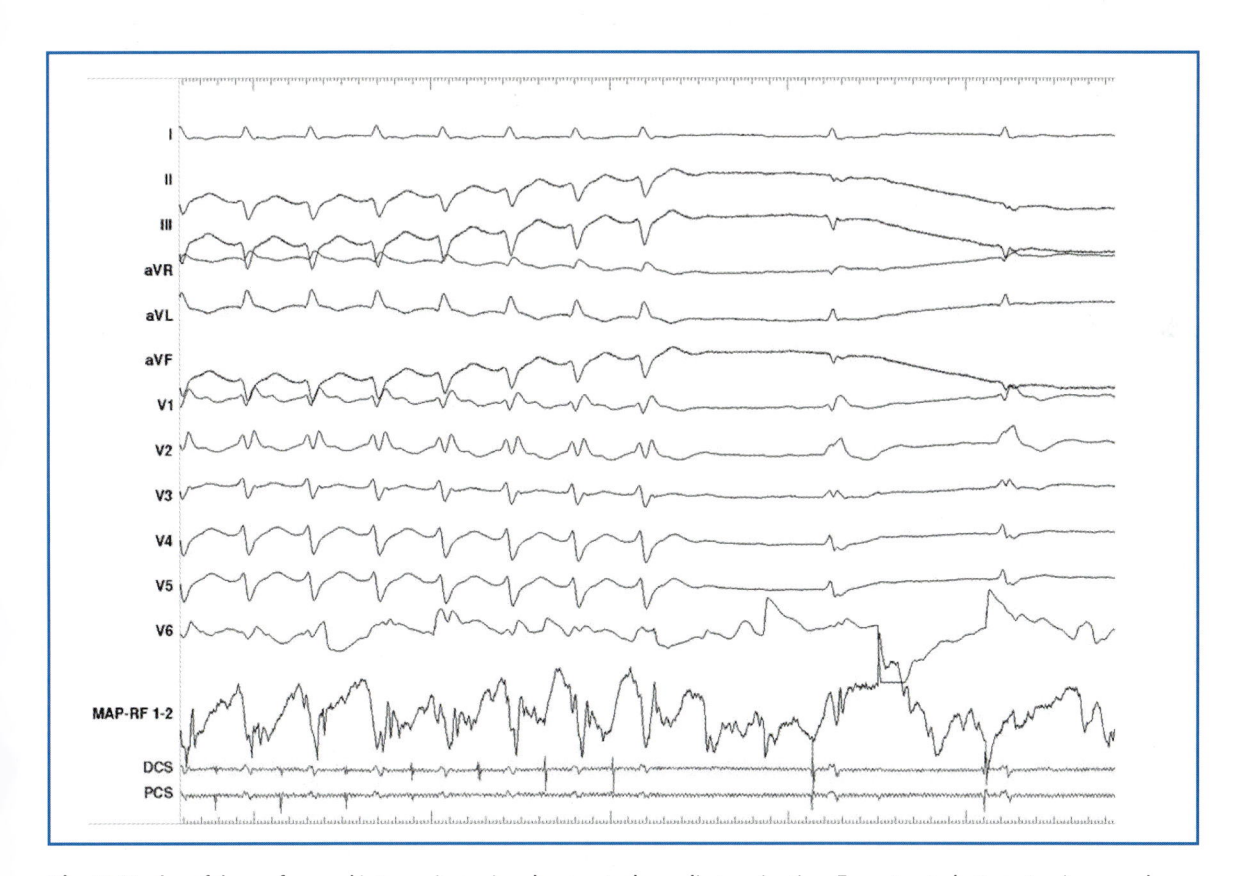

**Fig. 8.** Display of the surface and intracavitary signals upon tachycardia termination. From *top to bottom*, tracings are shown as follows: 12 surface leads, bipolar signal of the distal electrode pair from the ablation catheter (MAP-RF 1-2), and the bipolar signals of the distal (DCS) and proximal (PCS) electrode pairs from the coronary-sinus catheter. After the tachycardia cycle length had been prolonged by the first application with occurrence of 1:1 atrioventricular conduction, the arrhythmia was terminated by the second energy application. The very-low-voltage P wave in the 12 leads is particularly evident also during sinus rhythm

duced disappearance of local potentials. After ablation, an aggressive stimulation protocol induced sustained atrial fibrillation, which had not been previously documented in this patient and therefore was not treated. After restoration of sinus rhythm by electrical cardioversion, the procedure was terminated. Initially, the patient had no early arrhythmia recurrences. Subsequently, she was lost to follow-up. After 24 months, a phone contact revealed that the patient had been referred to another centre for recurrent atrial fibrillation and pulmonary-vein ablation was performed.

## Commentary

Prolongation of atrial conduction time and the effective refractory period, together with the finding of an altered electroanatomic pattern with low voltage, atrial scarring and delayed interatrial conduction, was described in patients with congestive heart failure without atrial arrhythmias [1]. This atrial remodelling in the settings of heart failure renders such patients particularly prone to develop atrial arrhythmias during follow-up. An altered atrial substrate is not unexpected in patients with severe organic heart disease and poor left ventricular function (left ventricular ejection fraction 25.5±6.0%), as was the case in patients studied by Sanders et al. [1], but it is certainly more impressive when found in a patient with a cardiomyopathy, the only expression of which is a mild impairment of left ventricular function, as in the present case. The severity of atrial alterations could be appreciated on surface P wave, during tachycardia and sinus rhythm, and, in a more sophisticated approach, during eletroanatomic mapping. At present, the disease, in this patient, has probably manifested mainly in the atrial myocardium, although the family history of sudden death and the observation of nonsustained ventricular arrhythmias suggest a strict follow-up to detect the appearance of life-threatening ventricular arrhythmias. Certainly, the occurrence of atrial fibrillation during follow-up was not unexpected.

One of the difficulties of this case was the poor definition of the P wave morphology on surface electrocardiograms, actually discernible only in lead V1. This, on the one hand, does not allow preprocedure prediction of the arrhythmia origin based on noninvasive criteria and, on the other, may prevent correct setting of the window of interest for macroreentry, which, according to our method, requires measurement of the maximal P wave duration on the simultaneously displayed 12 leads. Nevertheless, in this case the window of interest could be correctly set considering the P wave duration in lead V1 only.

Another difficulty was in the interpretation of right atrial activation to discriminate right from left tachycardia origin. In fact, in the absence of an indicative P wave morphology, the finding of a proximal to distal coronary sinus activation, a mid-diastolically activated area (as the one observed in the purple area in the dead-end channel in the posterolateral wall; see Figs. 2a and 4) and of an unusually prolonged right atrial activation time, spanning more than 60% of the tachycardia cycle length, could lead the electrophysiologist, using only conventional criteria, to prolong right atrial mapping to search for the missing part of the circuit. In our experience in patients with structural heart disease, by-stander right atrial activation time during a left macroreentrant tachycardia in the absence of cavotricuspid isthmus conduction block generally ranges between 105 and 145 ms and spans about 40% of the tachycardia cycle length. This is in accordance with the previously mentioned study [1], which reported a right atrial activation time of 125.3±14.9 ms during distal coronary sinus stimulation in patients with congestive heart failure and delayed atrial conduction. In spite of the unusually prolonged atrial activation time, the presence of a by-stander mid-diastolically activated area, enlarged right atrium and diffuse atrial scarring, electroanatomic reconstruction of the right atrium provided per se, in this as well as in other cases (Cases 9–11, 15–17), clear evidence of the left origin of the arrhythmia.

Therefore, in the discrimination of left-right origin, careful analysis of the right atrial electroanatomic pattern can be a valid alternative to entrainment, which has been shown to be useful to this prupose [2]. However, a definition based only on entrainment mapping has several limitations and exceptions. In fact, electrical stimulation during tachycardia may produce arrhythmia termination, morphology modification and/or degeneration into atrial fibrillation even if only a limited number of sites are sampled. Moreover, if a post-pacing interval of < 20 ms shows with certainty that the pacing site is part of the circuit, the finding of a post-pacing interval of 40–50 ms in the right atrium does not exclude the possibility, especially in enlarged atria with delayed conduction, that there are right atrial pacing sites not in the circuit, but the circuit is in any case in the right atrium, away from the sites usually tested by entrainment. This occurrence has been reported by very experienced electrophysiologists [3], and the failure to take this possibility into account might lead to unnecessary trans-septal catheterisation. Finally, it should never be assumed that the finding of a proximal to distal activation in the coronary sinus is indicative of a right atrial circuit. In fact, a focal tachycardia from the right superior pulmonary vein (Cases 4 and 5) and reentrant circuits with a counter-clockwise loop in the left atrium (macroreentrant tachycardia in Case 3, this case, and Cases 9, 11, and 16) are invariably responsible for a proximal to distal coronary sinus activation.

Once the right atrial origin was ruled out, the procedure is continued in the left atrium until the sum of the activation scale limits equalled the tachycardia cycle length. At this point, the electroanatomic map showed the entire reentry course and identify the mid-diastolic diastolic isthmus, independently from entrainment. In the present case, the limited extension of the isthmus and the presence of low-amplitude potentials, particularly in that area, rendered the isthmus very vulnerable to ablation and tachycardia abolition was relatively easy to achieve.

Finally, the possibility of an activation pattern showing an area with the same activation time as the one at the entrance of the mid-diastolic isthmus (purple areas in Fig. 4) should be carefully considered. In this case, the fact that this area was remote from the reentrant circuit clearly defines it as by-stander-activated. Nevertheless, it should be considered that by-stander mid-diastolic activation may occur in a dead-end channel in the same heart chamber and close to the isthmus of mid-diastolic activation (see Case 10). This may represent an additional difficulty; thus, careful mapping and annotation are a prerequisite in these cases for correct definition of the reentry course by electroanatomic mapping.

***Acknowledgement.*** *The images of this case were provided by Maurizio Del Greco, MD, Cardiology Department, S. Chiara Hospital, Trento, Italy.*

# References

1. Sanders P, Morton JB, Davidson NC et al. Electrical remodeling of the atrial in congestive heart failure: electrophysiological and electroanatomic mapping in humans. Circulation 2003; 108: 1461-1468.
2. Miyazaki H, Stevenson WG, Stephenson K et al. Entrainment mapping for rapid distinction of the left and right atrial tachycardias. Heart Rhythm 2006; 3: 516-523.
3. Jaïs P, Hocini M, Sanders P et al. An approach to noncavotricuspid isthmus dependent flutter. J Cardiovasc Electrophysiol 2005; 16: 666-673.

# Case 8
# Double-loop Reentry in the Right Atrium with a Shared Mid-Diastolic Isthmus in a Postsurgical Patient: Identifying and Targeting the Shared Isthmus

## Case Presentation

This is a 49-year-old male patient who five years earlier was operated on for mitral and aortic-valve replacement. The subsequent follow-up was uneventful until 1 month before the procedure described here, when the patient began complaining of dyspnea, which worsened in the following weeks. At his first examination, initial-stage congestive heart failure with regular 2:1 atrial flutter and a ventricular rate of 125 beats/min was diagnosed. The atrial flutter morphology (Fig. 1) resembled that of a typical reverse form (positive P waves in leads I, II, III, aVF, V3–V6, negative in aVR, V1–V2 and flat in aVL), although an isoelectric line was present between P waves. After appropriate therapy for congestive heart failure, the patient underwent an electrophysiologic procedure while in arrhythmia.

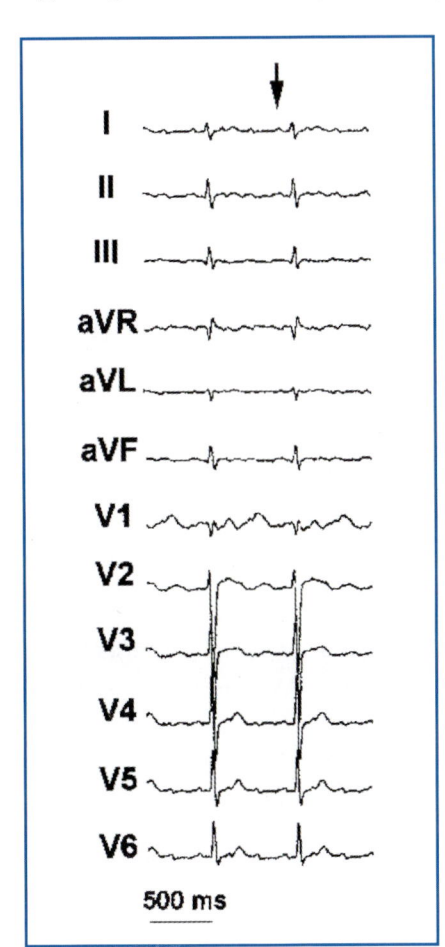

## Procedure

At the beginning of the procedure, clinical atrial flutter at a cycle length of 240 ms was still present. Two decapolar catheters were placed, one along the crista terminalis and one into the coronary sinus. The sequence recorded from the crista terminalis catheter was consistent with a clockwise circuit around the tricuspid annulus; the coronary sinus was activated from proximal to distal. The window of interest was set as for macroreentry, with a mid-coronary sinus atriogram as the reference signal. Right atrial mapping was started and activation of the right atrium was

**Fig. 1.** Twelve-lead electrocardiogram of the clinical arrhythmia, showing 3:1 atrioventricular conduction

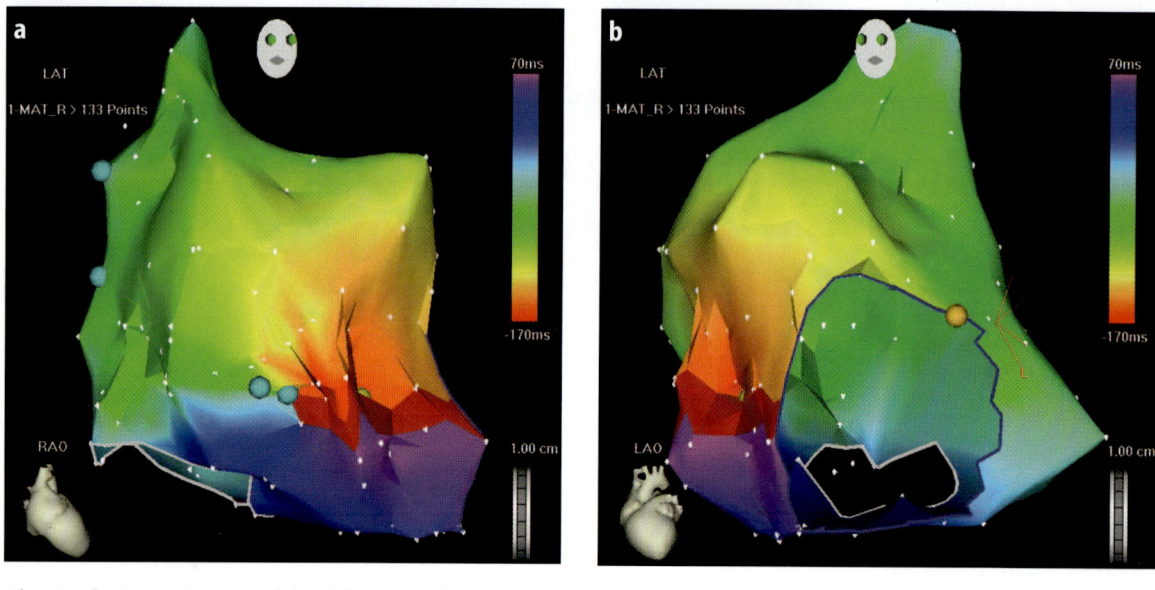

**Fig. 2a, b.** Activation map of the right atrium during tachycardia in right anterior oblique (RAO) (**a**) and left anterior oblique (LAO) (**b**) views. *Blue dots* indicate sites of double potentials; the *orange dot* indicates the His-bundle area, and the *yellow dot* the site of entrainment in the mid-diastolic isthmus. The similar colour distribution clockwise around the tricuspid annulus and counter-clockwise in the lateral wall around the double-potential area suggested the presence of a double-loop reentry, more intuitively visualised in Fig. 3

completely reconstructed. As shown in Fig. 2a, b, right atrial activation equalled the tachycardia cycle length. The right atrial volume was 138 ml. The mid-diastolic isthmus was identified in the lateral wall. It was bounded posteriorly by a small area of double potentials (possibly corresponding to prior atriotomy for insertion of a cannula in the right atrium) and anteriorly by the tricuspid annulus, at 9 o'clock. Analysis of both the colour distribution in the activation map and the propagation map (Fig. 3) identified the reentrant circuit as a double-loop reentry, with the two loops sharing the same mid-diastolic pathway, in a typical "figure of eight" reentry. In fact, the first loop, upon exiting from the mid-diastolic isthmus, rotated clockwise around the

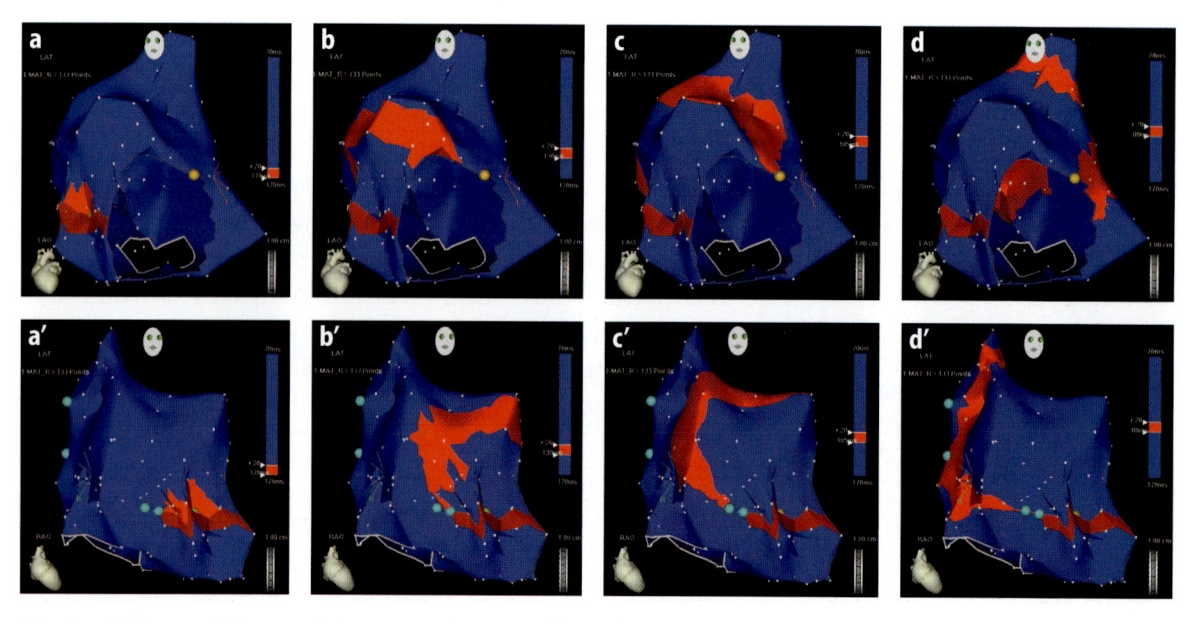

**Fig. 3a–h'.** Sequential frames of the propagation map of the right atrium during tachycardia, in LAO (**a–h**) and RAO (**a'–h'**) view, showing the presence of a double-loop reentry sharing the same mid-diastolic isthmus

tricuspid annulus (Fig. 3a–h). The second loop rotated counter-clockwise in the lateral wall around the small area of double potentials (Fig. 3a'–h'). It separated early from the first loop upon exiting the mid-diastolic isthmus and was directed posteriorly to the double-potential area (Fig. 3a'–d'), then engaged the isthmus between the double-potential area and the inferior vena cava (Fig. 3e'–f') and finally re-joined the first loop in the lower lateral wall (Fig. 3g') to re-enter the mid-diastolic isthmus (Fig. 3h'). The superior vena cava was activated as a dead-end pathway (Fig. 3d, d', e). The propagation map indicated that the two loops were equally dominant, since activation along each one spanned > 90% of the tachycardia cycle. Nevertheless, the lengths of the two loops were quite different, with the loop around the tricuspid annulus significantly longer (18.7 cm) than the lateral-wall loop (9.9 cm). Analysis of the conduction velocities showed slow conduction in the mid-diastolic isthmus (28 cm/s). In the outer part of the first loop, conduction velocities were 78, 100 and 74 cm/s in the anterior wall, medial wall and cavotricuspid isthmus, respectively. Conversely, conduction velocities over the second loop were considerably slower (65 and 66 cm/s in the superior and inferior part of the lateral wall, respectively) while that of a very short tract of the channel, between the double-potential area and the inferior vena cava os, was even slower (16 cm/s). Bipolar voltage mapping during atrial flutter (Fig. 4a, b), showed generally preserved voltage in the right atrium, whereas low-amplitude potentials (<0.5 mV) were recorded in the mid-diastolic isthmus, with the exception of a small channel where voltage was 0.9 mV. Low-voltage areas were also present around the venae cavae orifices and in the posterior wall. Entrainment stimulation in the mid-diastolic isthmus to validate its critical role resulted initially in no capture. However, repositioning the catheter in the only area of preserved voltage along the mid-diastolic isthmus (yellow dot in Figs. 2, 3 and 4), concealed entrainment with the post-pacing interval equalling the tachycardia cycle length was obtained. The ablation strategy was aimed at the mid-diastolic isthmus to simultaneously abolish both loops. Radiofrequency energy application with an irrigated-tip catheter (maximum power 40 W, cut-off temperature 43°C, duration 45 s) was started from the posterior area of the mid-diastolic isthmus, moving anteriorly. After 13 energy applications, the tricuspid annulus was reached (Fig. 5). Further energy deliveries produced tachycardia termination with conduction block over the diastolic isthmus, as assessed by the appearance of double potentials in sinus

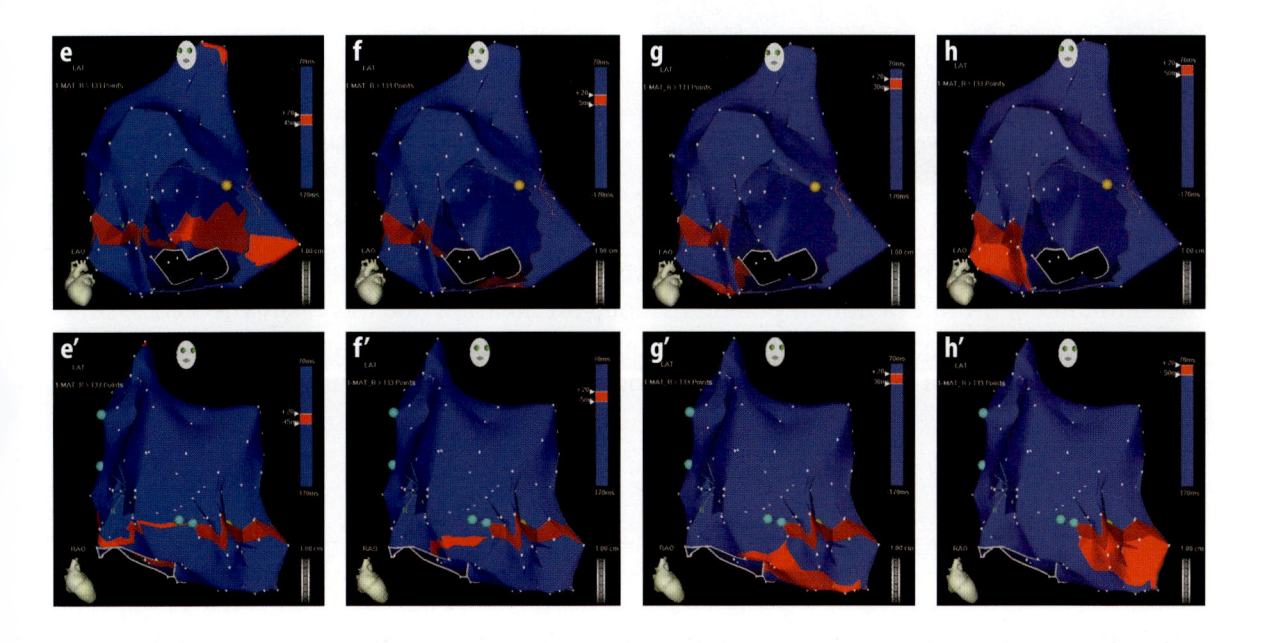

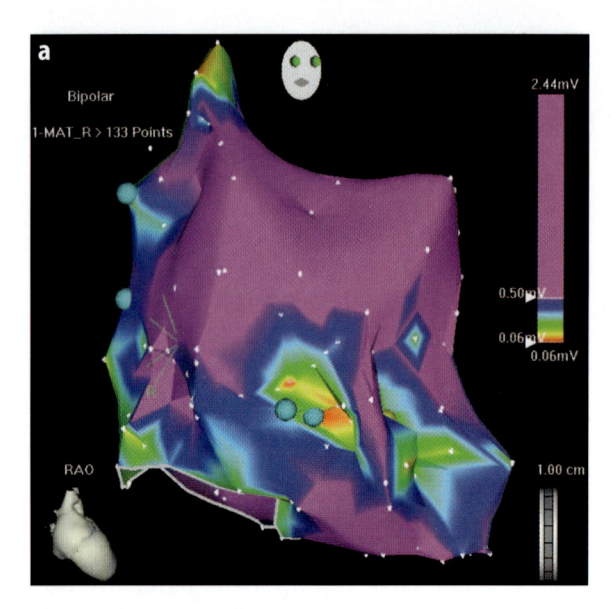

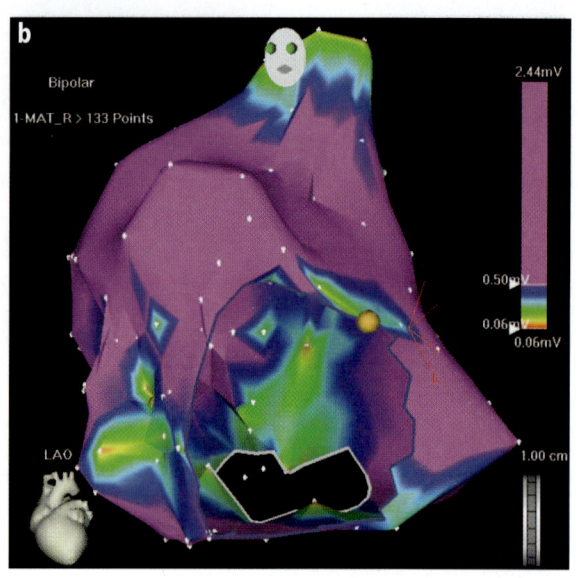

**Fig. 4a, b.** Bipolar voltage map of the right atrium during tachycardia in RAO (**a**) and LAO (**b**) views. According to the setting of the colour-coded scale, areas of preserved voltage are shown in *purple*

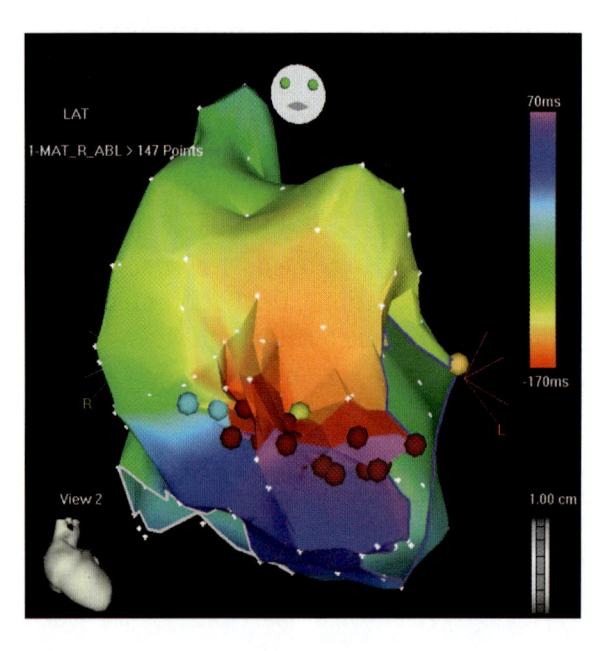

**Fig. 5.** Activation map of the right atrium during tachycardia in a caudal RAO view. Ablation tags in *red* indicate the line of ablation, aimed at the mid-diastolic isthmus

rhythm in the catheter positioned along the crista terminalis (Fig. 6). After ablation termination, the continuity of the line of double potentials along the ablation line was easily checked in sinus rhythm. Afterwards, aggressive atrial stimulation–also during isoprenaline infusion–did not induce arrhythmias. In a 30-month follow-up the patient was arrhythmia-free without antiarrhythmic drugs.

## Commentary

This is a typical "figure of eight" double-loop reentry, in which the two loops rotate in opposite directions and share the same mid-diastolic slow conduction isthmus, as originally described both experimentally [1] and clinically [2] by El Sherif et al. in macroreentrant ventricular ar-

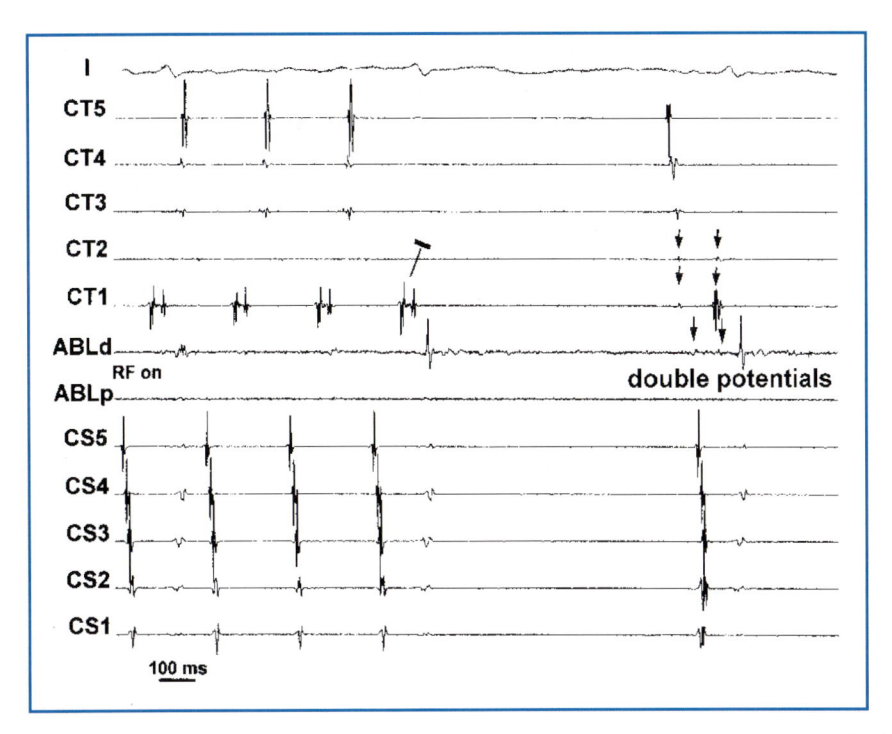

**Fig. 6.** Surface and intracavitary signals upon tachycardia termination. From *top to bottom*, tracings are displayed as follows: lead I, bipolar signals of the crista terminalis catheter from the upper to the lower part (CT5–1), bipolar signals from the distal (ABLd) and proximal (ABLprox) electrode pairs of the ablation catheter, bipolar signals of the coronary sinus catheter from proximal to distal (CS5–1). Radiofrequency energy is delivered and the ablation catheter is in the proximity of the tricuspid annulus, as demonstrated by the presence of a small atrial deflection and a higher ventricular deflection in ABLd. Tachycardia terminates in the mid-diastolic isthmus with conduction block between CT1 and CT2. In the first sinus beat, double potentials separated by approximately 100 ms are evident in the lower crista terminalis and in the distal electrode pair of the ablation catheter

rhythmias. In the present case and in the macroreentrant tachycardia in Cases 3, 9, 11, 13, 16, 18 and 22, two loops were simultaneously present, each one fulfilling the definition of a reentry circuit, i.e. the spatially shortest route of unidirectional activation spanning > 90% of the tachycardia cycle length and returning to the site of earliest activation. In typical "figure of eight" reentry, it is interesting to observe how the different lengths of each loop combine with different conduction velocities to synchronise both loops. Therefore, the two rings of the "eight" do not necessarily have the same size.

In our experience, this form of double-loop reentry with a shared mid-diastolic isthmus is by far the most common. Only rarely are there two independent loops in the same heart chamber, each with its own mid-diastolic isthmus, as in the non-clinical tachycardia of Case 18.

Double-loop reentry in the right atrium can be a frequent finding, especially in postsurgical patients [3, 4]. The ablation strategy of aiming at the shared mid-diastolic isthmus seems more parsimonious than targeting each loop separately by ablating an anatomically defined critical isthmus for each loop. In fact, this strategy can be simpler and faster than independent ablation of each loop, since the time needed for remapping and ablation of the "second" tachycardia, which becomes apparent after conversion of the first one following ablation of the first loop, is spared. Moreover, this strategy aims at what is expected to be the weakest part of both reentrant loops, where very-low-amplitude potentials are combined with slow conduction velocity–as observed in the vast majority of the cases in our experience. In this site, conduction block can be obtained with limited energy delivery and conduction resumption is less likely to occur, thus increasing the short-term success rate and limiting recurrences during follow-up.

A superficial approach to this case would have diagnosed this arrhythmia as a clockwise peritricuspid reentry, with a surface electrocardiogram slightly different from the classic typical reverse atrial flutter. As a result, the cavotricuspid isthmus would have been targeted, which in turn would have only transformed the first tachycardia without an interventional pause in the other, sustained by reentry around the second loop, as frequently occurs when the two loops are separately targeted. This would have prolonged the procedure time and endangered successful ablation. The lesson from this case is that apparently simple arrhythmias in postsurgical patients have to be carefully evaluated.

Demonstration of conduction block by double potentials separated by >100 ms in a site other than the cavotricuspid isthmus is not common, in our experience. In this particular patient, the perpendicular direction of the sinus wavefront with respect to the isthmus together with the presence of preserved voltage areas superior and inferior to the isthmus could have contributed to the easy demonstration of an interrupted line of double potentials during sinus rhythm. In other cases, when the target isthmus is surrounded by a low-voltage area (as in the macroreentrant tachycardia in Case 3 and in the arrhythmias presented in Cases 7, 9, 10, 11, 15, 16 and 17), ablation results in the diffuse disappearance of electrical activity without evidence of double potentials, even during pacing from different sites.

## References

1. El Sherif N, Mehra R, Gough WB, Zeiler RH. Reentrant ventricular arrhythmias in the late myocardial infarction period: interruption of reentrant circuits by cryothermal techniques. Circulation 1983; 8: 644-656.
2. El Sherif N, Restivo M, Gough WB. The figure of eight model of reentrant ventricular rhythms in the subacute phase of myocardial infarction. In: Shenasa M, Borggrefe M, Breithardt G, eds. Cardiac Mapping. Mount Kisco, NY, Futura Publishing Co; 1993: 159-182.
3. Shah D, Jaïs P, Takahashi A et al. Dual-loop intra-atrial reentry in humans. Circulation 2000; 101: 631-639
4. Magnin-Poull I, De Chillou C, Miljoen H et al. Mechanism of right atrial tachycardia occurring late after surgical closure of atrial septal defects. J Cardiovasc Electrophysiol 2005; 16: 681-687.

# Case 9
# Double-loop Reentry in the Left Atrium with a Shared Mid-Diastolic Isthmus in a Non-surgical Patient with Left Atrial Scarring: a More Common than Expected Arrhythmia?

## Case Presentation

This is an 80-year-old female patient with dilated cardiomyopathy and poor left ventricular function (ejection fraction 25%) as well as moderate mitral regurgitation. Prior coronary angiography showed no critical stenosis. Four years earlier, she had experienced episodes of persistent atrial fibrillation, thus worsening her congestive heart failure. After cardioversion, oral amiodarone prevented recurrences of atrial fibrillation in the following years. In the months before the current procedure, while still on amiodarone, the patient complained again of palpitations. Persistent atrial tachycardia with a cycle length of 300 ms and 2:1 atrioventricular conduction with left bundle branch block was documented. Since the arrhythmia recurred after electrical cardioversion and caused worsening of her clinical conditions, the patient was referred for ablation, in spite of her age. Before the procedure, an intravenous bolus of adenosine helped identify the surface P wave morphology, which showed diffuse low voltage (Fig. 1) and was positive in V1–V4, biphasic (-/+) in the inferior leads and flat in all other leads.

## Procedure

At the beginning of the procedure, clinical tachycardia was present, with a cycle length of 310 ms and 2:1 atrioventricular conduction. A decapolar catheter was inserted into the coronary sinus, and a tetrapolar catheter in the His bundle area. A third catheter for electroanatomic mapping was inserted in the right atrium. Mapping commenced after the window of interest had been set as for macroreentry. Right atrial activation (Fig. 2a, b) corresponded to only 35% of the tachycardia cycle length, with early activation in a relatively wide area around the coronary sinus. The latest activated area in the right atrium was located diametrically opposite that of the earliest, in the middle part of the crista terminalis. At the site of earliest activation, in the right atrium, the chronology of the local bipolar signal was presystolic, while, as expected, the local unipolar atriogram showed an initial positive deflection. All these findings strongly favoured a left atrial origin. Therefore, after transseptal catheterisation, mapping was continued in the left atrium. Left atrial enlargement, especially when compared to the right atrium (94 vs. 52 ml, respectively), was evident. No diastolic potential was found until the anterior left atrial wall was mapped. After careful mapping of the anterior wall, left atrial activation was reconstructed for 96% of the tachycardia cycle length. The activation map is shown in Fig. 3. The isthmus of mid-diastolic activation was located between an electrically silent area in the anterior wall and the mitral annu-

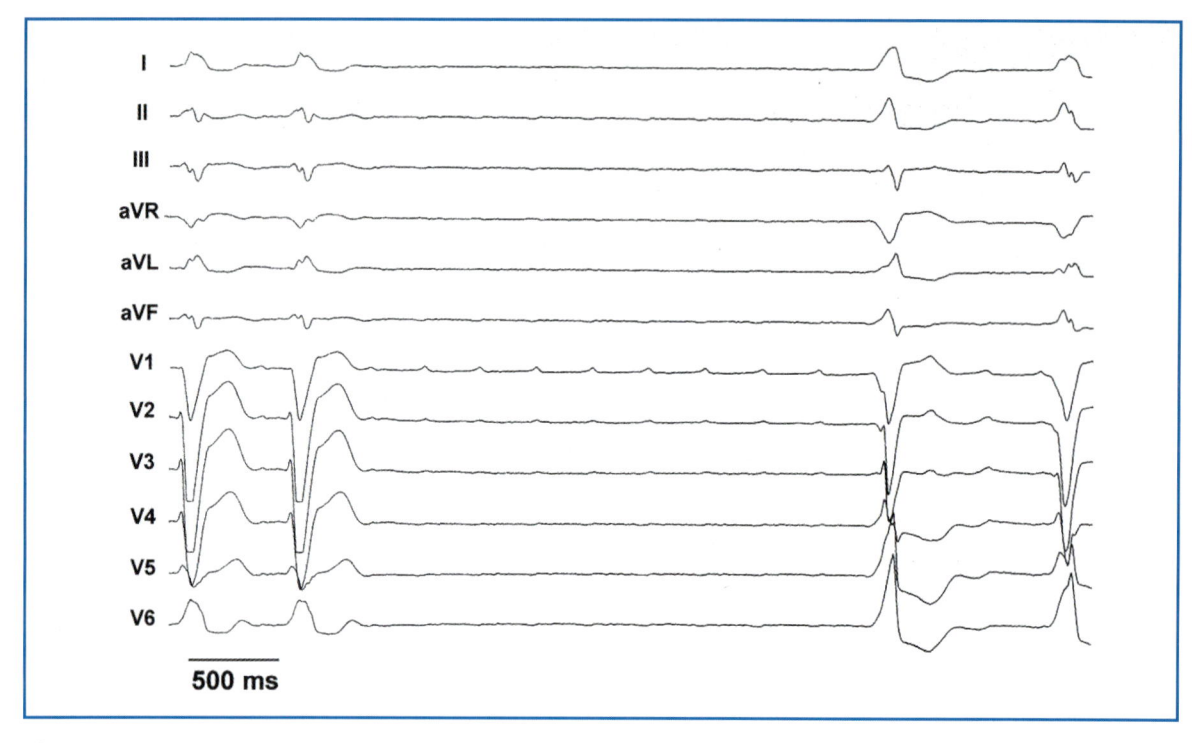

**Fig. 1.** Twelve-lead electrocardiogram of the clinical tachycardia showing 2:1 atrioventricular conduction and left bundle branch block at baseline. Transient atrioventricular block was observed after an intravenous bolus of adenosine, thereby allowing identification of the low-voltage P waves

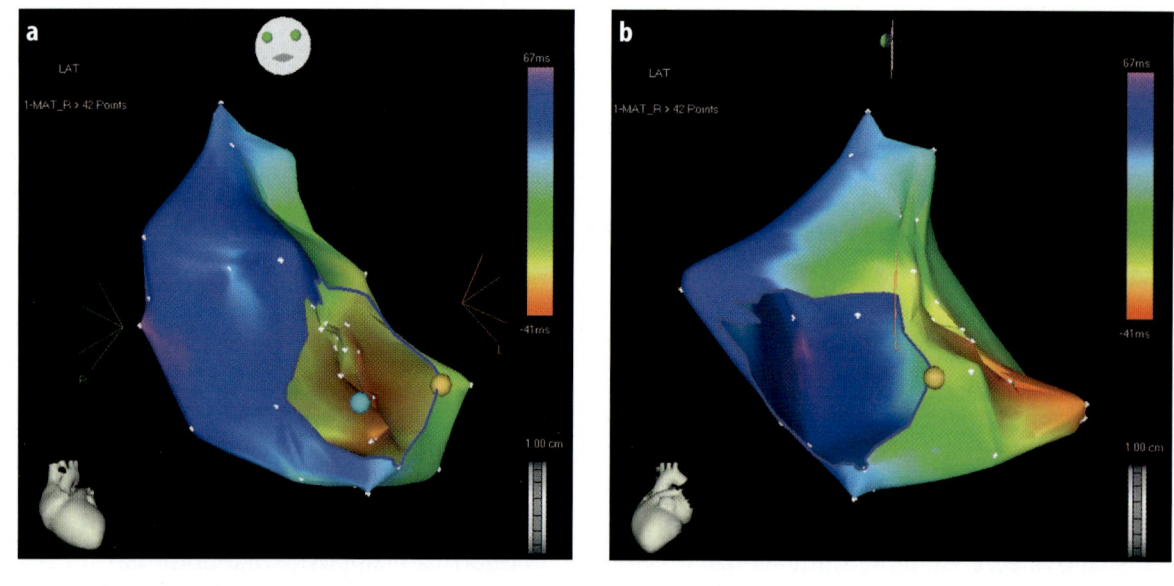

**Fig. 2a, b.** Activation map of the right atrium during tachycardia in caudal AP (**a**) and left lateral (**b**) views. The *orange dot* indicates the His-bundle area, while the site marked by a *blue dot* shows double potentials. In **b**, it is particularly evident that, although the entire atrial septum is activated early, the earliest activated right atrial site is around the coronary sinus os

lus at 12 o'clock. This isthmus measured 5 mm. The bipolar signals recorded in the mid-diastolic isthmus (Fig. 4) were fragmented, with low-amplitude, and lasted 70–80 ms. As usual, the first sharp deflection was annotated in the electroanatomic map (arrow in Fig. 4). Interatrial propagation, as shown in the biatrial propagation map (Fig. 5a–d), occurred preferentially over the

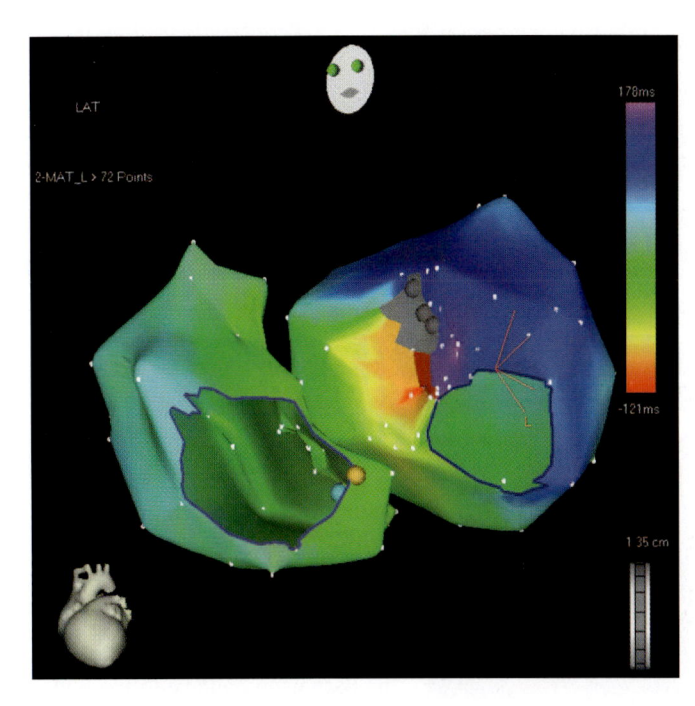

**Fig. 3.** Activation map of the right and left atria during tachycardia in a left anterior oblique (LAO) view. The electrically silent area in the left atrium is marked by *grey dots*

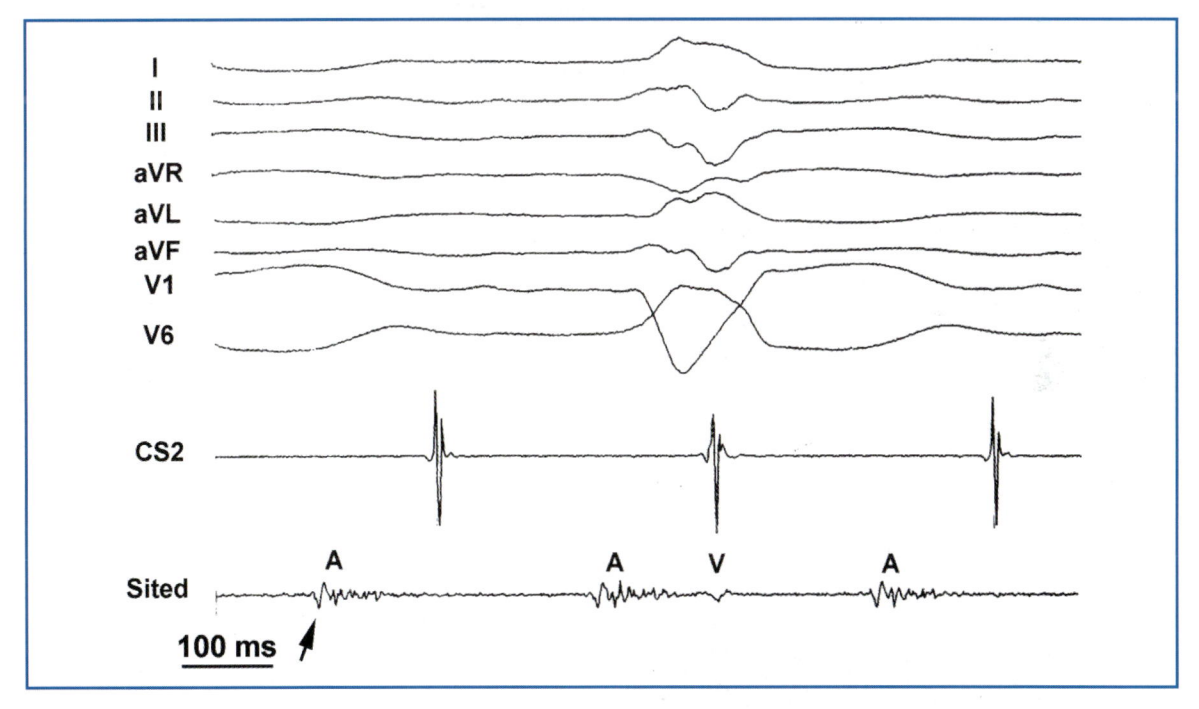

**Fig. 4.** Surface and intracavitary signals during tachycardia. From *top to bottom*, limb and V1, V6 leads, a bipolar coronary sinus signal (CS2) and the bipolar signal from the distal electrode pair of the mapping catheter (Sited) are shown. The mapping catheter is positioned in the mid-diastolic isthmus, where a fragmented, multicomponent, low-amplitude long-lasting signal is recorded. Annotation was made on the first negative deflection (indicated by the *arrow*)

coronary sinus and the fossa ovalis rather than over Bachmann's bundle, although the exit site from the mid-diastolic pathway was located close to the insertion in the left atrium of Bachmann's bundle. As a result, the atrial septum activated from inferior to superior. Analysis of the bipolar voltage map on tachycardia (Fig. 6) showed a relatively preserved voltage in the right atrium (with the exception of the area around the venae cavae and the lower atrial septum), whereas a very low (between 0.06 and 0.14 mV) voltage area was present in the mid-diastolic

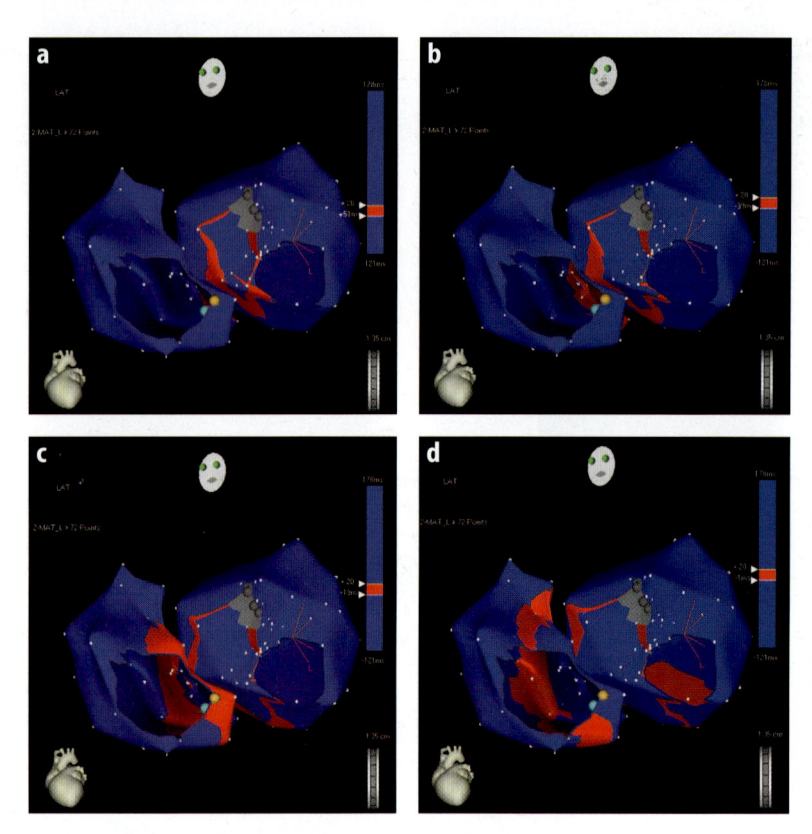

**Fig. 5a-d.** Sequential frames of the propagation map of both atria during tachycardia in LAO view. Interatrial propagation occurs during tachycardia mainly over the coronary sinus fibres with early activation also of the area of the fossa ovalis (**a**, **b**). The insertion of the Bachmann's bundle in the upper medial right atrium is activated late and from the septal area (**c**, **d**), suggesting delayed conduction over Bachmann's bundle

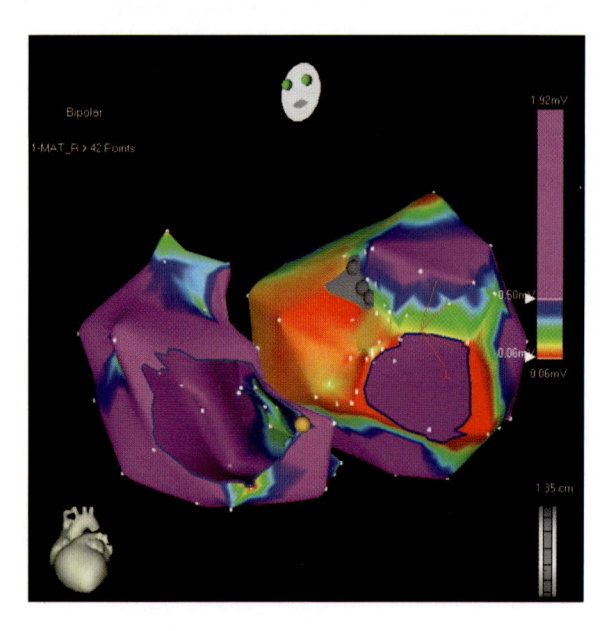

**Fig. 6.** Bipolar voltage map of both atria in LAO view during tachycardia. According to the setting of the colour-coded scale, areas of preserved voltage are shown in *purple*

isthmus and in the medial part of the anterior left atrium. The analysis of both colour distribution in the activation map and propagation in the left atrium showed that the tachycardia was sustained by a double-loop reentry, with the first loop rotating counter-clockwise around the mitral annulus (Fig. 7a–f) and the second one rotating clockwise in the roof around the electrically silent and low-voltage area (Fig. 7a'–f'). The two loops shared the mid-diastolic isthmus in a typical "figure of eight" morphology and parted upon exiting the isthmus (Fig. 7b'), rejoining in the area of the appendage (Fig. 7d), just before reentering the mid-diastolic isthmus (Fig. 7e, f). The two loops were of approximately the same length: 14.5 cm for the perimitral loop and

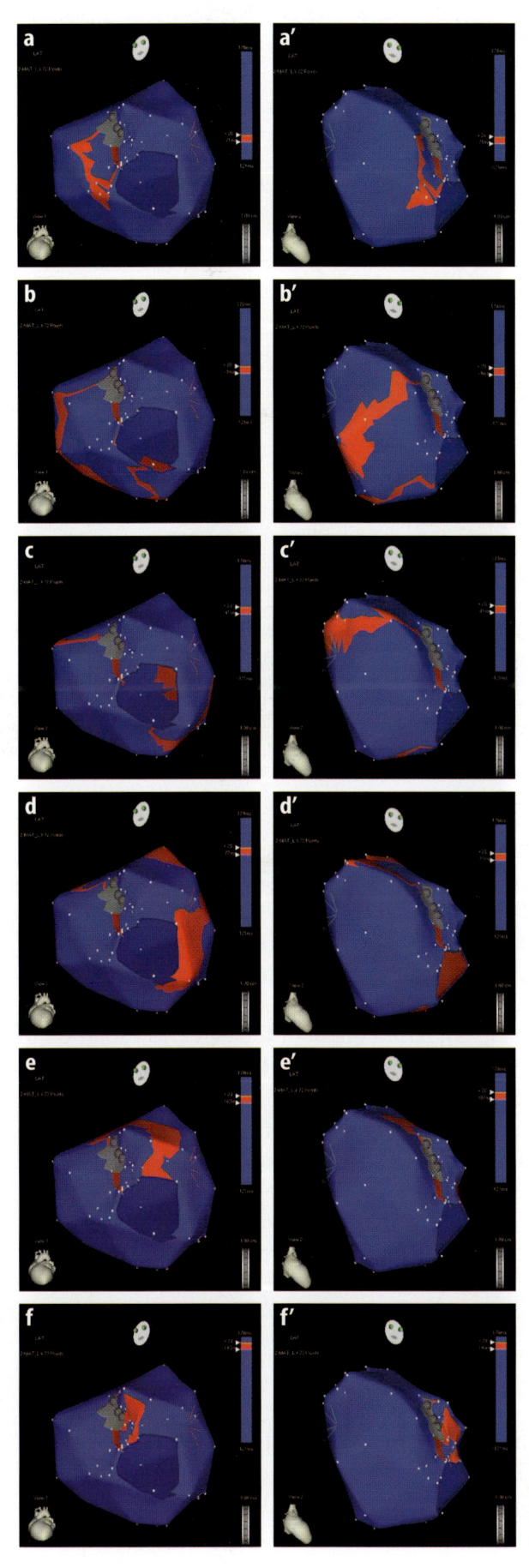

**Fig. 7a-f'.** Sequential frames of the propagation map of the left atrium during tachycardia in caudal LAO (**a–f**) and caudal RAO (**a'–f'**) views, showing the course of the double-loop reentry

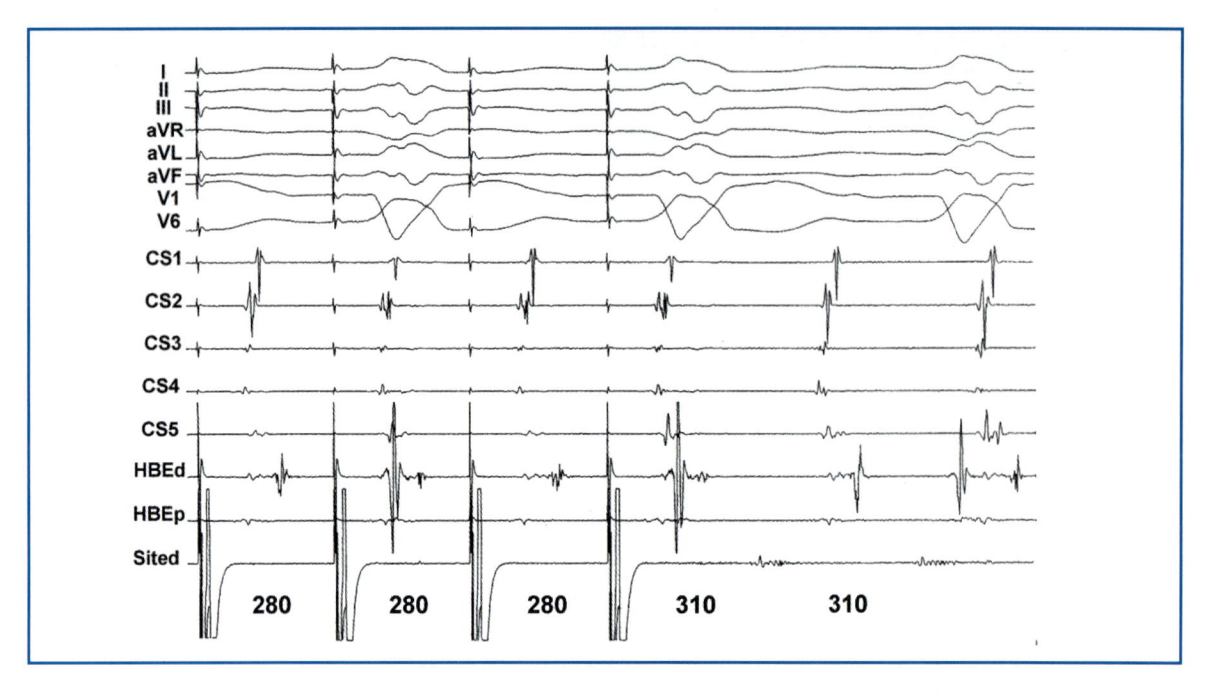

**Fig. 8.** Surface and intracavitary signals during entrainment of the tachycardia. From *top to bottom*, the signals are displayed as follows: limb and precordial leads V1 and V6, bipolar signals of the coronary sinus catheter from distal to proximal (C1–5), bipolar signals from the distal (HBEd) and proximal (HBEp) electrode pairs of the His-bundle catheter and bipolar signal of the distal (Sited) electrode pair of the mapping catheter, positioned in the miad-diastolic isthmus. From this site, the tachycardia is entrained at a cycle length corresponding to 90% of the tachycardia cycle length (280 ms). During stimulation, the atrial activation sequence in the coronary sinus and His-bundle area is unchanged and the post-pacing interval equals the tachycardia cycle length (310 ms)

15.4 cm for the roof loop. Conduction velocity was very low in the mid-diastolic isthmus (13 cm/s); the velocities measured in three segments of the outer part of each loop were comparable (63, 74 and 100 cm/s for the perimitral loop and 58, 97 and 79 cm/s for the roof loop). Electrical stimulation at the mid-diastolic isthmus with a cycle length of 280 ms resulted in concealed entrainment, with an intracavitary activation sequence superimposable on that of the tachycardia (the P wave morphology was difficult to analyse, even at baseline) and a postpacing interval equalling the tachycardia cycle length (Fig. 8). Based on all of the evidence, ablation of the mid-diastolic isthmus was expected to proceed with ease. Indeed, the first radiofrequency energy application with an irrigated-tip catheter (maximum power 35 W, cut-off temperature 43°C, duration 60 s) initially prolonged the tachycardia cycle to 400 ms and soon after terminated the arrhythmia (Fig. 9). As shown in Fig. 10, another two applications during sinus rhythm caused complete disappearance of the potentials in the isthmus. Subsequently, no other arrhythmia was inducible by S2S3 stimulation; therefore, the procedure was terminated with a total duration of 120 min. During a 2-year follow-up, while on amiodarone for prior atrial fibrillation, the patient was asymptomatic on sinus rhythm.

## Commentary

In the left atrium, the presence of electrically silent areas was previously reported in nonsurgical patients with rheumatic or nonrheumatic heart disease, such as hypertrophic or dilated cardiomyopathies and coronary artery disease [1–3]. In these studies, which included patients with left atrial macroreentrant tachycardias, the electrically silent areas had a different location, ex-

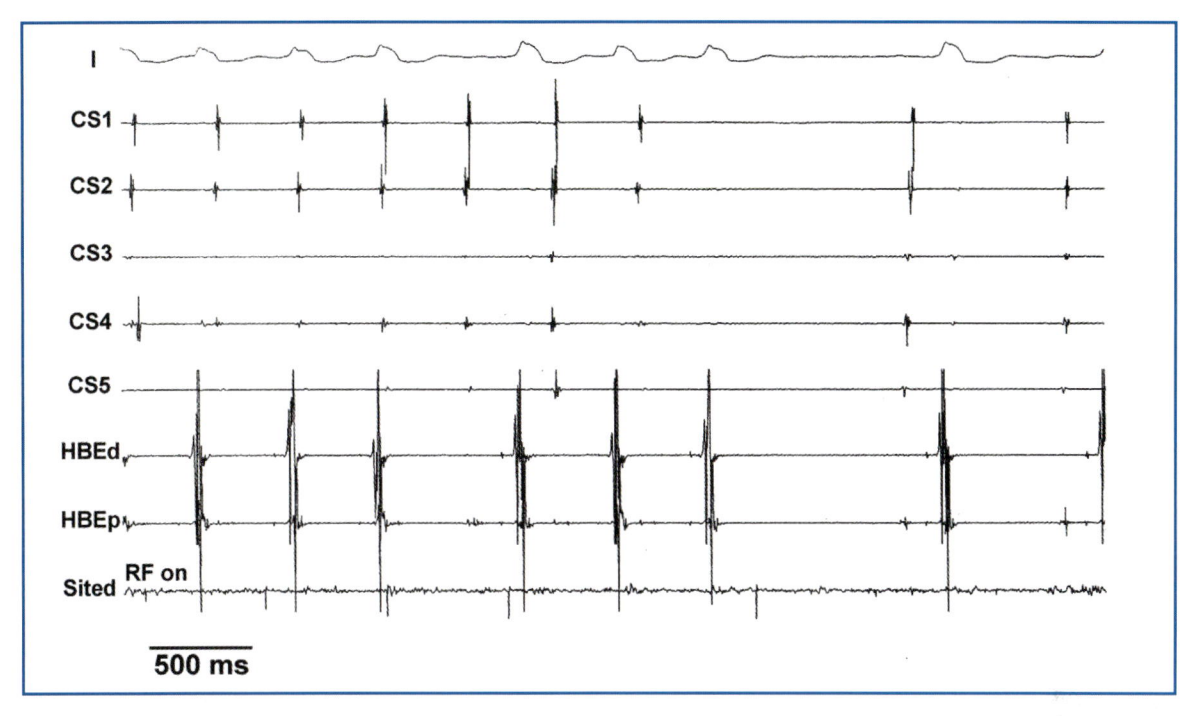

**Fig. 9.** Surface and intracavitary signals upon termination of the tachycardia by radiofrequency energy delivery. Same tracing display and catheter positioning as in the Fig. 8 with the exception that only surface lead I is shown. The first energy application is ongoing and a progressive prolongation of the tachycardia cycle is observed, until the arrhythmia terminates and sinus rhythm is restored

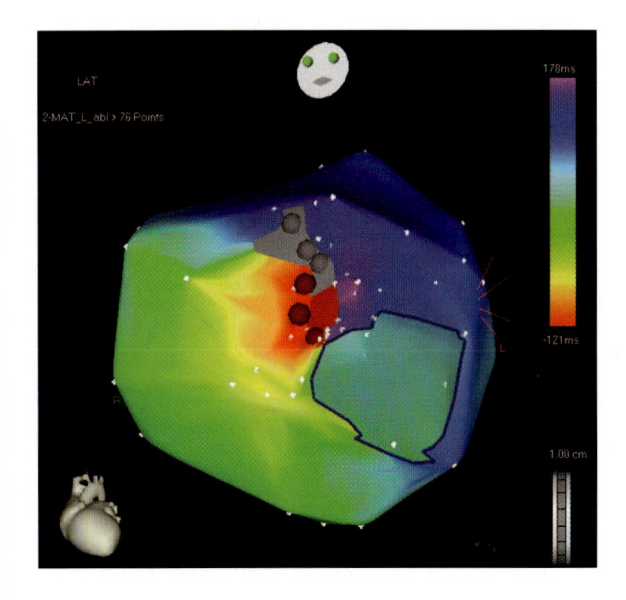

**Fig. 10.** Activation map of the left atrium during tachycardia in caudal LAO view. *Red tags* indicate the sites of ablation, aimed at the shared mid-diastolic isthmus

tension, and distribution, even in patients affected by the same disease. Possibly, the pathogenesis of this alteration is related not only to a "jet" lesion, observed especially in patients with mitral regurgitation, but also to a myopathy predominantly affecting the atrial myocardium, such as in Case 7. In any event, the location and extension of the electrically silent area and the type of macroreentrant circuit presented in this case are not very rare and are almost identical to the ones observed in Case 3.

In spite of the complexity of the reentrant circuit, this tachycardia could be easily ablated by targeting (as in the previous case and in Cases 3, 11, 13 and 16) the shared mid-diastolic isthmus, which in this patient was particularly narrow, with very-low-amplitude potentials and very slow conduction velocity. Particularly in this patient, a quickly successful procedure was important due to her age and the severe associated heart disease. Especially in female patients with structural heart disease, impaired atrial conduction and prior pulmonary-vein ablation for chronic atrial fibrillation with associated ablation of the isthmus between the left inferior pulmonary vein and mitral annulus, this arrhythmia may "survive" as a single clockwise loop reentry in the left atrial roof, requiring further ablation of the mid-diastolic isthmus [4].

Biphasic (-/+) P wave morphology in the inferior leads is not expected in a macroreentrant arrhythmia with an exit from the mid-diastolic isthmus located at the left atrial roof. In fact, in Case 3, a similar macroreentrant circuit gave origin to positive P waves in the inferior leads in the index tachycardia morphology. The peculiar interatrial propagation in the present case, possibly related to conduction delay over Bachmann's bundle, may explain this morphology. As a corollary, not only in postsurgical patients but also in patients with severe structural heart disease, the P wave morphology may not be indicative of the site of origin of the tachycardia.

## References

1. Jaïs P, Shah DC, Haïssaguerre M et al. Mapping and ablation of left atrial flutters. Circulation 2000; 101: 2928-2934.
2. Ouyang F, Ernst S, Vogtmann T et al. Characterization of reentrant circuits in the left atrial macroreentrant tachycardia: critical isthmus block can prevent atrial tachycardia recurrence. Circulation 2002; 105: 1934-1942.
3. Shah D, Sunthorn H, Burri H, Gentil-Baron P. How to ablate left atrial flutter. Heart Rhythm 2005; 2: 1153-1157.
4. Jaïs P, Sanders P, Hsu L et al. Flutter localized to the anterior left atrium after catheter ablation of atrial fibrillation. J Cardiovasc Electrophysiol 2006; 17: 279-285.

# Case 10
## Macroreentrant Atrial Tachycardia in a Left Atrium With a Prosthetic Mitral Valve (Example 1): a Reentrant Circuit Confined to the Left Atrial Roof and the Need for Reconstruction of the Entire Reentrant Circuit

### Case Presentation

This is a 67-year-old female patient who underwent mitral and aortic valve replacement with mechanical prosthesis for a postrheumatic disease. No detailed report of surgical intervention was available. She had associated systemic hypertension and diabetes. Seven years after valvular replacement, the patient began complaining of palpitations. The surface electrocardiogram showed atrial tachycardia with a cycle length of 450 ms and positive P waves in the inferior and precordial leads, while a flat/negative P wave was present in leads I and aVL (Fig. 1). At electrocardiographic monitoring, 1:1 atrioventricular conduction was frequently observed. The ar-

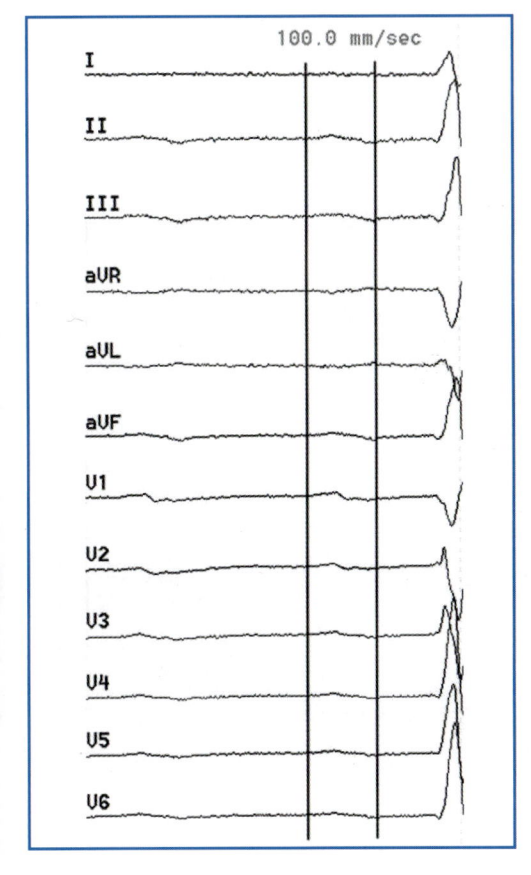

**Fig. 1.** Twelve-lead electrocardiogram of the clinical tachycardia at a sweep speed of 100 mm/s. The two *vertical lines* indicate the P wave duration and help to identify the P wave morphology

rhythmia was persistent and highly symptomatic and it recurred early after electrical cardioversion, even after intravenous and oral amiodarone administration. A transthoracic echocardiogram showed normal function of the prosthetic valves, mild impairment of left ventricular function and an enlarged left atrium. The patient was on oral anticoagulation and a transesophageal echocardiogram showed no endocavitary thrombi. Since the arrhythmia was drug-refractory and highly symptomatic, an ablation procedure was planned with the expectation of a left atrial origin of the arrhythmia and the need for transseptal catheterisation in the presence of a mechanical mitral prosthetic valve.

## Procedure

At the time of the electrophysiologic procedure, the clinical arrhythmia persisted with unchanged cycle length. A coronary-sinus atriogram was set as the reference signal, and electroanatomic mapping of the right atrium was commenced with a window-of-interest setting as for macroreentry. As shown in Fig. 2a, b, right atrial activation spanned 33% of the tachycardia cycle length, with the site of earliest activation in the medial high right atrium, corresponding to the putative site of Bachmann's bundle insertion. Here, a bipolar signal inscribing just after the onset of the surface P wave with an initially positive unipolar deflection was recorded (Fig. 3). The findings were consistent with breakthrough in the right atrium of a left-sided arrhythmia. Transseptal catheterisation was performed using a sheath with a 30° distal curve. This was accomplished with difficulty due to posterior displacement of the fossa ovalis and to the presence of an atrial septum particularly resistant to puncture. Once the transseptal sheath was correctly placed in the left atrium (Fig. 4a), a left atrial angiogram visualised the limits of the enlarged left atrium (Fig. 4b). Left atrial mapping was then started, with the intention of limiting catheter manipulation and trying to keep the catheter as posterior as possible, in order to avoid interference with the prosthetic mechanical mitral valve. In this way, electroanatomic mapping limited to the very cranial part of the left atrium was performed, as shown in Fig. 5a, b. Apparently, the activation map showed a "head-meets-tail" pattern, with a critical isthmus identified in the medial part of the left atrial roof, as a narrow conducting channel between two electrically silent ar-

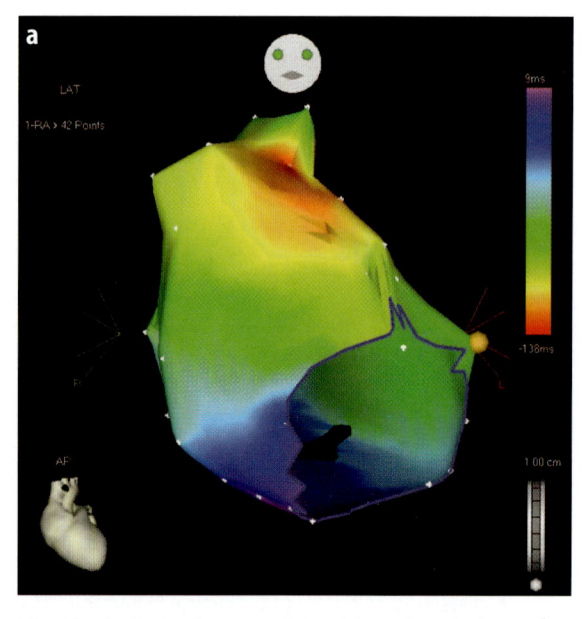

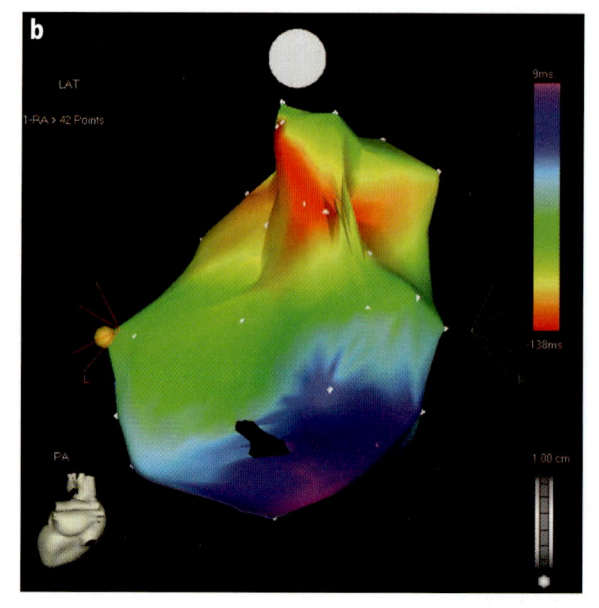

**Fig. 2a, b.** Activation map of the right atrium during tachycardia in AP (**a**) and PA (**b**) views. The *orange dot* indicates the His-bundle area

Case 10    89

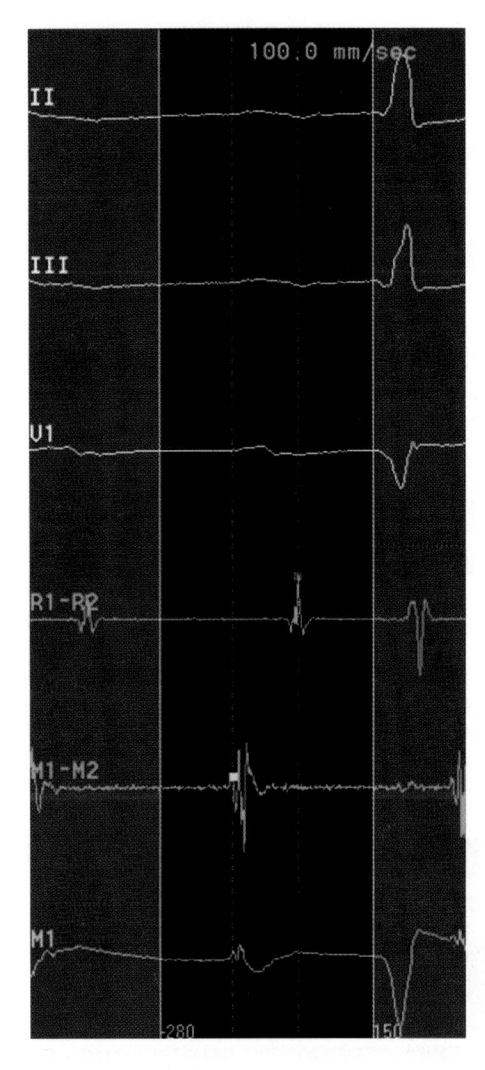

**Fig. 3.** Surface and intracavitary signals during tachycardia at the earliest activated area in the right atrium. From *top to bottom*, tracings are displayed as follows: leads II, III, V1, reference coronary sinus signal (R1–R2), bipolar signal from the distal electrode pair of the mapping catheter (M1–M2) and unipolar signal from the distal electrode of the mapping catheter (M1). *Red dot* and *yellow dot* indicate, respectively, where the coronary sinus signal and the signal from the mapping catheter were annotated

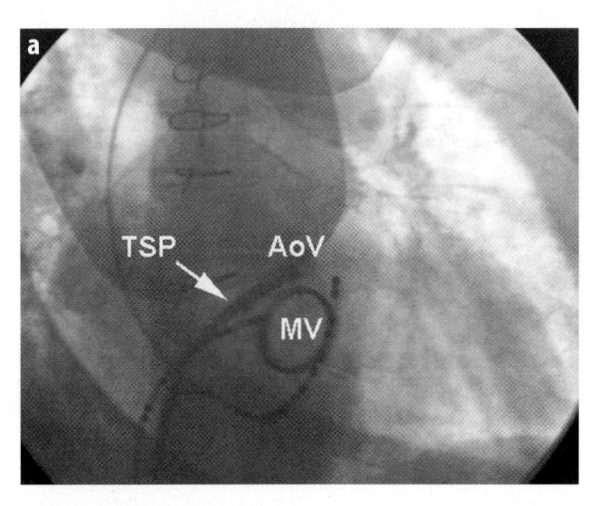

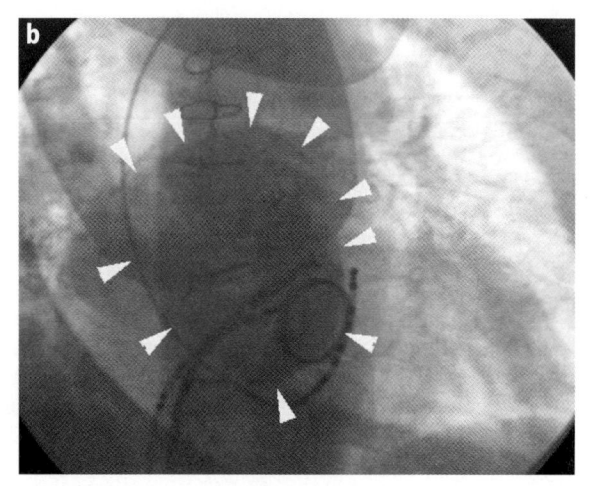

**Fig. 4a, b.** Fluoroscopic image in AP projection of the positioning of the transseptal sheath (**a**) and during left atrial angiogram (**b**). One decapolar catheter is positioned in the coronary sinus and another in the His-bundle area. In **b**, *arrows* indicate the limits of the left atrium, visualised during dye injection. *AoV* Prosthetic aortic valve, *MV* prosthetic mitral valve, *TSP* transseptal sheath

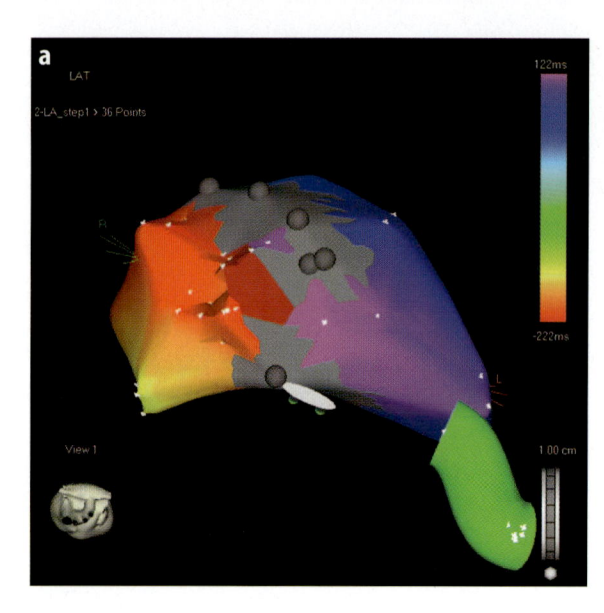

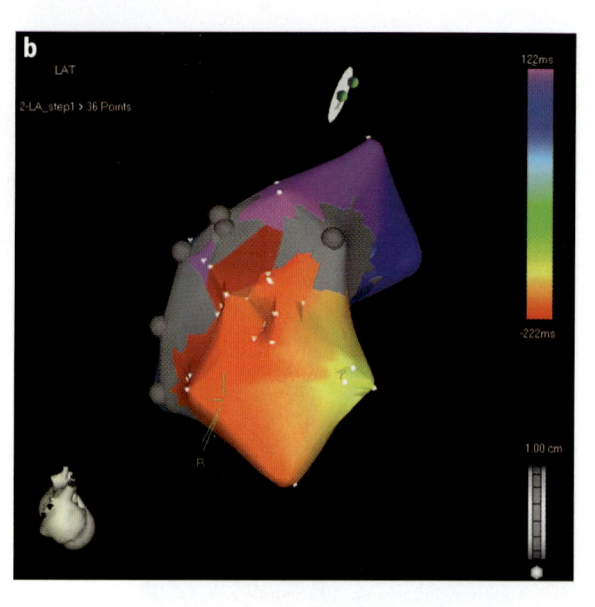

**Fig. 5a, b.** Activation map of a partially reconstructed left atrium during tachycardia in cranial (**a**) and cranial RAO (**b**) views. The *green tubular tag* in **a** indicates the position of the left superior pulmonary vein; electrically silent areas are tagged in *grey*. As shown by the limits of the colour-coded scale, only 76% of the tachycardia cycle was mapped. The "early-meets-late" option was active by default and set at 90%. In this phase, the *dark red band* between the "earliest" and "latest" activated site incorrectly indicated the channel between the two electrically silent areas as the mid-diastolic isthmus. In fact, after further mapping (Fig. 6), the red area became yellow, denoting presystolic activation, while the purple area remained purple, reflecting late activation in a dead-end channel outside the circuit

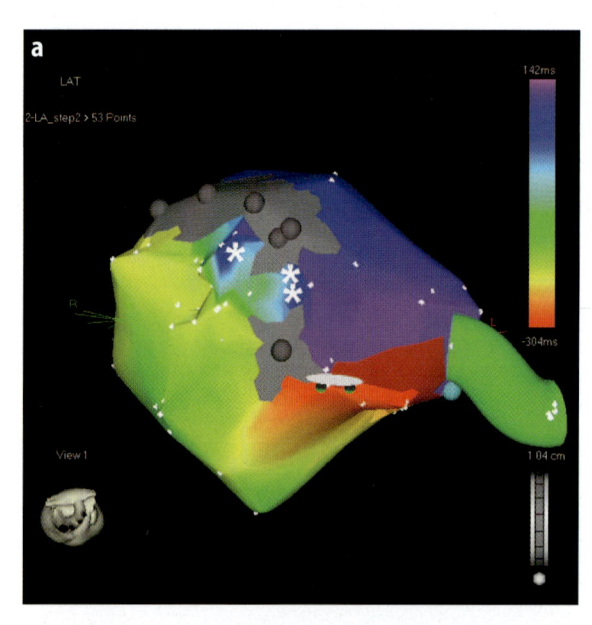

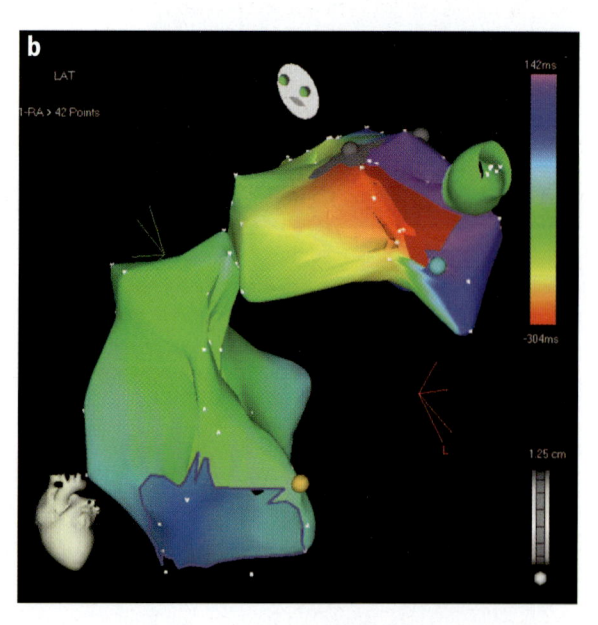

**Fig. 6a, b.** Activation map of the cranial part of the left atrium during tachycardia in cranial view (**a**) and biatrial activation map during tachycardia in cranial left anterior oblique (LAO) view (**b**) when the entire course of reentry has been reconstructed. In **a**, the area marked by a single *asterisk* can be clearly identified as a dead-end channel activated from anterior to posterior. The two sites at the end of the channel and anterior to the largest electrically silent area have a mid-diastolic chronology, indicated in *purple*. In the area marked by two asterisks, which faces the entrance of the mid-diastolic isthmus, conduction block is likely to occur

eas. However, the map reconstructed only 76% of the tachycardia cycle length and this was considered insufficient for proceeding to ablation. Therefore, the left atrial roof was further mapped circularly until the entire reentrant circuit was reconstructed, avoiding positioning of the mapping catheter around or close to the prosthetic valve. Once the activation map was reconstructed (99% of the tachycardia cycle; Fig. 6a, b), it turned out that the arrhythmia was sustained by

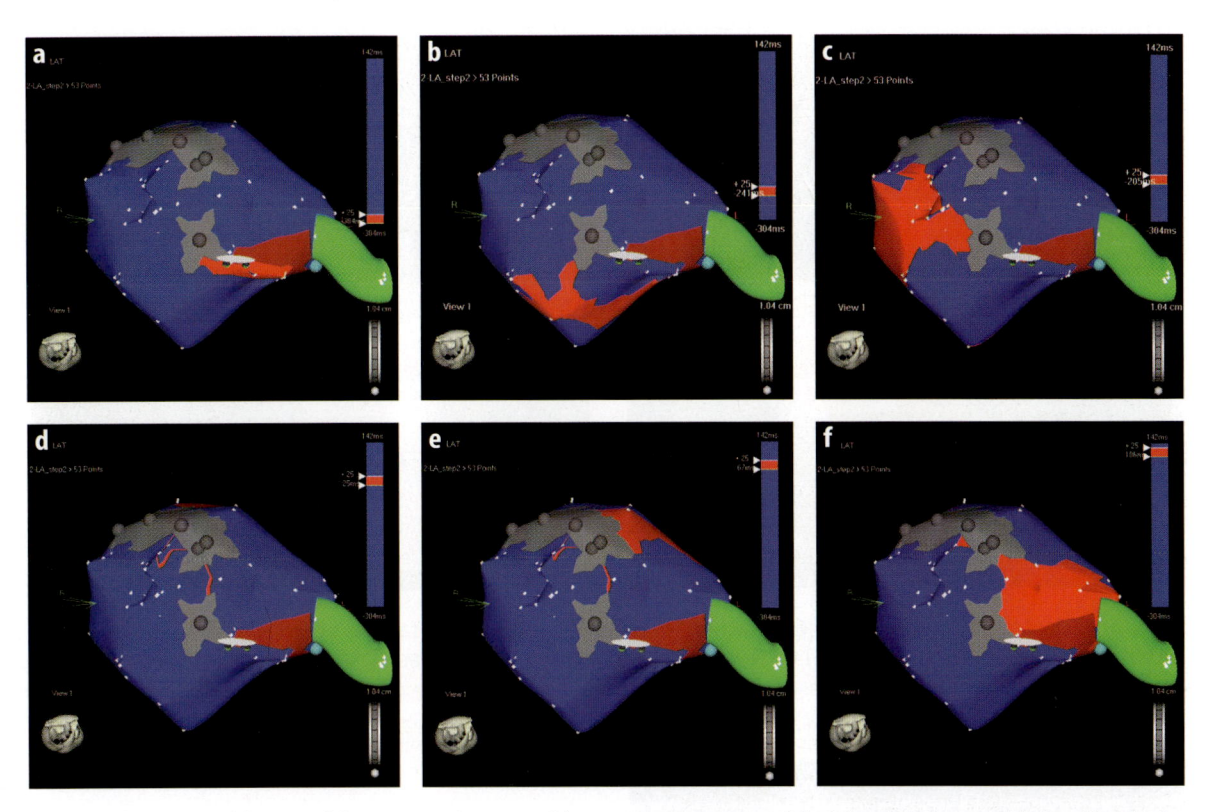

**Fig. 7a–f.** Sequential frames of the propagation map of the reconstructed part of the left atrium in a cranial view. The single-loop counter-clockwise reentry in the left atrium with dead-end activation of the region medial to the electrically silent areas is evident

a larger counter-clockwise reentry confined to the cranial part of the left atrium. Unlike the previous map (Fig. 5a, b), the mid-diastolic isthmus was now correctly localised in the lateral region of the left atrial roof, between an electrically silent area and a site of double potentials close to the left superior pulmonary vein os, corresponding to an area of conduction block and activation detour possibly related to prior surgery. Careful analysis of the propagation map (Fig. 7a–f) confirmed the presence of a single-loop counter-clockwise reentry. In fact, upon exiting from the mid-diastolic isthmus (Fig. 7a), the propagating wavefront quickly moved medially (Fig. 7b) and posteriorly (Fig. 7c) and then travelled to the posterior wall (Fig. 7d) and around the larger electrically silent area (Fig. 7e) to finally reenter the mid-diastolic isthmus (Fig. 7f). It also was clear (Fig. 7d–f) that the channel between the two electrically silent areas, previously thought to be the mid-diastolic isthmus when the tachycardia was incompletely mapped, was in fact a dead-end pathway with by-stander activation. As shown in Figs. 6a and 7f, the posterior part of the dead-end channel had the same diastolic chronology as the entrance of the mid-diastolic isthmus. Analysis of the bipolar voltage map (Fig. 8a) showed diffusely very low voltage (0.07 mV) at the left atrial roof, especially in the dead-end channel, while the right atrium (Fig. 8b) showed wide areas of preserved voltage. The bipolar voltage amplitude of the mid-diastolic isthmus was between 0.07 and 0.20 mV. Ablation aimed at the mid-diastolic isthmus and sequential radiofrequency energy pulses using an irrigated-tip catheter (maximum power 35 W, cut-off temperature 43°C, duration 45 s) were delivered from the electrically silent area, proceeding along the mid-diastolic isthmus in the anterolateral direction towards the site of double potentials (Fig. 9). After the posterior part of the ablation line was completed, the tachycardia terminated and the anterior part of the line was accomplished in sinus rhythm, with complete disappearance of electrical activity in this area. Afterwards, no arrhythmia was inducible. The

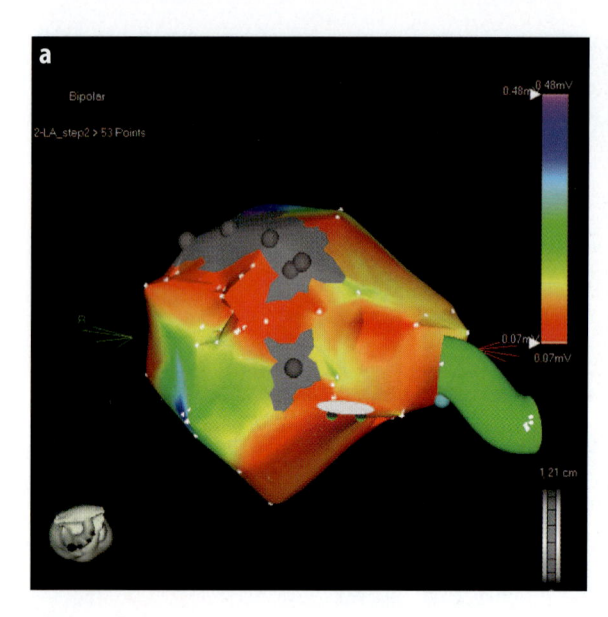

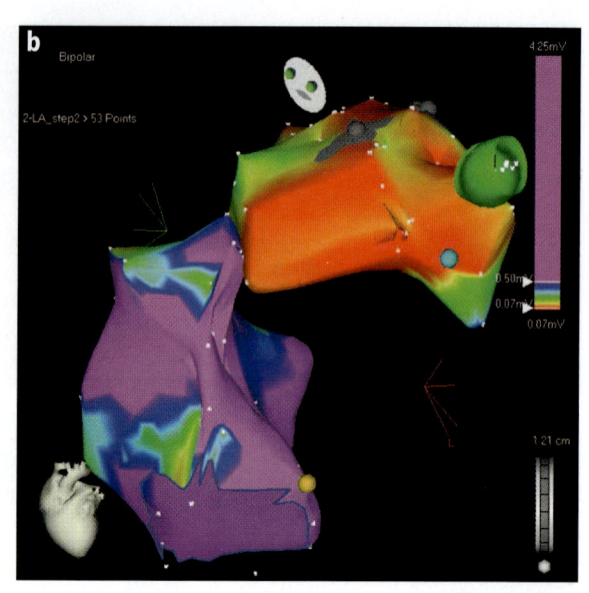

**Fig. 8a, b.** Bipolar voltage map of the reconstructed part of the left atrium during tachycardia in a cranial view (**a**) and bipolar voltage map of both atria in a cranial LAO view (**b**). According to the colour-coded scale, areas with preserved voltage are shown in *purple*

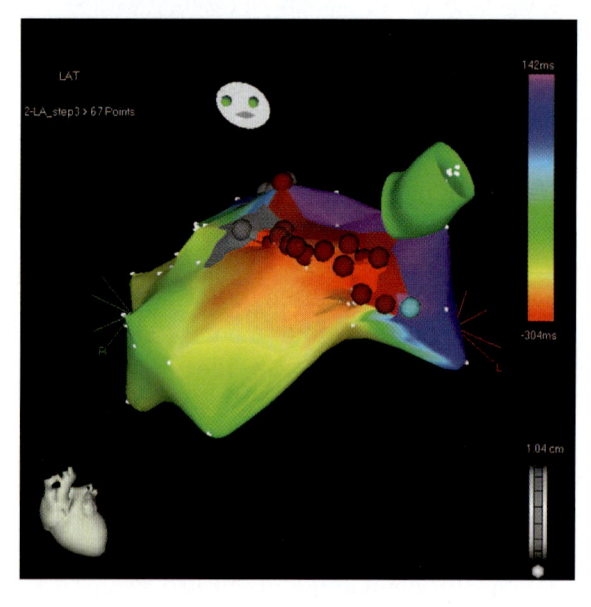

**Fig. 9.** Activation map of the reconstructed part of the left atrium in a cranial AP view. The *red dots* indicate the ablation line

result persisted after 30 min from ablation and therefore the procedure was terminated. During a 24-month follow-up, the patient had two recurrences of atrial fibrillation, subsequently prevented by increased dosage of oral amiodarone.

## Commentary

Transseptal catheterisation, in the presence of a prosthetic mechanical mitral valve, with the purpose of directly recording the transvalvular pressure gradients in patients with heart failure was reported as a safe and useful procedure more than 20 years ago [1].

In cases with a prosthetic mitral valve, a transseptal sheath with a small distal angle (30°) is preferable to the classic Mullins sheath with a 180° distal curve, to avoid interference of the tip with the prosthesis. Certainly, when a mapping catheter is introduced in the left atrium, it should be very carefully manipulated to avoid catheter entrapment in the prosthetic valve; there should be no attempt to cross the valve. When left atrial enlargement is present, the creation of large loops in the left atrium with the mapping catheter should also be avoided, to prevent catheter entrapment if the loop inadvertently releases or displaces. Obviously, the clinical conditions and the arrhythmia-related symptoms should justify a left atrial procedure in the presence of a mechanical mitral prosthetic valve. It is interesting that in some cases, such as the one presented here and in Case 11, the circuit and the mid-diastolic isthmus may be relatively remote from the prosthetic valve, which may further increase safety in these patients.

As already observed in Case 7, another difficulty in this patient was the presence of a dead-end activated area close to an electrically silent area with mid-diastolic activation (purple colour) at the end of a dead-end pathway. When only a part of the reentry was mapped, the relative early activation just anterior to the dead-end channel and the relative late activation at the end of the channel yielded a map with a misleading colour pattern, in which the dead-end pathway appeared as the mid-diastolic isthmus. The entire course of the reentrant circuit was correctly reconstructed only after acquisition of other sites circularly distributed around the roof of the left atrium. Therefore, if the mid-diastolic isthmus is identified based on electroanatomic criteria, it is mandatory to reconstruct the entire reentry course, or not less than 90–95%, in order to correctly identify the critical isthmus, especially in patients with an enlarged atrium showing areas of delayed conduction.

This case also demonstrates the typical electroanatomic pattern of by-stander activation of the right atrium during a left macroreentrant arrhythmia. In fact, although limited atrial mapping was performed (only 42 points), it was clear that: (1) the right atrium had a wider area of earliest activation, corresponding to the breakthrough in the right atrium of one (in other cases more than one) interatrial conduction pathway; (2) the latest activated area in the right atrium, in the absence of conduction block of the cavotricuspid isthmus (as in Case 11) and/or other lines of block (as in Case 15), was diametrically opposite to the earliest activated area; (3) the right atrial activation time was < 40% of the tachycardia cycle length. That the area of earliest activation is due to the presence of a focal tachycardia originating from the septum can be ruled out by the finding of a wide area with multiple sites showing similar activation times, a bipolar signal synchronous with the P wave onset or inscribing in the first part of the P wave and a unipolar signal with an initial positive deflection.

## References

1. Schoenfeld MH, Palacios IF, Hutter AM et al. Underestimation of prosthetic mitral areas: role of transseptal catheterization in avoiding unnecessary repeat mitral valve surgery. J Am Coll Cardiol 1985; 5: 1387-1392.

# Case 11
## Macroreentrant Atrial Tachycardia in a Left Atrium With a Prosthetic Mitral Valve (Example 2): the Problem of Minimal Amplitude Potentials

## Case Presentation

This is a 43-year-old male patient who had rheumatic disease during childhood and developed mitral stenosis associated with regurgitation. At the age of 39, he underwent mitral valve replacement with a mechanical prosthesis. Since he suffered from episodes of atrial fibrillation before surgical intervention, intraoperative ablation of the pulmonary vein was carried out as well, but a detailed description of the procedure was missing. At the age of 41, 2 years prior to our observation, he had recurrent typical atrial flutter, for which he underwent ablation of the cavotricuspid isthmus conduction at another centre. Subsequently, he suffered from very frequently recurring episodes of atrial tachycardia, which usually showed a long cycle length (570 ms) with positive P waves in the inferior leads and in the precordial leads V1–V5, flat in I and V6 and negative in aVL (Fig. 1). The arrhythmia recurred in spite of antiarrhythmic drug therapy with flecainide, sotalol and amiodarone, which was withdrawn 9 months prior to our observation for thyroid dysfunction. Then, the patient was referred for catheter ablation. Transthoracic echocardiogram showed an enlarged left atrium with preserved left ventricular function; the transesophageal echocardiogram showed no intracavitary thrombus. The procedure was performed 1 week after withdrawal of the last antiarrhythmic drug therapy (combination of flecainide and sotalol).

## Procedure

At the beginning of the procedure, the patient was in sinus rhythm. Two decapolar catheters were positioned, one in the coronary sinus and the other along the lower crista terminalis. A tetrapolar catheter was positioned in the His-bundle area. A coronary sinus atriogram served as the electrical reference signal. Persistence of a complete bidirectional block of the cavotricuspid isthmus conduction was first assessed. Subsequently, the clinical tachycardia was easily and reproducibly induced by incremental and by programmed atrial stimulation. Upon induction, the tachycardia had a relatively short cycle length (375 ms) for a limited time period, then shifted to a longer cycle length (575 ms) without modification of the intracavitary activation sequence (Fig. 2) and then remained stable. Consequently, electroanatomic mapping of the form with a longer cycle length was started with a window of interest setting as for macroreentry. Right atrial activation was consistent with left to right propagation of a left-sided arrhythmia, in the presence of cavotricuspid isthmus conduction block. As shown in Fig. 3a, b, in the right atrium the

# Macroreentrant Atrial Tachycardia/Flutter

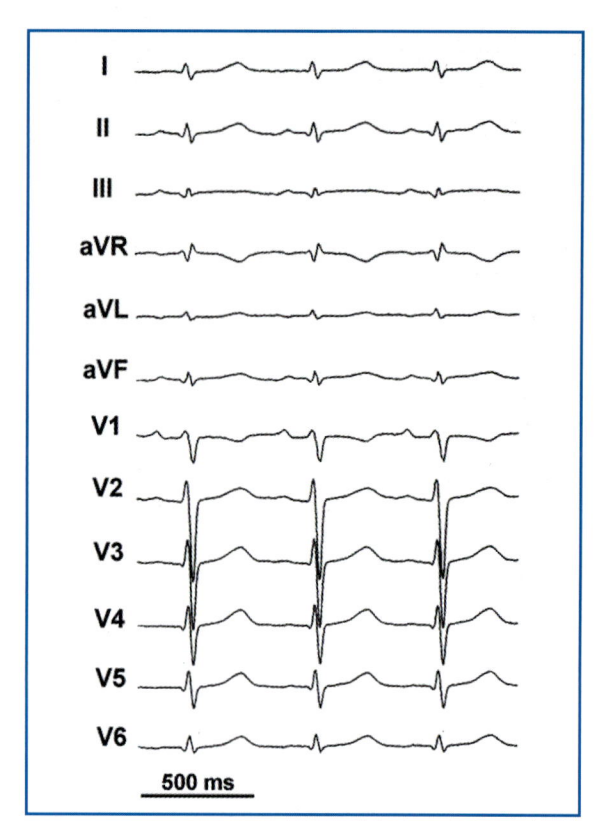

**Fig. 1.** Twelve-lead electrocardiogram of the tachycardia with longer cycle length

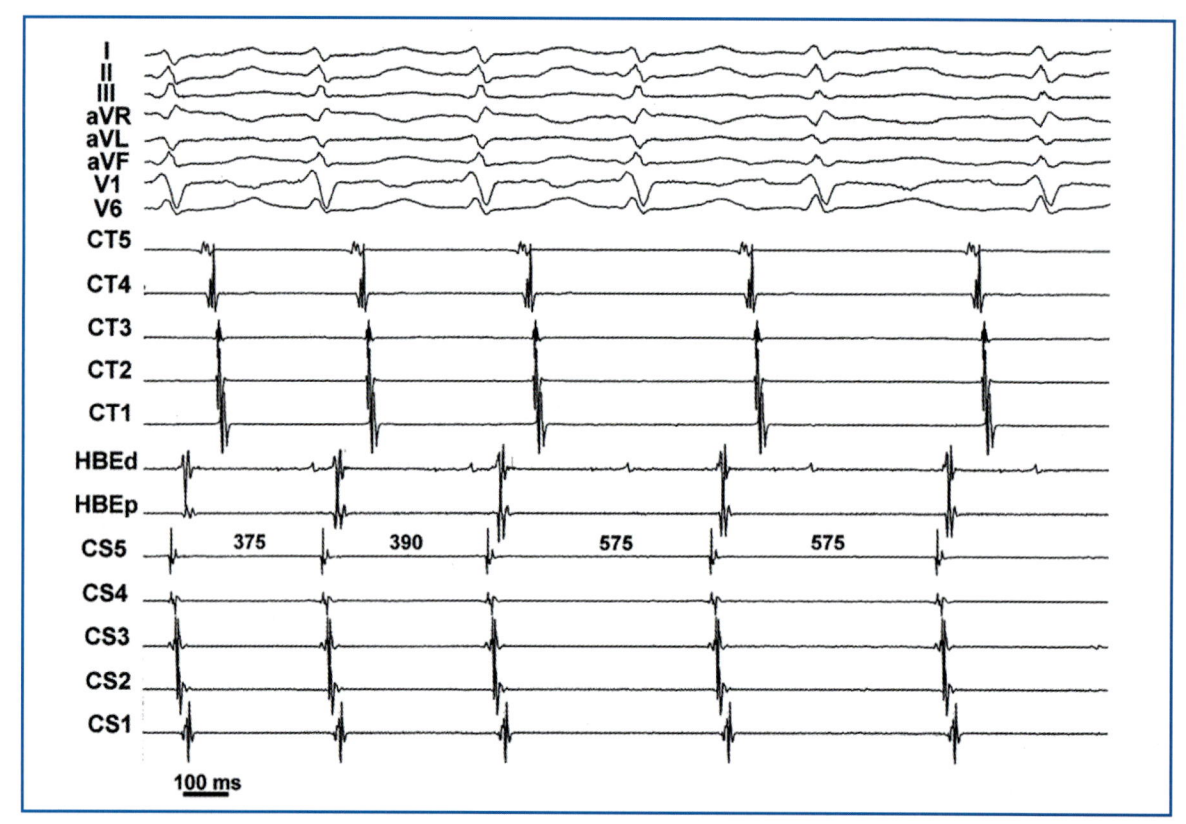

**Fig. 2.** Surface and intracavitary signals during spontaneous conversion from a tachycardia with a shorter cycle length to one with a longer cycle length. From *top to bottom*, tracings are displayed as follows: limb leads and precordial leads V1 and V6, bipolar signals of the decapolar catheter positioned along the crista terminalis, from the upper to the lower part (CT5–CT1), bipolar signals from the distal (HBEd) and proximal (HBEp) electrode pairs of the tetrapolar catheter placed in the atrioventricular node/His-bundle area, bipolar signals of the decapolar catheter, placed in the coronary sinus, from proximal to distal (CS5–CS1). Numbers indicate the cycle length in ms

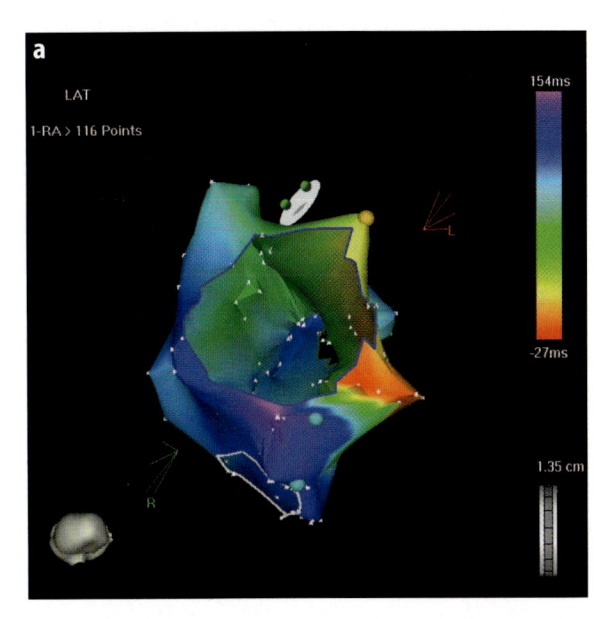

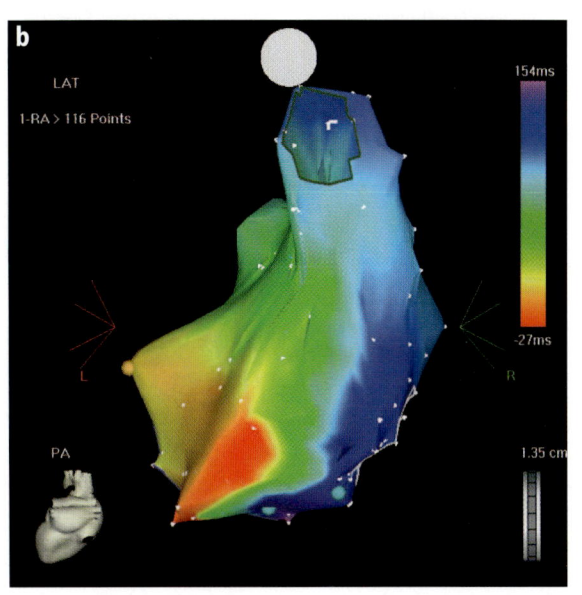

**Fig. 3a, b.** Activation map of the right atrium during tachycardia in caudal (**a**) and PA (**b**) views. The *orange dot* indicates the His-bundle area; the *blue dots* in the cavotricuspid isthmus indicate the anterior and posterior limits of the line of double potentials, corresponding to the line of previous ablation

earliest activation was observed around the coronary sinus os, propagated from medial to lateral rotating counter-clockwise around the tricuspid annulus and extinguished lateral to the prior ablation line in the cavotricuspid isthmus (blue dots in Fig. 3a). By preventing a fast propagation from medial to lateral, the cavotricuspid isthmus conduction block was mainly responsible for a prolonged right atrial activation time (181 ms). However, it represented only 31% of the tachycardia cycle length. Although the rainbow of colours was distributed around the tricuspid annulus in a "head-meets-tail" – like pattern, a reentrant circuit around the tricuspid annulus was easily excluded for the limited duration of the right atrial activation. After transseptal catheterisation, mapping was continued in the left atrium, while avoiding the area of the anterior wall, close to the mechanical prosthetic valve. An approximate estimate of the left atrial volume was 141 ml. Mapping was continued in the left atrium untill reconstruction of activation corresponded to 95% of the tachycardia cycle length (Fig. 4a, b). The main difficulty encountered during mapping was signal analysis in the posteromedial left atrium, where very-low-voltage (close to 0.06 mV) diastolic potentials were found (Fig. 5a, b). The minimal voltage amplitude may have been related to the underlying heart disease and to the previous intraoperative ablation of the pulmonary vein. However, every effort was made to analyse and annotate these signals on the first sharp deflection, instead of tagging this area as electrically silent. In fact, in the posteromedial left atrium, between the oses of the right pulmonary veins, a distinct bipolar signal of very low amplitude (0.06 mV), which preceded the reference signal by 212 ms (Fig. 6a), was reproducibly recorded and, consequently, annotated with a late mid-diastolic (red colour) chronology, according to the setting of the window of interest. Similarly, about 1 cm more medially, another very low (0.08 mV) bipolar signal that followed the reference signal by 332 ms (Fig. 6b) was detected and annotated with an early mid-diastolic chronology (purple colour), according to the setting of the window of interest. This signal analysis allowed clear identification of the mid-diastolic isthmus in the posteromedial wall, in the area between the two right pulmonary vein ostia (Fig. 4). Nevertheless, in the mid-diastolic isthmus, high-density mapping could not be performed, since positioning of the catheter in this site rendered the tachycardia cycle length unstable and repeatedly terminated the tachycardia, which in any case was easily

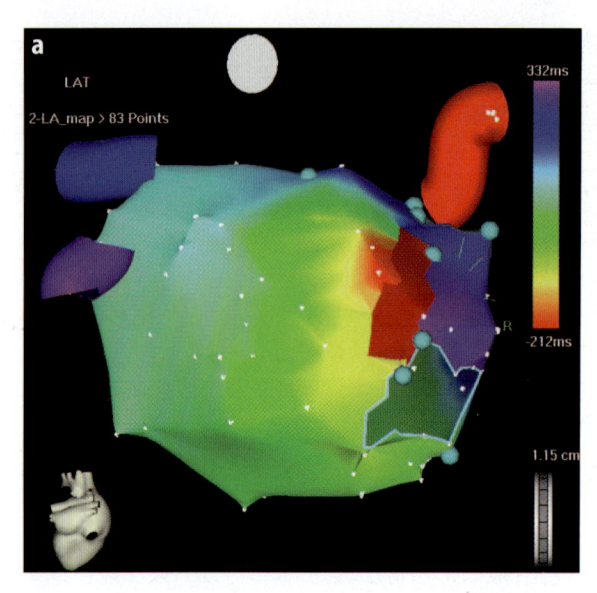

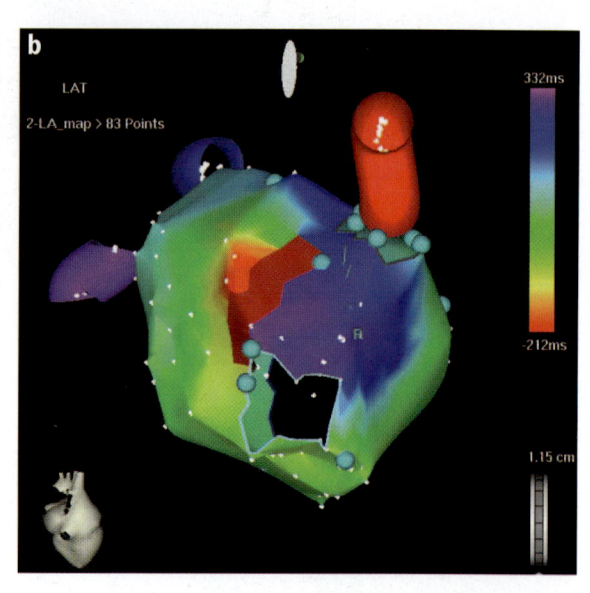

**Fig. 4a, b.** Activation map of the left atrium during tachycardia in caudal PA (**a**) and right lateral (**b**) views. The left and the right superior pulmonary veins are shown as tubular icons, while the os of the right inferior pulmonary vein is identified by the circular line. *Blue dots* indicate multiple sites of double potentials, found especially around the right pulmonary veins

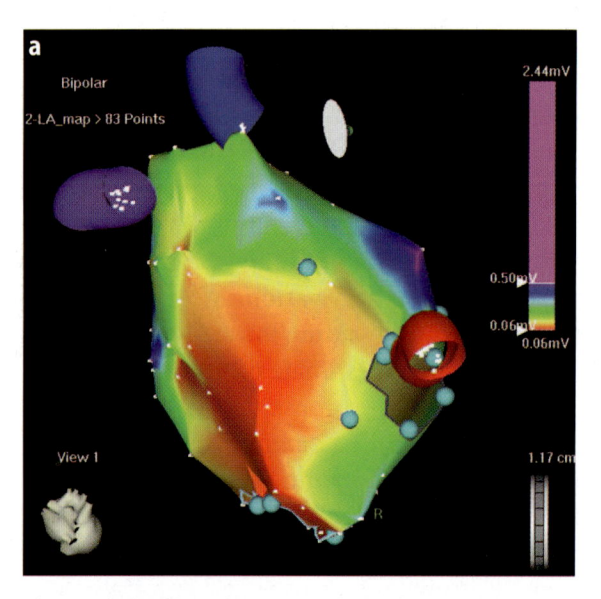

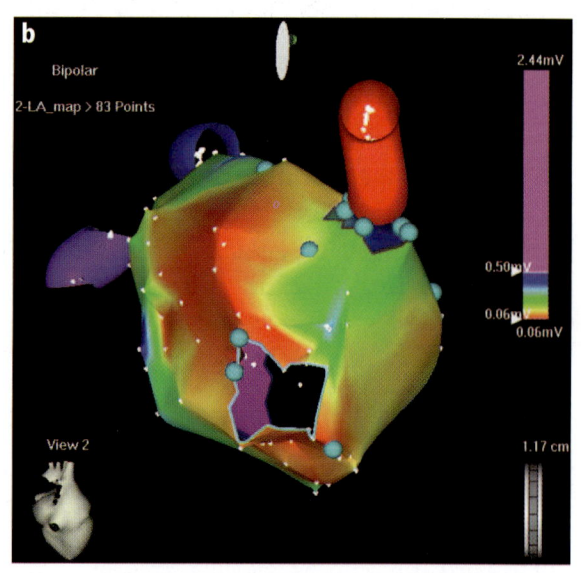

**Fig. 5a, b.** Bipolar voltage map of the left atrium during tachycardia in cranial right lateral (**a**) and right lateral (**b**) views. According to the setting of the colour-coded scale, areas with preserved voltage are shown in *purple* and are of very limited extent in this patient

reinducible at the same cycle length. Another peculiarity of this case, as shown in Fig. 4, was the diffuse presence of double potentials (separated by at least 70 ms), tagged by blue dots around the os of the right pulmonary veins, the atrial septum and the left atrial roof, which could have been related to prior atriotomy and/or prior intraoperative ablation, since it was less likely that functional conduction block could occur at this tachycardia cycle. Analysis of the propagation map showed that the tachycardia was sustained by a double-loop reentry. In fact, the first loop

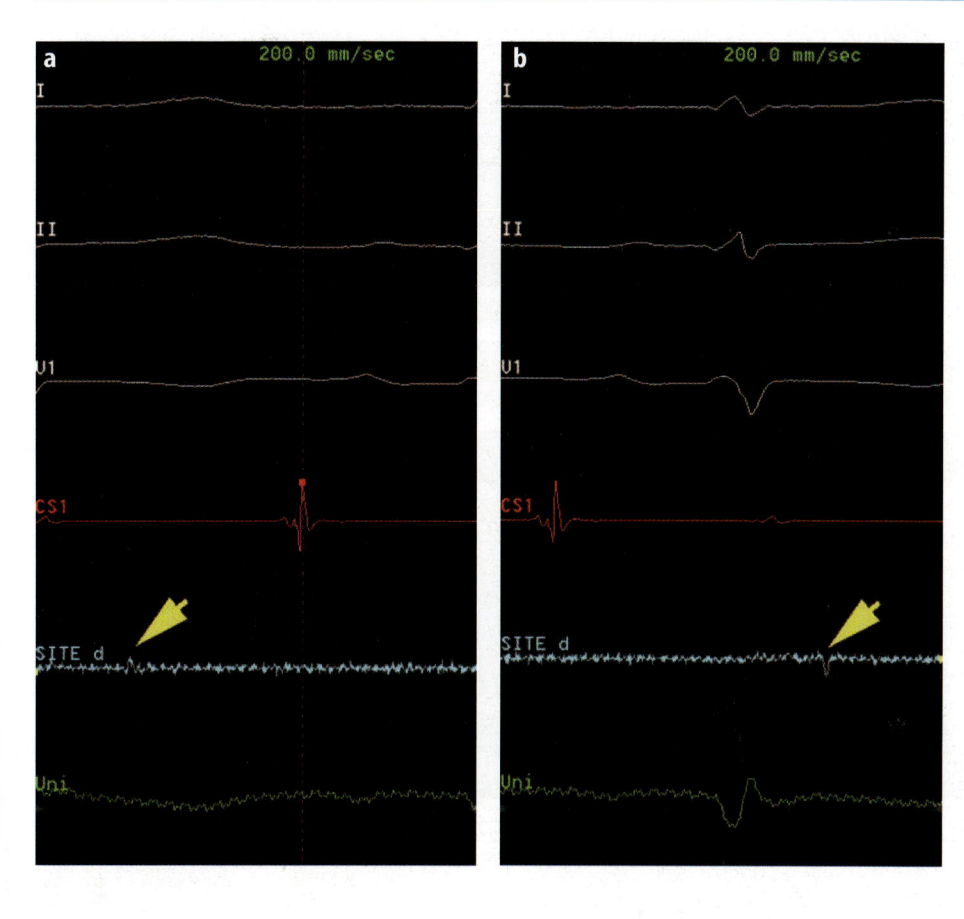

**Fig. 6a, b.** Surface and intracavitary signals at the exit (**a**) and entrance (**b**) of the mid-diastolic isthmus. From *top to bottom*, surface leads I, II, V1, reference coronary sinus signal (CS1) and bipolar (Sited) and unipolar (Uni) signals from the mapping catheter are shown. The *arrows* indicate where the very-low-amplitude fragmented signals (0.06 and 0.08 mV in **a** and **b**, respectively) were annotated for activation mapping

(Fig. 7a–f), upon exiting the mid-diastolic isthmus (Fig. 7a), activated the posterior wall (Fig. 7b–d) from proximal to distal (activation was also recorded conventionally from the proximal to the distal coronary sinus, as shown in Fig. 2), rotated around a conduction block area at the left atrial roof and rejoined the second loop (Fig. 7e) before reentering the mid-diastolic isthmus (Fig. 7f). The second loop (Fig. 7a'–f') rotated counter-clockwise in the left atrial septum, moving initially inferior to the right inferior pulmonary vein os (Fig. 7a, b), then anteriorly to a line of block in the atrial septum (Fig. 7c', d') to finally activate the anteromedial left atrium (Fig. 7e') before joining the first loop and entering the mid-diastolic isthmus (Fig. 7f'). Figure 8a–f shows the biatrial propagation with the differences in activation times between the two atria. In fact, right atrial activation began relatively late (Fig. 8a) and, as noted above, was prolonged by the cavotricuspid isthmus conduction block (Fig. 8b, d). However, when right atrial activation ended (Fig. 8d), the reentrant circuit had activated roughly half of the left atrium and a considerable time interval was required to end left atrial activation (Fig. 8e, f). An analysis of the conduction velocity showed that slow conduction was present not only in the mid-diastolic isthmus (25 cm/s), but also in a 24 mm tract at the exit of the mid-diastolic isthmus, corresponding to the area of very-low-amplitude potentials and delayed propagation in the posteromedial wall (area in red in the voltage map in Fig. 5 and area with a narrow band of propagation in Fig. 7a–c), where conduction velocity was persistently around 20 cm/s. In the outer part of both loops, the conduction velocity was normal (68 cm/s). The tachycardia was easily terminated by radiofrequency energy application with an irrigated-tip catheter (maximum power 30 W, cut-off temperature 43°C and duration 60 s) in the mid-diastolic isthmus and was non-inducible after the first energy application. Nonetheless, ablation along the entire mid-diastolic isthmus was per-

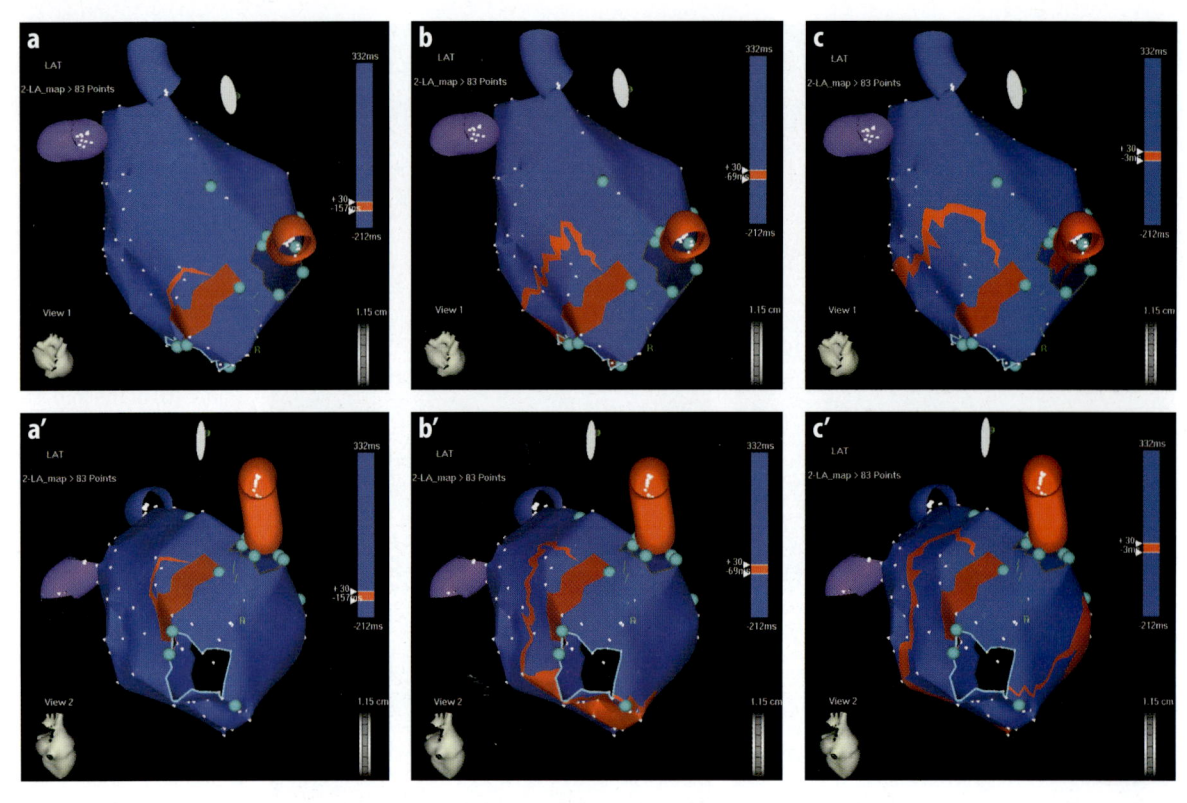

**Fig. 7a–f'.** Propagation map of the left atrium during tachycardia in cranial right lateral (**a–f**) and right lateral (**a'–f'**) views. The double-loop reentry in the left atrium is evident ▶

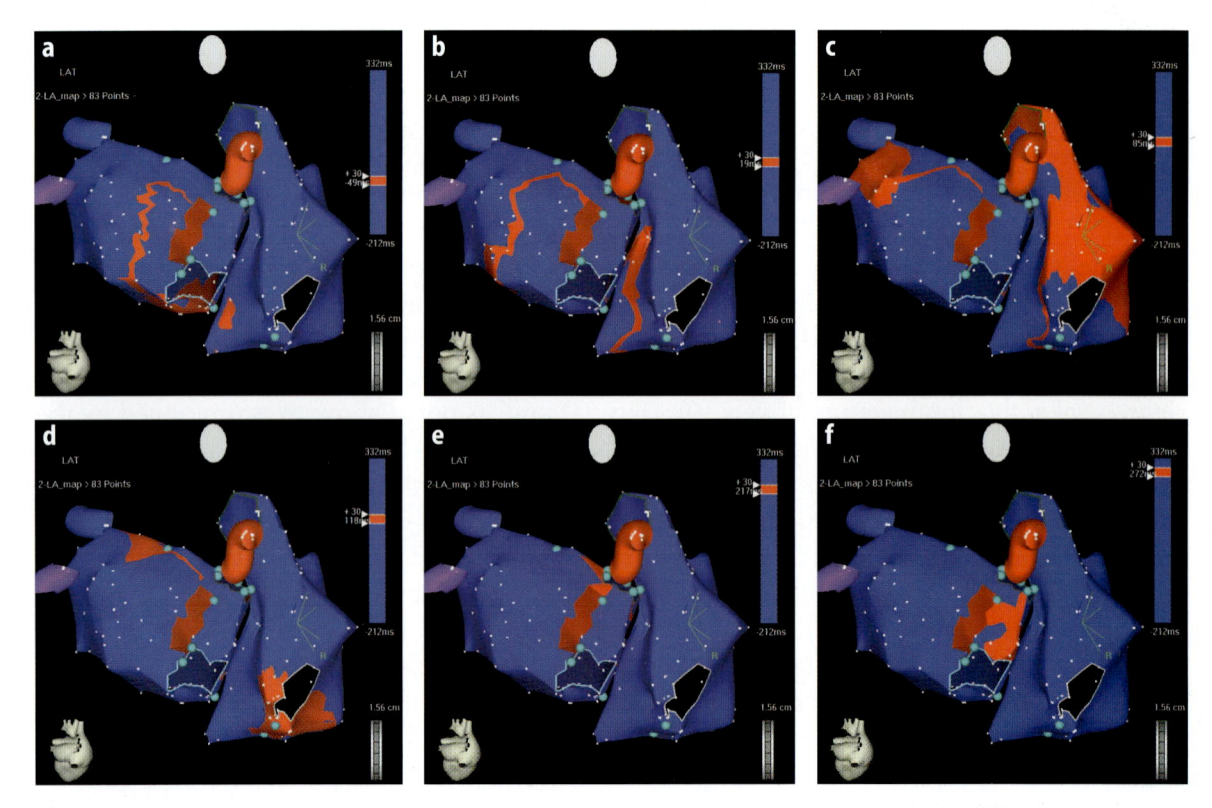

**Fig. 8a–f.** Biatrial propagation map during tachycardia in a posteriorly tilted right lateral view. The difference between the duration of right and left atrial activation is evident

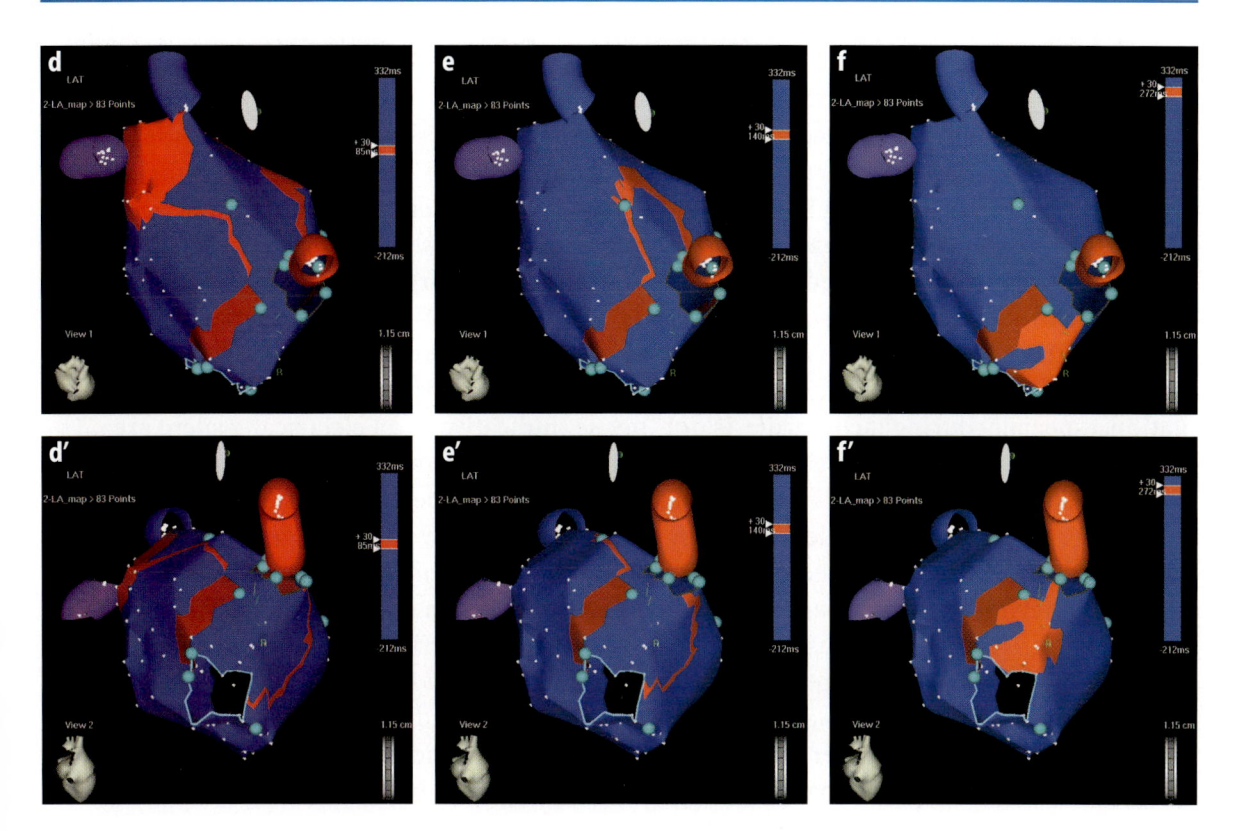

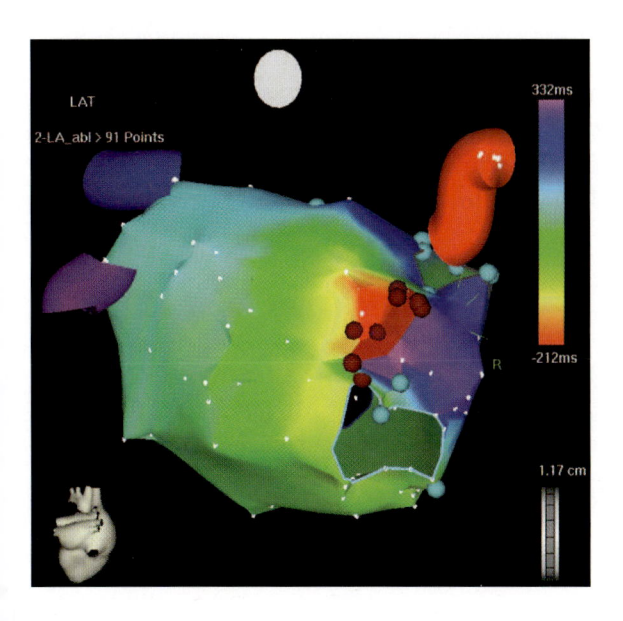

**Fig. 9.** Activation map of the left atrium in a caudal PA view. *Red dots* indicate the ablation line between the oses of the right pulmonary vein, corresponding to the mid-diastolic isthmus

formed (Fig. 9) until the local signal had completely disappeared. Afterwards, no other arrhythmia was induced (surprisingly, not even atrial fibrillation) by programmed atrial stimulation with multiple extrastimuli and bursts up to 260 ms also during isoprenaline infusion. After a 1-year follow-up, the patient was arrhythmia-free without antiarrhythmic drugs.

## Commentary

The difficulty of this case resided mainly in the fact that analysis of the signals, and therefore of activation, was difficult in a very-low-voltage area with a signal amplitude close to the baseline noise value of 0.05 mV. Classifying such areas as electrically silent and tagging it as "scar" early during mapping may be misleading. In these cases, mapping should commence in an area of preserved or relatively preserved voltage and, after the major part of the reentry circuit has been grossly identified, every effort should be made to analyse very-low-voltage areas with bipolar signal identification, which can usually be done at the standard filter setting (10–400 Hz) of the Carto system, with adequate increases in the gain setting. Lack of capture during electrical stimulation, especially during tachycardia, is not "per se" indicative of an electrically silent area. The finding of very-low-voltage areas should be expected in patient with structural heart disease and prior surgery, intraoperative ablation and repeated prior percutaneous ablation. Nonetheless, the arrhythmia in this patient was easy to ablate, since very-low-voltage areas are oversensitive to heating during radiofrequency energy delivery and even catheter pressure during mapping may interfere with tachycardia. However, as pointed out in a previous study [1], the entire extension of the critical isthmus should be ablated in order to minimise recurrences.

It remains unclear what the reentrant circuit might have been in the tachycardia with a shorter (375 ms) cycle length. This was observed both clinically and during the procedure, albeit only for a very short period after induction, since this form quickly converted into one with a longer cycle length, without changing the activation sequence in conventional recordings. For this reason, electroanatomic mapping of the shorter cycle length form was not even attempted, as it was felt that it might have been the same arrhythmia with a different cycle length. Moreover, the form with the longer cycle length recurred more frequently during spontaneous episodes. In the form with the shorter cycle length, the reentrant course might have been shorter (i.e. around the right inferior pulmonary vein os) and/or involved a channel of faster conduction in the posteromedial left atrium, which became functionally blocked after a limited time period. However, it can be assumed that the tachycardia with a shorter cycle length shared the mid-diastolic isthmus with the longer cycle length form, since after ablation of this area the arrhythmia was not inducible, nor did it recur during follow-up without antiarrhythmic drug therapy.

## References

1. Ouyang F, Ernst S, Vogtmann T et al. Characterization of reentrant circuits in left atrial macroreentrant tachycardia: critical isthmus block can prevent atrial tachycardia recurrence. Circulation 2002; 105: 1934-1942.

# Case 12
## Counter-clockwise Isthmus-Dependent Peritricuspid Reentry with an Atypical Electrocardiographic Pattern: what Should Be Complex is not Always Actually Complex

## Case Presentation

This is a 79-year-old-female patient with hypertensive heart disease without previous cardiac or thoracic surgery. Two years before the procedure described here, she presented with recurrent episodes of atrial fibrillation, which was treated with oral amiodarone at a dose of 1.4 g per week. An echocardiogram in sinus rhythm showed a hypertrophic left ventricle with impaired systolic function (ejection fraction of 44%), enlargement of both atria and moderate mitral and tricuspid regurgitation. On antiarrhytmic therapy, she had no recurrence of atrial fibrillation, but six months before the procedure she exhibited recurrent episodes of persistent atypical atrial flutter. These were poorly tolerated and required electrical cardioversion for their termination. As shown in Fig. 1, surface P wave morphology during the clinical arrhythmia was pos-

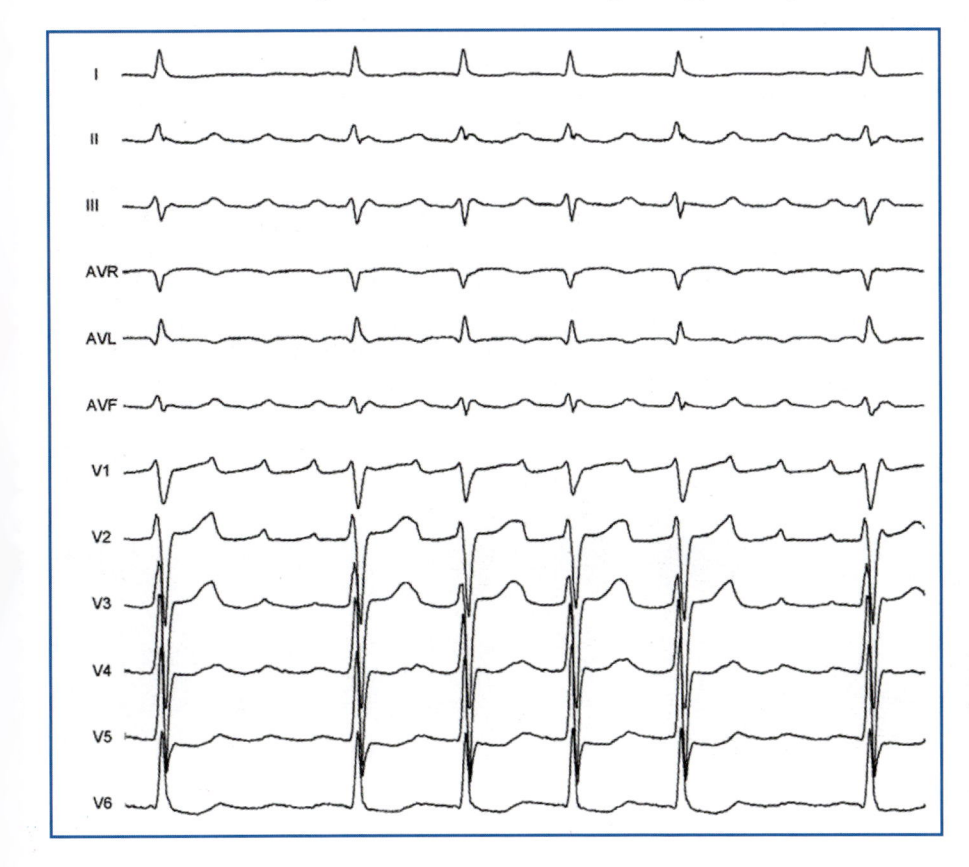

**Fig. 1.** Twelve-lead electrocardiogram of the clinical arrhythmia with a 250 ms cycle length and variable atrioventricular conduction

itive in the inferior leads and in all precordial leads, flat in I and negative in aVL, suggesting a left atrial arrhythmia. The procedure described below was performed during hospitalisation for arrhythmia recurrence.

## Procedure

During the procedure, the clinical arrhythmia showed a cycle length of 250 ms. Two multipolar catheters were placed, one in the coronary sinus and the other in the His-bundle area. Bipolar recordings from the coronary sinus had a proximal to distal activation with a diastolic chronology, suggesting, together with the surface P wave morphology, a left atrial circuit. Before transseptal catheterisation, the right atrium was mapped, with the window of interest set as for a macroreentrant arrhythmia. Early during mapping, the right atrium showed enlargement (104 ml) and a distorted anatomy. Unexpectedly, the right atrial activation spanned 98% of the tachycardia cycle length, showing a clear "head-meets-tail" pattern with a counter-clockwise circuit around the tricuspid annulus and a mid-diastolic area in the medial cavotricuspid isthmus (Fig. 2a, b) that had a "pouch" anatomy. An area of double potentials separated by > 70 ms of isoelectric line, suggesting conduction block and activation detour, was found around the coronary sinus os and extended to the inferior vena cava. An unusual pattern of propagation (Fig. 3a–f) was noted, and, with respect to the classic isthmus-dependent counter-clockwise reentry, it appeared to be affected by the line of block around the coronary sinus os. In fact, the activation wavefront, exiting from the medial cavotricuspid isthmus (Fig. 3a, a'), proceeded upward, but the propagation towards the posterior atrial septum and the coronary sinus os was blocked by the line of double potentials (Fig. 3b, b'). This was very likely to considerably modify left atrial activation as well. Subsequently, the main propagating wavefront rotated counter-clockwise around the tricuspid annulus (Fig. 3c-f), whereas, as a consequence of the line of block/activation detour, propagation around the inferior vena cava and in the posterior right wall (Fig. 3b'–e') resulted only in a delayed and minor wavefront. This formed an incomplete clockwise loop around the inferior vena cava, which collided in the low lateral wall with the prevailing wavefront,

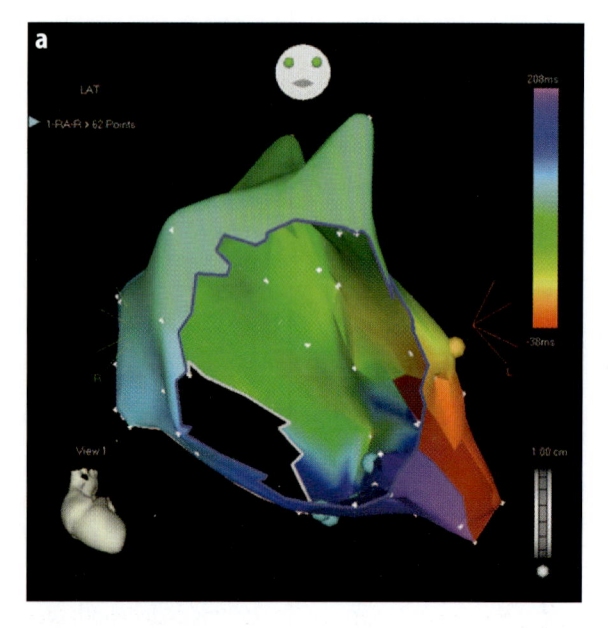

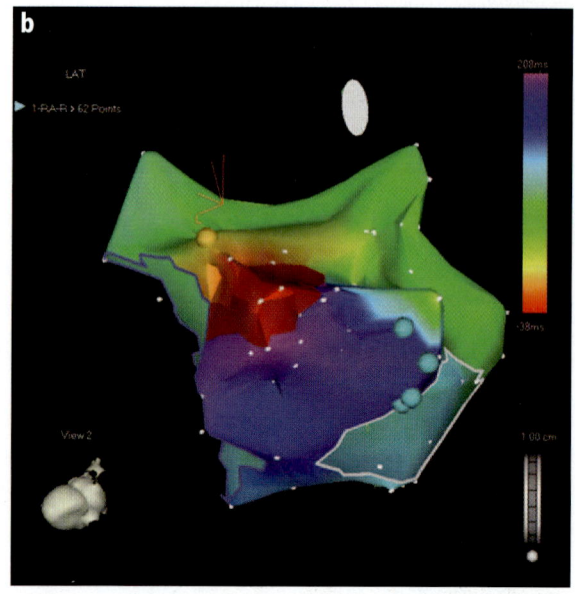

**Fig. 2a, b.** Activation map of the right atrium during flutter in left anterior oblique (LAO) (**a**) and caudal left lateral (**b**) views. The *orange dot* indicates the site of His-bundle recording and the *blue dots* indicate the line of double potentials

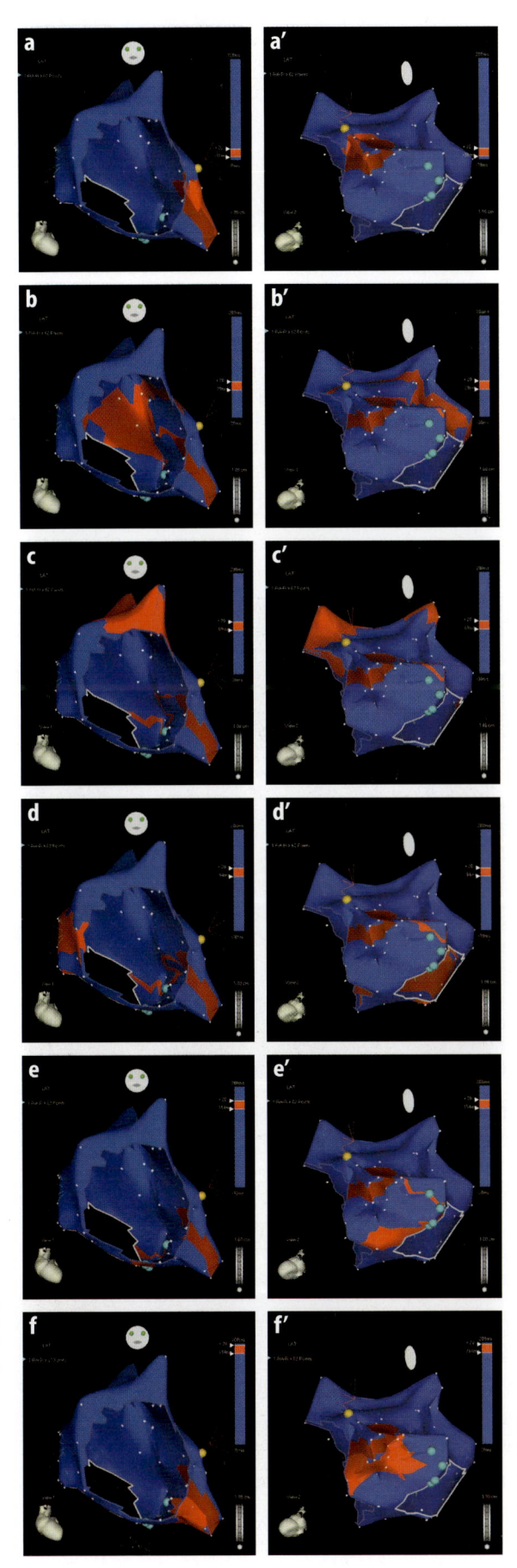

**Fig. 3a-f'.** Sequential frames of the propagation map during flutter in LAO (**a–f**) and caudal left lateral (**a'–f'**) views. The counter-clockwise loop spanning the entire tachycardia cycle length around the tricuspid annulus and the line of block and activation detour corresponding to the *blue dot* line are evident

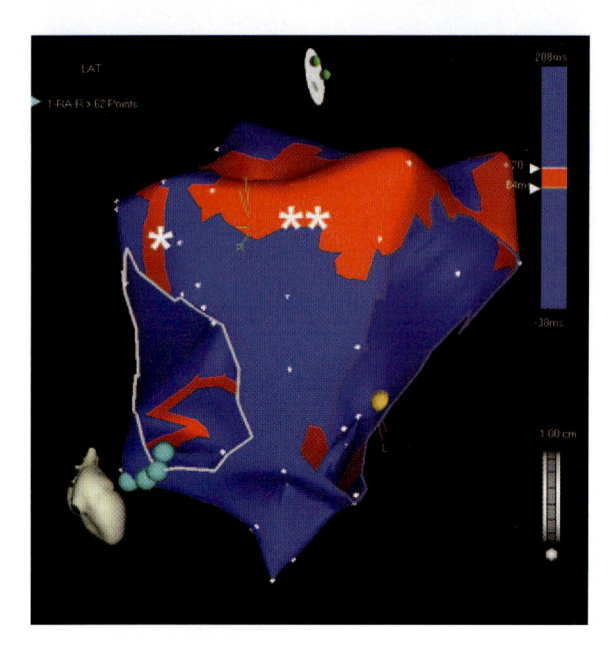

**Fig. 4.** Single frame of the propagation map of the right atrium in caudal RAO projection showing the collision in the low lateral region between the main wavefront of the counter-clockwise loop around the tricuspid annulus (marked by *two asterisks*) and the minor wavefront of the incomplete clockwise loop around the inferior vena cava (marked by a *single asterisk*) before entering the lateral part of the cavotricuspid isthmus

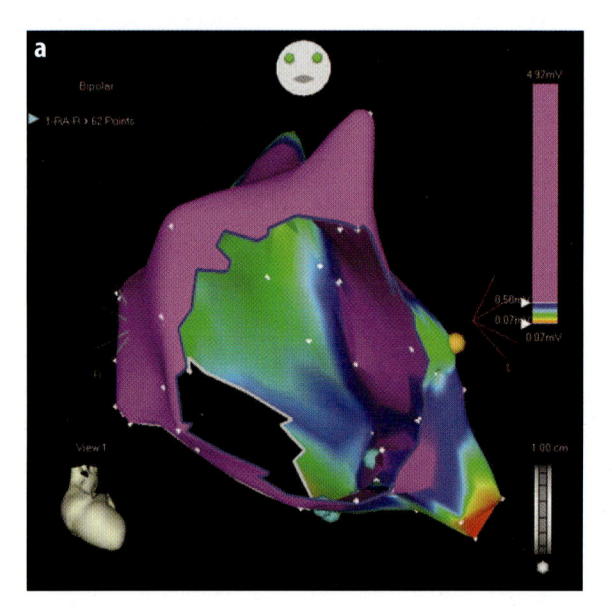

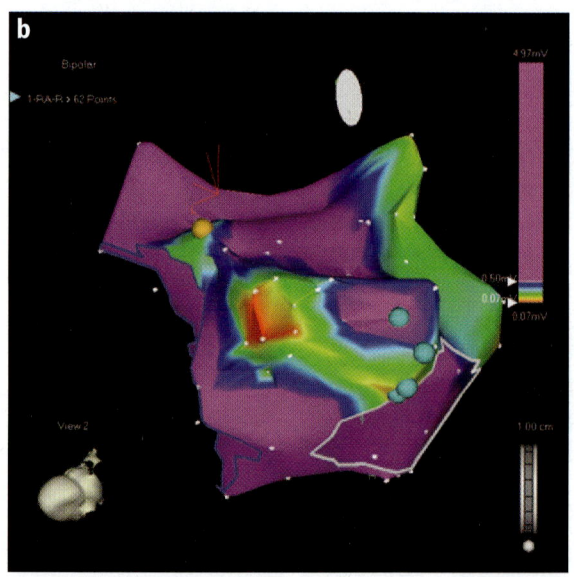

**Fig. 5a, b.** Bipolar voltage map of the right atrium during the clinical arrhythmia in LAO (**a**) and caudal left lateral (**b**) views. According to the setting of the colour-coded scale, areas with preserved voltage area shown in *purple*

rotating counter-clockwise around the tricuspid annulus (Fig. 4). The bipolar voltage map (Fig. 5a-b) during the arrhythmia showed that the area of low voltage was confined to the medial cavotricuspid isthmus and the posterior right atrium. Based on the activation mapping data of the right atrium, it was considered unnecessary to proceed to left atrial mapping. Further mapping into the coronary sinus to clarify its diastolic activation implied a high risk of displacing the reference catheter, due to the unusual anatomy. Therefore, radiofrequency energy using an irrigated-tip catheter (maximum power 40 W, cut-off temperature 43°C, duration 45 s) was sequentially delivered in the mid-diastolically activated area (Fig. 6), in the medial cavotricuspid isthmus, starting from the tricuspid annulus. When the ablation line reached the line of double potentials, close to the inferior vena cava os, the arrhythmia terminated, with restoration of sinus rhythm (Fig. 7). Conduction block along the cavotricuspid isthmus was demonstrated by

**Fig. 6.** Activation map of the right atrium during the clinical arrhythmia in left lateral view. The ablation line (*red dots*) extends from the tricuspid annulus to the double potential line, close to the inferior vena cava os

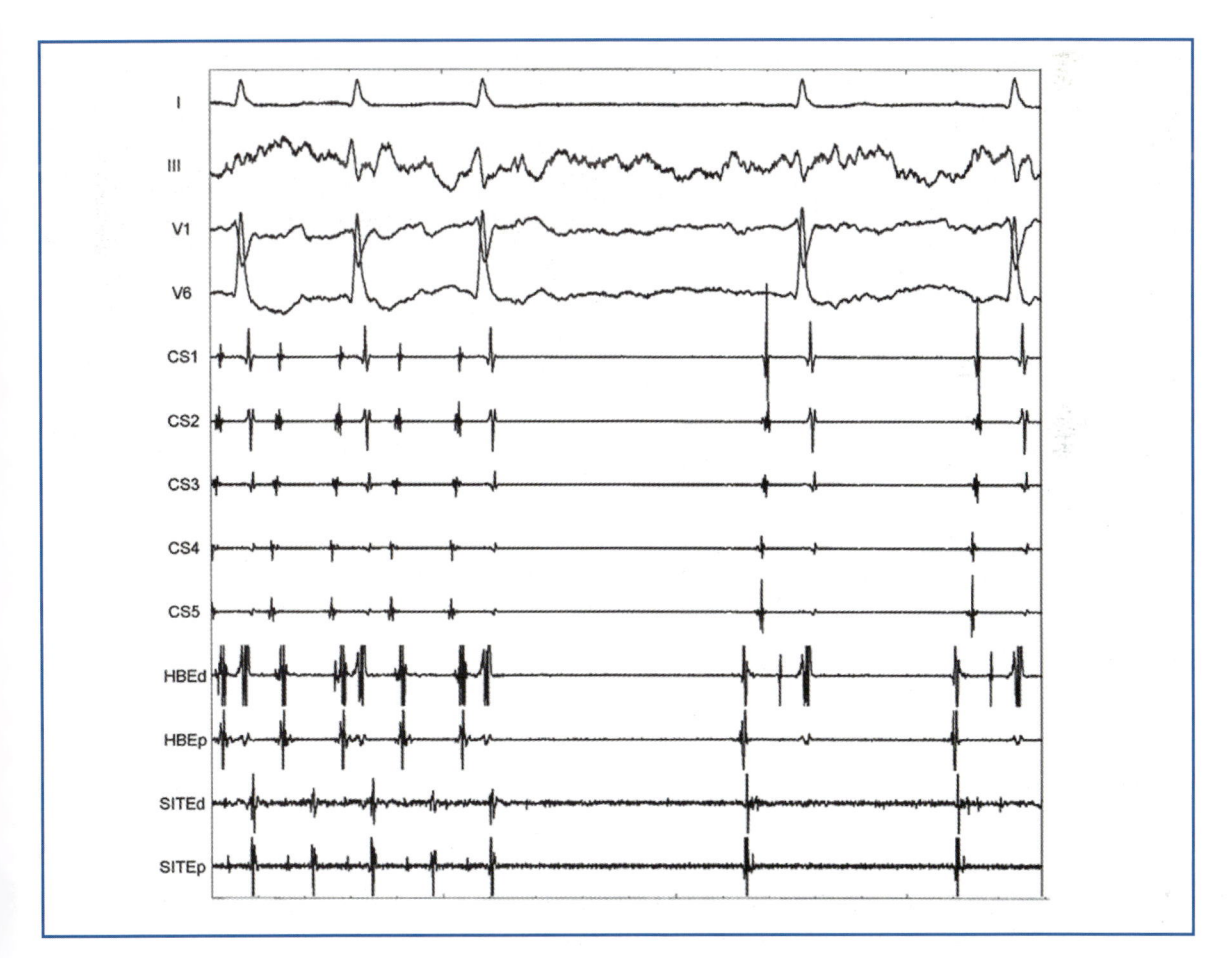

**Fig. 7.** Surface and intracavitary recordings during arrhythmia termination by radiofrequency energy delivery. From *top to bottom*, tracings are displayed as follows: surface leads I, III, V1, V6, bipolar recordings of the coronary-sinus catheter from distal to proximal (CS1–5), bipolar recordings from the distal (HBEd) and proximal (HBEp) electrode pairs of the His-bundle catheter and bipolar recording from the distal (SITEd) and proximal (SITEp) electrode pairs of the ablation catheter. The ablation catheter is positioned at the posterior end of the ablation line, close to the inferior vena cava, and radiofrequency energy delivery is ongoing. Conduction interrupts at this ablation site and stable sinus rhythm is restored

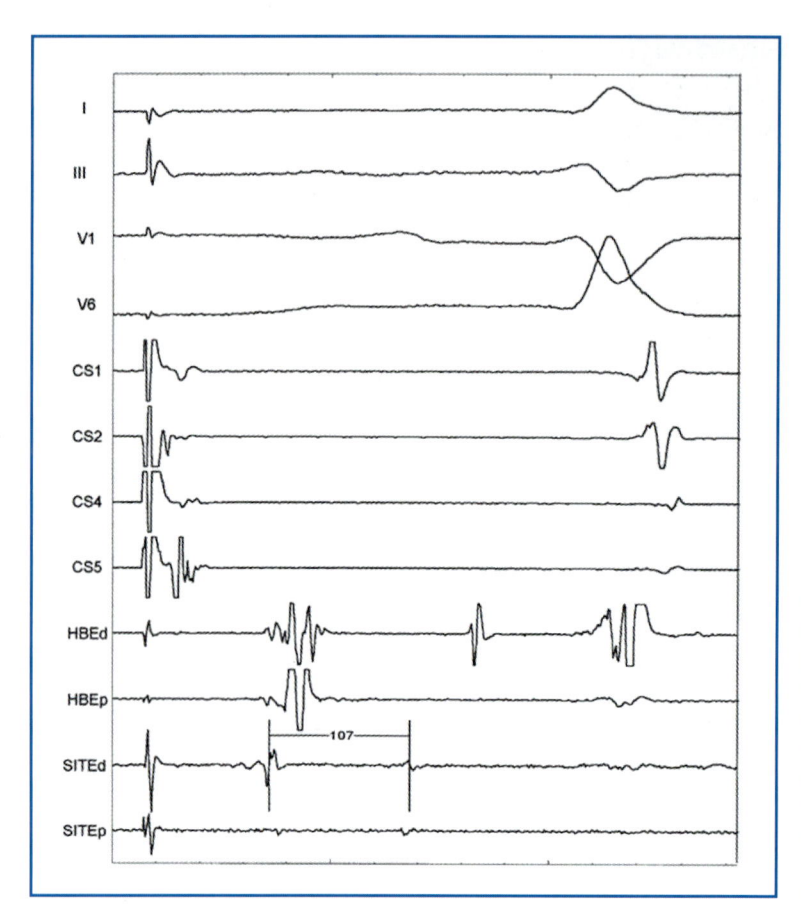

**Fig. 8.** Surface and intracavitary recordings during coronary-sinus pacing at 600 ms after arrhythmia termination. Tracings are displayed as in the Fig. 7. Double potentials separated by > 100 ms are recorded in the cavotricuspid isthmus (SITEd and SITEp) to demonstrate the conduction block produced by ablation. A prolonged interval between the atrial deflection at the pacing site and the one in the His-bundle area is evident and suggests delayed conduction, even at this pacing rate

the presence of an uninterrupted line of double potentials along the isthmus during coronary-sinus pacing (Fig. 8). Of interest, during coronary-sinus pacing there was a prolonged interval (200 ms) between the stimulus and the end of the P wave, which showed an abnormally flat morphology in the inferior leads. No other arrhythmia was inducible. The cavotricuspid isthmus conduction block persisted after 30 min; accordingly, the procedure was terminated. During follow-up, the patient continued on amiodarone and she had only one recurrence of persistent atrial fibrillation two years after this procedure, with sinus rhythm restoration by electrical cardioversion.

## Commentary

It was previously reported [1] that in typical counter-clockwise isthmus-dependent atrial flutter, left atrial activation is initiated adjacent to the coronary sinus ostium in the inferior atrial septum. From this site, propagation proceeds in two directions: (1) along the inferior left atrial wall with a septal-to-posterior orientation, and (2) up to the atrial septum towards the superior left atrium. Synchronous inferosuperior septal and left atrial activation are thought to cause the negative polarity of the flutter waves in the inferior leads.

The case presented here is an example of how a counter-clockwise isthmus-dependent circuit may exhibit an atypical P wave pattern, even in patients without prior thoracic or cardiac surgery, or prior ablation. It is likely that the line of block and activation detour, observed in the right atrium around the coronary sinus ostium, was the major determinant in modifying the surface P wave pattern from the typical one, by altering the septal and initial phases of left atrial propagation. However, it cannot be excluded that other lines of conduction block in the left atrium, enlarged atrial size, left atrial scarring and delayed atrial conduction (well evident in this patient during coronary-sinus pacing) significantly contributed to modification of the surface P wave pattern during flutter. This hypothesis is corroborated by previous data [2], in which an atypical ECG pattern during cavotricuspid isthmus-dependent atrial flutter was reported in patients with prior left atrial ablation for atrial fibrillation. In fact, prior ablation is responsible in such cases for altered left atrial activation, with a debulking effect by left atrial ablation and thus a marked reduction in left atrial voltage.

Based on this experience, P wave morphology may not be indicative of the site of arrhythmia not only in postsurgical patients, who may have large scars and prior atriotomy, but also in elderly patients with associated structural heart disease and possibly delayed atrial conduction. In all such cases, the presence of a right atrial reentry should be ruled out before proceeding to left atrial mapping, even if the surface P wave pattern strongly suggests a left atrial origin.

# References

1. Rodriguez LM, Timmermans C, Nabar A et al. Biatrial activation in isthmus-dependent atrial flutter. Circulation 2001; 104: 2545-2550.
2. Chugh A, Latchamsetty R, Oral H et al. Characteristics of cavotricuspid isthmus-dependent atrial flutter after left atrial ablation of atrial fibrillation. Circulation 2006; 113: 609-615.

# Case 13
## Recurrence of Typical Counter-clockwise Atrial Flutter in a Postsurgical Patient: an Unexpected Trap

## Case Presentation

This is a 49-year-old male patient with prior surgery for mitral valve replacement at the ages of 33 and 47. The surgical interventions comprised right atrial atriotomy and direct suture of an atrial septal defect. After the second intervention, the patient began complaining of palpitations. Initially, the episodes were short-lasting and self-terminating, but they later became persistent, were documented in all cases as typical common atrial flutter (Fig. 1a) and invariably recurred

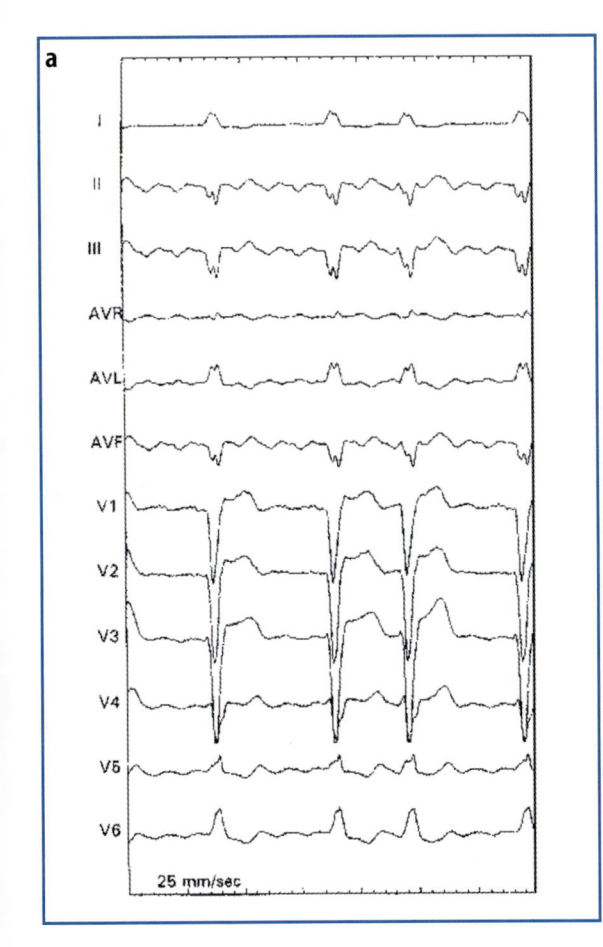

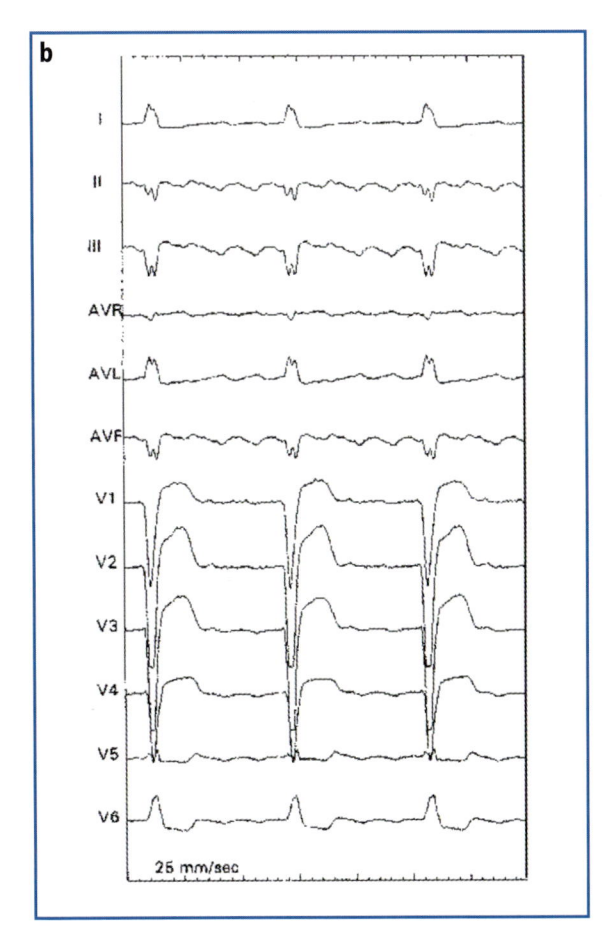

**Fig. 1a, b.** Twelve-lead electrocardiogram of the index arrhythmia (**a**) and of the postablation recurrence (**b**)

after DC-shock cardioversion in spite of therapy with oral amiodarone. During the year before undergoing the procedure described here, the patient developed left bundle branch block, initially rate-dependent and subsequently permanent. Echocardiogram showed enlarged right and left atria, normal functioning of the prosthetic mechanical mitral valve and preserved left ventricular function. While experiencing counter-clockwise typical atrial flutter at 250 ms cycle length, the patient was admitted to our institution. Cavotricuspid isthmus ablation terminated the arrhythmia and produced bidirectional conduction block, restoring stable sinus rhythm. However, two weeks later, the patient had recurrence of palpitations. Surface ECG showed recurrence of what appeared to be the same arrhythmia (Fig. 1b), but with a longer cycle length (305 ms), most likely due to conduction resumption over the cavotricuspid isthmus, delayed by previous ablation. For the recurrent arrhythmia, the patient was re-admitted for a second electrophysiologic procedure.

## Procedure

At the time of the procedure, the clinical arrhythmia persisted with unchanged cycle length. Two decapolar catheters were positioned, one in the lower part of the crista terminalis close to the tricuspid annulus and the other in the coronary sinus. Diastolic activation of the crista terminalis and a proximal to distal activation in the coronary sinus were observed. Interestingly, mapping of the cavotricuspid isthmus identified an uninterrupted line of double potentials separated by > 70 ms, suggestive of conduction block and inconsistent with an isthmus-dependent atrial flutter. For this reason, extensive electroanatomic mapping of the right atrium was performed by acquiring 159 sites. The right atrial volume was 106 ml. Right atrial activation spanned the entire tachycardia cycle length with a clear "head-meets-tail" pattern in the lateral wall (Fig. 2a, b). In fact, the mid-diastolic isthmus was located in the middle of the crista terminalis, boundered anterosuperiorly by a line of double potentials (possibly related to prior atriotomy in the area of the right atrial appendage) and posteroinferiorly by a small area of double potentials in the posteroinferior right atrium (arrow in Fig. 3a"). Analysis of the propagation map showed that reentry in the right atrium was sustained by two loops that shared the same mid-diastolic isthmus. The first loop (Fig. 3a–g) rotated counter-clockwise in the right atrium; upon exiting the mid-diastolic isthmus (Fig. 3a), its wavefront propagated inferoposteriorly towards the posterior wall (Fig. 3b, c) and then towards the upper medial right atrium (Fig. 3d, e) and the upper crista terminalis (Fig. 3f), to finally reenter the mid-diastolic isthmus (Fig. 3g). The second loop (Fig. 3a'–g' and a"–d") rotated counter-clockwise in the anterosuperior right atrium. In fact, from the mid-diastolic isthmus (Fig. 3a', a") it propagated anterosuperiorly in the anterolateral right atrium towards the tricuspid annulus (Fig. 3b'–d' and 3b"–d"), passing anteriorly to the atriotomy in the area of the right atrial appendage. It then directed posteriorly to the superior vena cava os before joining the first loop in the upper crista terminalis (Fig. 3e') and finally moved down along the crista terminalis (Fig. 3f', g') to reenter the mid-diastolic isthmus. The first loop measured 15.7 cm and the second 18 cm. Analysis of conduction velocities showed that the mid-diastolic isthmus was slower (38 cm/s). In the outer part of both loops, values were higher; specifically, in the first loop the conduction velocities were 83 and 56 cm/s in the central and final parts of the outer loop, respectively, whereas in the initial part of the outer loop (low medial right atrium) the conduction velocity remained slow (34 cm/s). As expected, in the second and longer loop, conduction velocities were higher, 105 and 77 cm/s in the initial and final parts of the outer loop, respectively, with the exception of a small segment in the central part of the outer loop (Fig. 3c'), where the velocity decreased to 16 cm/s. Further propagation analysis (Fig. 3a"–g") confirmed by-stander activation of the cavotricuspid isthmus. In this area,

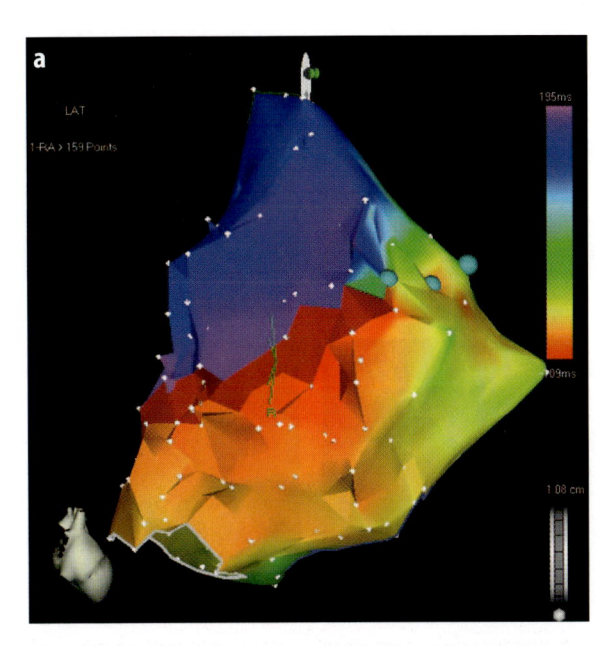

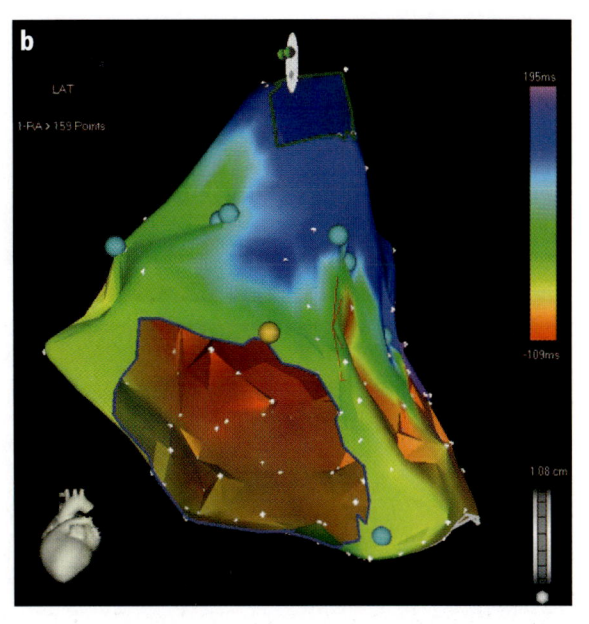

**Fig. 2a, b.** Activation map of the right atrium during atrial flutter in right lateral (**a**) and left anterior oblique (LAO) (**b**) views. *Orange dot* indicates the site of His-bundle recording; the *blue dots* indicate the site where double potentials were recorded

the collision of two wavefronts, lateral and medial, was observed (Fig. 3a"–d"). The lateral wavefront was generated by the second loop and propagated anteriorly just after exiting the mid-diastolic isthmus. The medial one derived from the first loop, coming from the propagation in the posteromedial wall and then moving counter-clockwise around the inferior vena cava. Analysis of the bipolar voltage map (Fig. 4) showed that the anterosuperior part of the mid-diastolic isthmus had low-amplitude potentials, while the posterior part included points with voltage amplitudes >1 mV. However, the average voltage value in the mid-diastolic isthmus was low (0.78±0.85 mV) and the voltage range was between 0.12 and 1.8 mV. The extension of the mid-diastolic isthmus was longer, i.e. 4.6 cm from anterosuperior (line of double potentials close to the right appendage area) to posteroinferior (small area of double potentials indicated by the arrow in Fig. 3a"). After alternative ablation strategies were considered and in spite of the extent of the planned line of ablation, the mid-diastolic isthmus was considered the best ablation target in this case. The other possible ablation approach consisted of separately targeting each loop at the site of its narrower anatomic isthmus. The location of the two anatomic isthmi were identified as follows: (1) anterior (red arrow in Fig. 5), to transect the second loop between the double potential line close to the right atrial appendage and the tricuspid annulus, and (2) posterior (green arrow in Fig. 5), to transect the first loop between the small double potential area and the inferior vena cava. It was calculated that the anterior isthmus measured 3.1 cm, with a voltage of 2.3±1.2 mV on average and a voltage range between 1.4 and 3.5 mV, while the posterior isthmus measured 2.3 cm, with an average voltage of 2.6±1.8 mV, ranging between 0.4 and 4.9 mV. Therefore, in this alterative strategy, the extension of the two ablation lines was longer than the mid-diastolic isthmus; moreover, the presence of extended areas with a voltage value > 2 mV and up to 4 mV represented a substrate likely to be very resistant to ablation even using an irrigated-tip catheter. For this reason, after it was determined that stimulation in this area at 10 mA output would not result in phrenic nerve capture, ablation was aimed at the mid-diastolic isthmus. Sequential radiofrequency energy using an irrigated-tip catheter (maximum power 45 W, cut-off temperature 43°C, duration 60 s) was delivered from the anterosuperior to the inferoposterior part of the mid-diastolic isthmus (Fig. 5). When the posterior part of the mid-diastolic isthmus was targeted, the tachycardia cycle prolonged by 50 ms and soon after was interrupted, with restoration of stable sinus rhythm (Fig. 6). Further applications were delivered along the lesion line, until a line of conduction block was obtained, as assessed by recording of double potentials, separated by > 100 ms on sinus rhythm, and by the consistent change in right atrial activation during sinus rhythm (Fig. 7). Persistence of bidirectional conduction block along the cavotricuspid isthmus was also assessed by stimulation of the coronary sinus and the lower crista terminalis. No arrhythmia was inducible thereafter. The results achieved during the procedure persisted after 30 min; hence, the procedure was terminated. The patient continued to be arrhythmia free 6 months after the procedure.

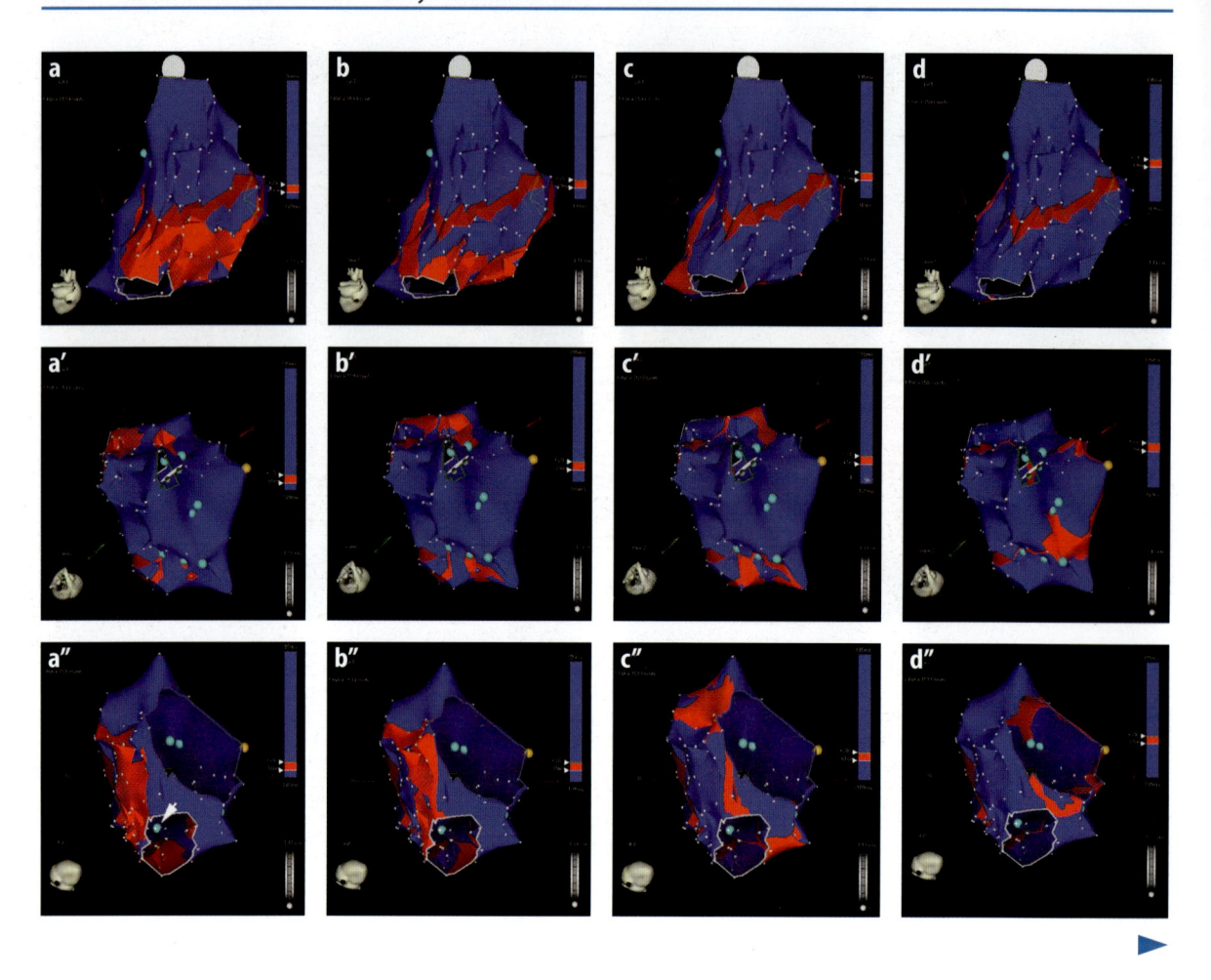

## Commentary

The electrocardiographic pattern of typical atrial flutter, especially in patients with prior surgery for congenital or acquired heart disease, is not "per se" predictive of a reentry circuit dependent on cavotricuspid isthmus conduction. Moreover, an electrocardiographic pattern of typical atrial flutter not associated with an isthmus-dependent circuit has been already reported also in patients without prior surgery, congenital heart disease, or prior ablation [1]. Interestingly, even an atrial tachycardia originating from the inferoseptal portion of the right atrium and with a short cycle length may mimic typical atrial flutter, due to functional block in the clockwise direction of the cavotricuspid isthmus [2].

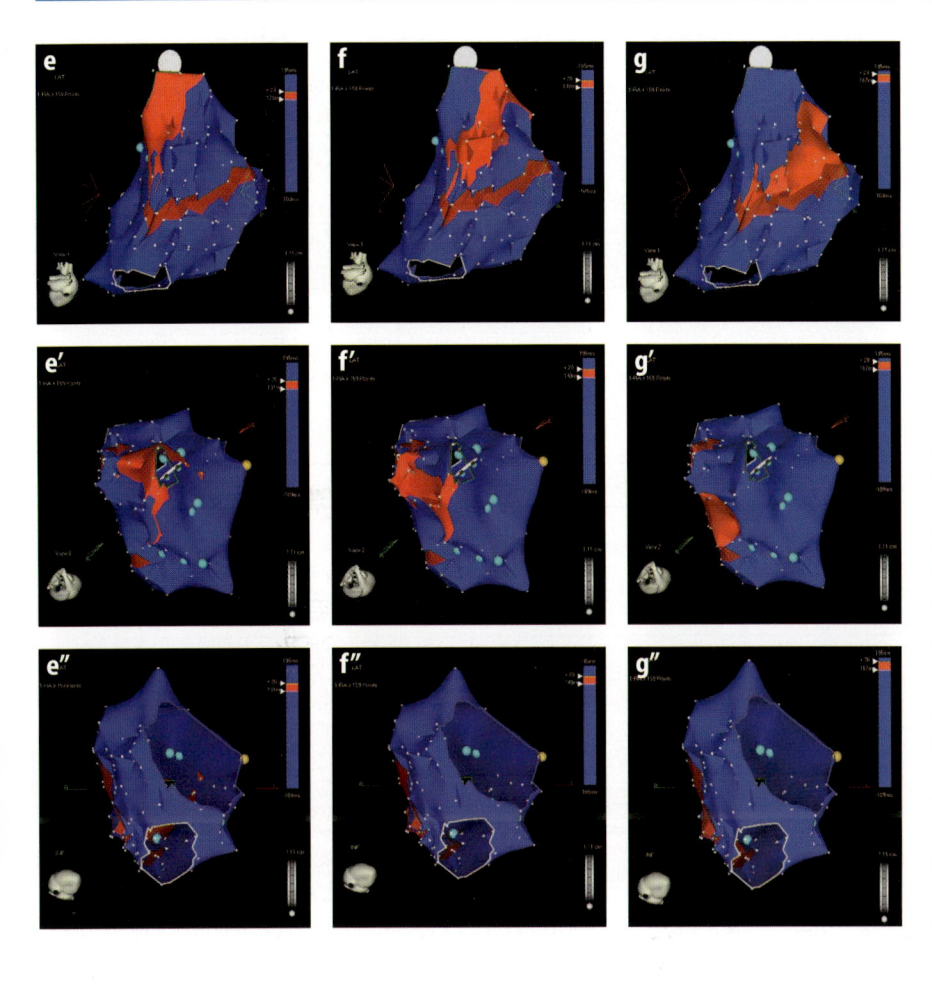

**Fig. 3a-g.** Sequential frames of the propagation map of the right atrium during atrial flutter in posterolateral (**a–g**), cranial (**a′–g′**) and inferior (**a″–g″**) views. The course of the two loops in the right atrium is evident, together with bystander activation of the cavotricuspid isthmus. In (**a″**), the *white arrow* indicates the small area of double potentials, which represented the posterior boundary of the mid-diastolic isthmus. It is not visible in Fig. 2

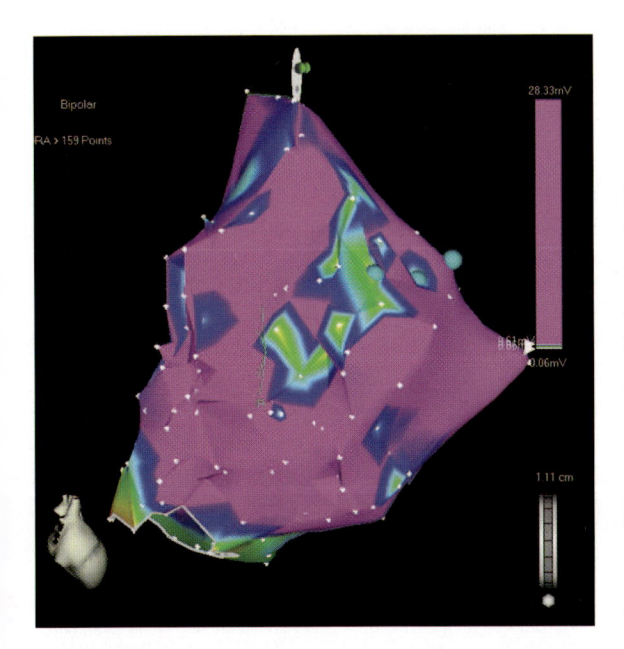

**Fig. 4.** Bipolar voltage map of the right atrium during atrial flutter in right lateral view. According to the setting of the colour-coded scale, areas with preserved voltage are shown in *purple*

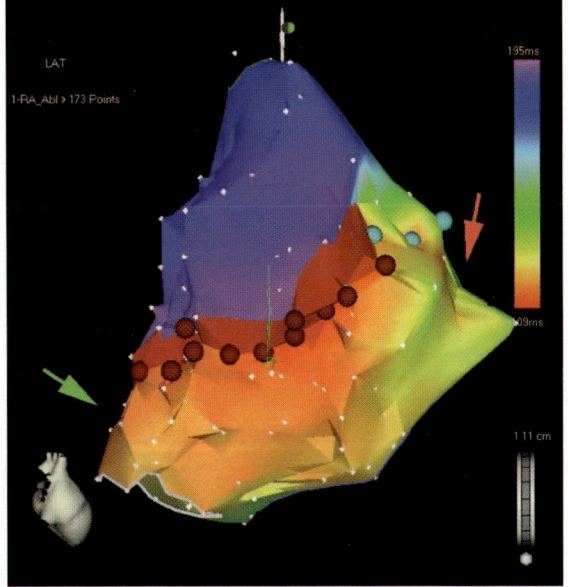

**Fig. 5.** Activation map of the right atrium during atrial flutter in right lateral view. *Red dots* indicate the ablation line along the mid-diastolic isthmus. *Red and green arrows* indicate the anatomically defined isthmi, possible candidates for ablation in an alternative ablation strategy

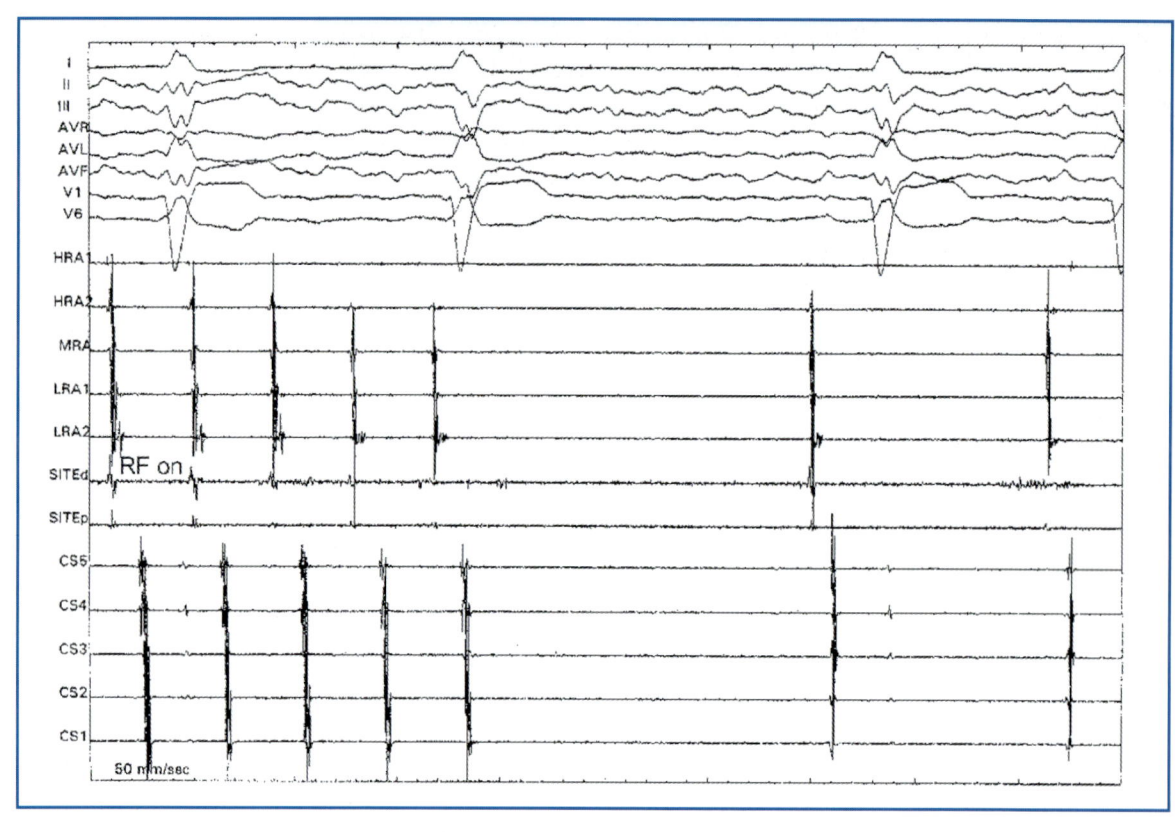

**Fig. 6.** Surface and intracavitary signal upon flutter termination during radiofrequency energy delivery. From *top to bottom*, tracings are displayed as follows: limb leads and precordial leads V1 and V6, bipolar signals of the decapolar catheter positioned along the crista terminalis, from the upper to the lower part (HRA1–LRA2), bipolar recordings from the distal (SITEd) and proximal (SITEp) electrode pairs of the ablation catheter and bipolar recordings of the decapolar coronary sinus catheter, from proximal to distal (CS5–CS1). The ablation catheter is positioned in the posterior part of the mid-diastolic isthmus, since the anterior portion has been already ablated. Radiofrequency energy is delivered and interrupts the arrhythmia, restoring stable sinus rhythm

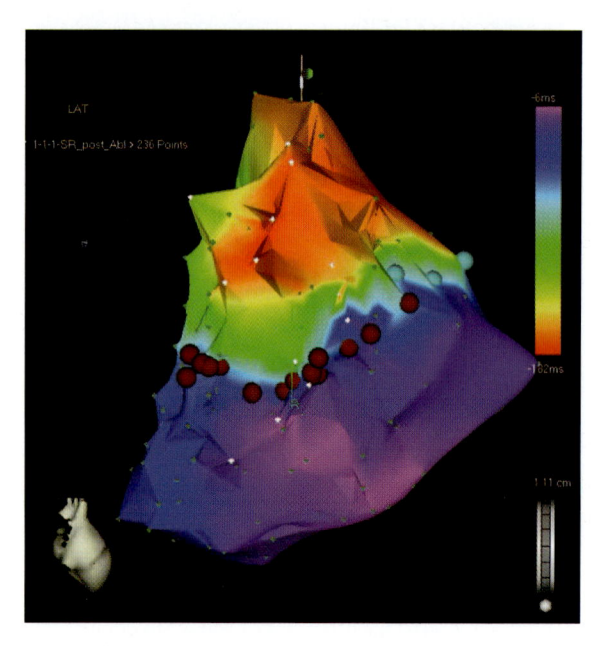

**Fig. 7.** Activation map of the right atrium during remapping in sinus rhythm, after arrhythmia ablation, in right lateral view. *Red dots* indicate the ablation line. Ablation prolonged right atrial activation to 176 ms. The latest activated site is in the lateral wall, specifically, in the central area of the region inferior to the ablation line

In this case, the right atrium was activated counter-clockwise by the first loop, with presystolic activation of the coronary sinus os, possibly resulting in left atrial activation starting in the inferomedial region, as in typical isthmus-dependent atrial flutter (as already discussed in the previous case). This sequence of events may have been the major determinant of a morphology that mimicked typical counter-clockwise atrial flutter on surface electrocardiogram. The "trap" in this case was that the index arrhythmia was actually an isthmus-dependent atrial flutter and, hence, recurrence of the same arrhythmia was expected in the second procedure. The lesson to be learned here is that recurrence of typical atrial flutter after successful ablation in postsurgical patients with structural heart disease and enlarged atria should be carefully considered during the repeated procedure, to exclude the presence of other reentry circuits mimicking the surface P wave pattern of the typical form. Accordingly, the repeated procedure should be planned while the patient is still in arrhythmia, to avoid a useless procedure if cavotricuspid isthmus conduction block persists and no arrhythmia is inducible.

## References

1. Lickfett L, Calkins H, Nasir K et al. Clinical prediction of cavotricuspid isthmus dependence in patients referred for catheter ablation of "typical" atrial flutter. J Cardiovasc Electrophysiol 2005; 16: 969-973.
2. Ito S, Tada H, Nogami A et al. Atrial tachycardia arising from the right atrial inferoseptum masquerading as common atrial flutter. Circ J 2007; 71: 160-165.

# Case 14
## Two Macroreentrant Tachycardias in a Patient after Fontan Surgery: the Difference between "Isthmic" and "Rotational" Atrial Macroreentry

## Case Presentation

This is a 21-year-old male patient with complex congenital heart disease that included a single ventricle, transposition of the great vessels, pulmonary valve stenosis and persistence of the left superior vena cava. At the age of four, he underwent a Fontan operation, consisting of insertion of the left superior vena cava in the left pulmonary artery and of the right superior vena cava in the right pulmonary artery, with direct closure of its orifice in the right atrium. The right atrium was connected through a conduit to the pulmonary artery. In the same intervention, the tricuspid orifice was closed by a prosthetic patch in order to separate venous from arterial blood flow. Six months before the procedure, the patient had episodes of typical atrial flutter (Fig. 1) with a cycle length of 285 ms and 2:1 atrioventricular conduction. In spite of amiodarone therapy, the arrhythmia recurred and was responsible for syncope and initial-stage congestive heart failure. Therefore, the patient was admitted for an electrophysiologic procedure.

## Procedure

At the beginning of the procedure, the spontaneous rhythm had a cycle length of 750 ms with negative P waves in the inferior leads. The coronary sinus was impossible to cannulate as it was likely that its orifice had been excluded from the right atrium by prior surgery. Stable intracavitary recordings from a catheter positioned in the right atrium to be used as reference signal were unlikely to be obtained in this enlarged chamber. Therefore, a bipolar catheter was positioned in the esophagus to record a left atrial electrogram, which then served as the electrical reference. Right atrial mapping was initiated using a long sheath to support the roving catheter during spontaneous rhythm, to define the chamber geometry. This rhythm was found to originate in the inferomedial part of the right atrium, presumably close to the os of the coronary sinus (Fig. 2a, b). The volume of the atrium was extremely enlarged (265 ml), and bipolar voltage mapping (Fig. 3a, b) showed low voltage around the inferior vena cava, the area of the prosthetic patch in the anterior wall and along the crista terminalis. The size of the prosthetic patch in the anterior wall, as visualised by voltage mapping, was very small. This suggested that the atrium had progressively and considerably enlarged since positioning of the patch, when the patient was 4 years old. The clinical arrhythmia, which had a cycle length of 285 ms, was easily induced by programmed atrial stimulation. High-density electroanatomic mapping was performed after the window of interest was set as for a macroreentrant arrhythmia. As shown in

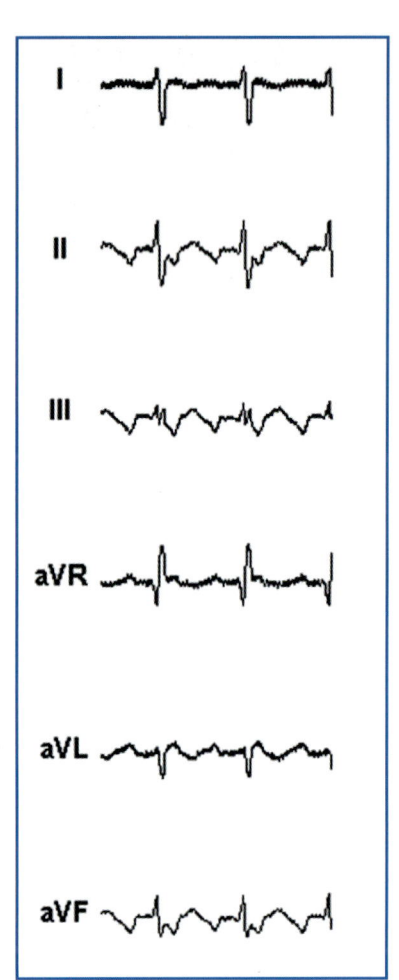

**Fig. 1.** Surface electrocardiogram of the clinical arrhythmia, showing the P wave pattern of counter-clockwise typical atrial flutter

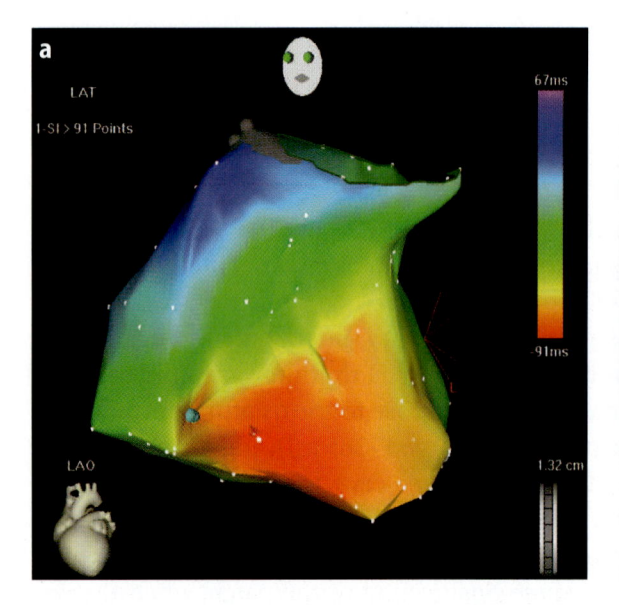

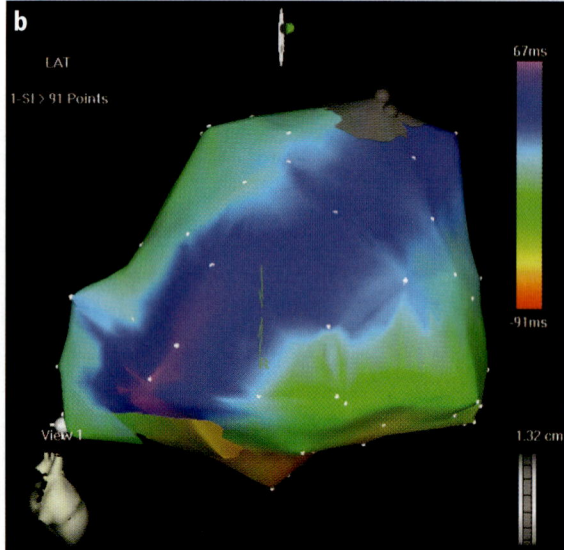

**Fig. 2a, b.** Activation map of the right atrium during spontaneous rhythm in left anterior oblique (LAO) (**a**) and right lateral (**b**) views. This rhythm originated from the inferomedial region. The His-bundle potential could not be recorded; the *blue dot* indicates a site of double potentials. The circular line defines the orifice in the upper right atrium of the conduit to the pulmonary artery; a small electrically silent area is present in the anterolateral region of the orifice (*grey dots*).

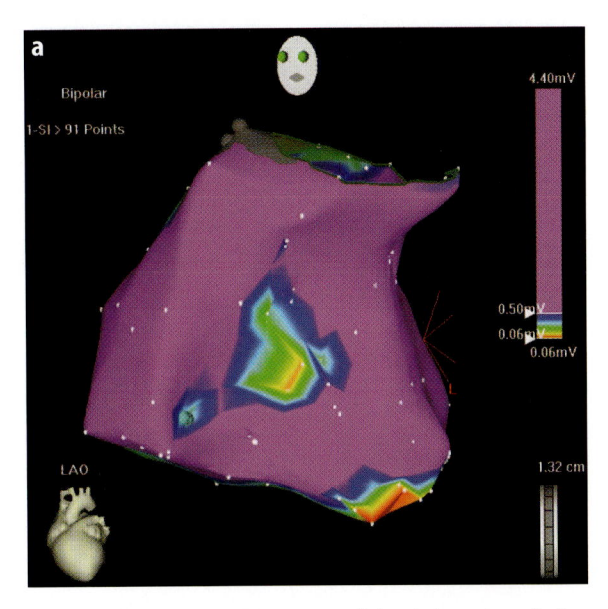

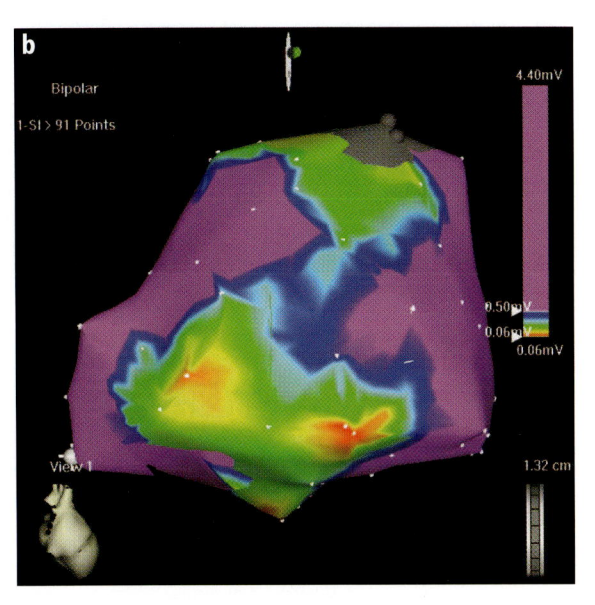

**Fig. 3a, b.** Bipolar voltage map of the right atrium during spontaneous rhythm in LAO (**a**) and right lateral (**b**) views. According to the setting of the colour-coded scale, areas with preserved voltage are shown in *purple*

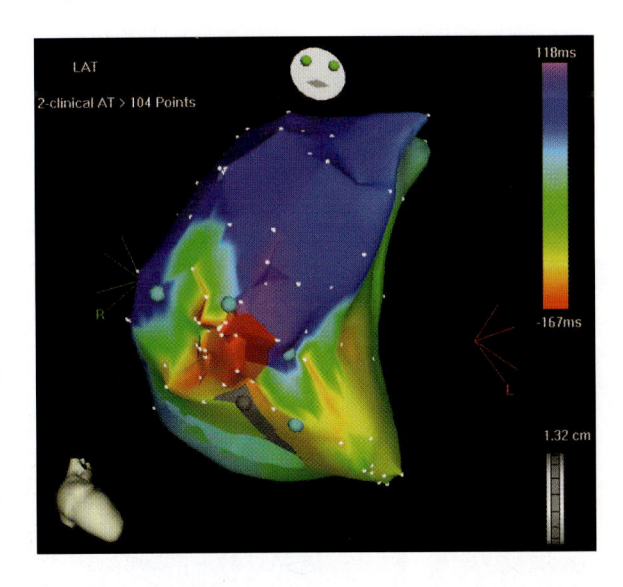

**Fig. 4.** Activation map of the right atrium during the clinical flutter in caudal right anterior oblique (RAO) view. *Blue dots* indicate sites of double potentials forming the anterior and posterior limits of the mid-diastolic isthmus, the extension of which measured 2.0 cm

Fig. 4, right atrial activation spanned the entire flutter cycle length, and the mid-diastolic isthmus was localised in the low lateral right atrium. Double potentials were identified at the anterior and posterior limits of this isthmus, which measured 20 mm. The complete course of these double potential lines was difficult to track due to the difficulties encountered in positioning the catheter in this area, despite the fact that a long sheath was used. Bipolar voltage mapping during flutter (Fig. 5a, b) showed the diastolic pathway as a channel of relatively low voltage (<1 mV, ranging from 0.65 to 0.38 mV), limited anteriorly and posteriorly by areas of preserved voltage (up to 5 mV). Analysis of the propagation map (Fig. 6) showed that, as suggested by the surface P wave morphology, the main reentrant wavefront resembled that of typical counter-clockwise atrial flutter, although only an anatomic equivalent of the cavotricuspid isthmus was present in this patient, due to positioning of the prosthetic patch. From the mid-diastolic isthmus (Fig. 6a, a'), the propagation moved anteromedially (Fig. 6b, b') and then superiorly (Fig. 6c, d) in a counter-clockwise single-loop circuit around an area of block corresponding to the prosthetic

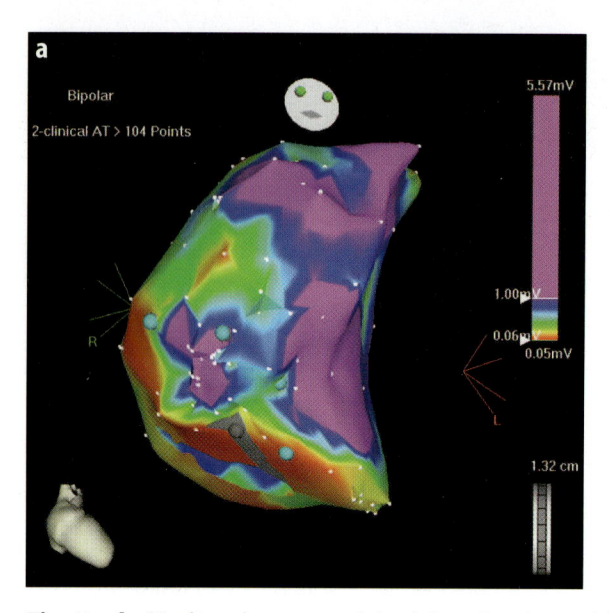

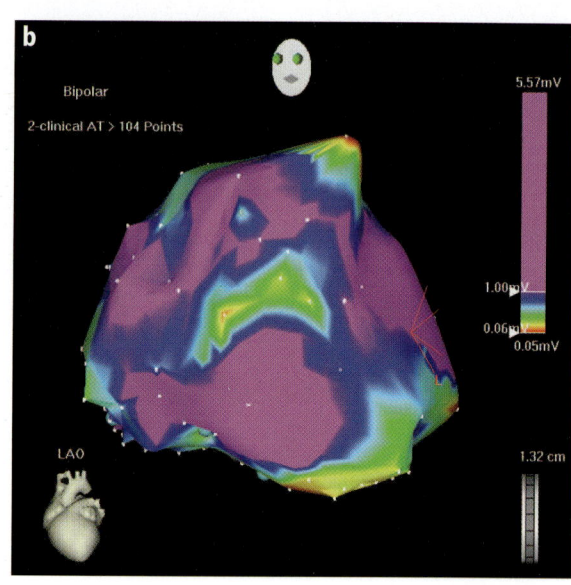

**Fig. 5a, b.** Bipolar voltage map of the right atrium in caudal RAO (**a**) and LAO (**b**) views. According to the setting of the colour-coded scale, areas with voltage > 1.0 mV are shown in *purple*. The difference in voltage between the mid-diastolic isthmus (<1.0 mV) and the anterior and posterior adjacent areas (>1.0 mV) is evident

patch. In the cranial right atrium, the flutter wavefront split into two components (Fig. 6e') due to the presence of the conduit to the pulmonary artery and surgical suture of the superior vena cava os. Subsequently, the two wavelets rejoined and directed inferolaterally towards the entrance of the mid-diastolic isthmus (Fig. 6f, f'). A wide area posterior to the mid-diastolic isth-

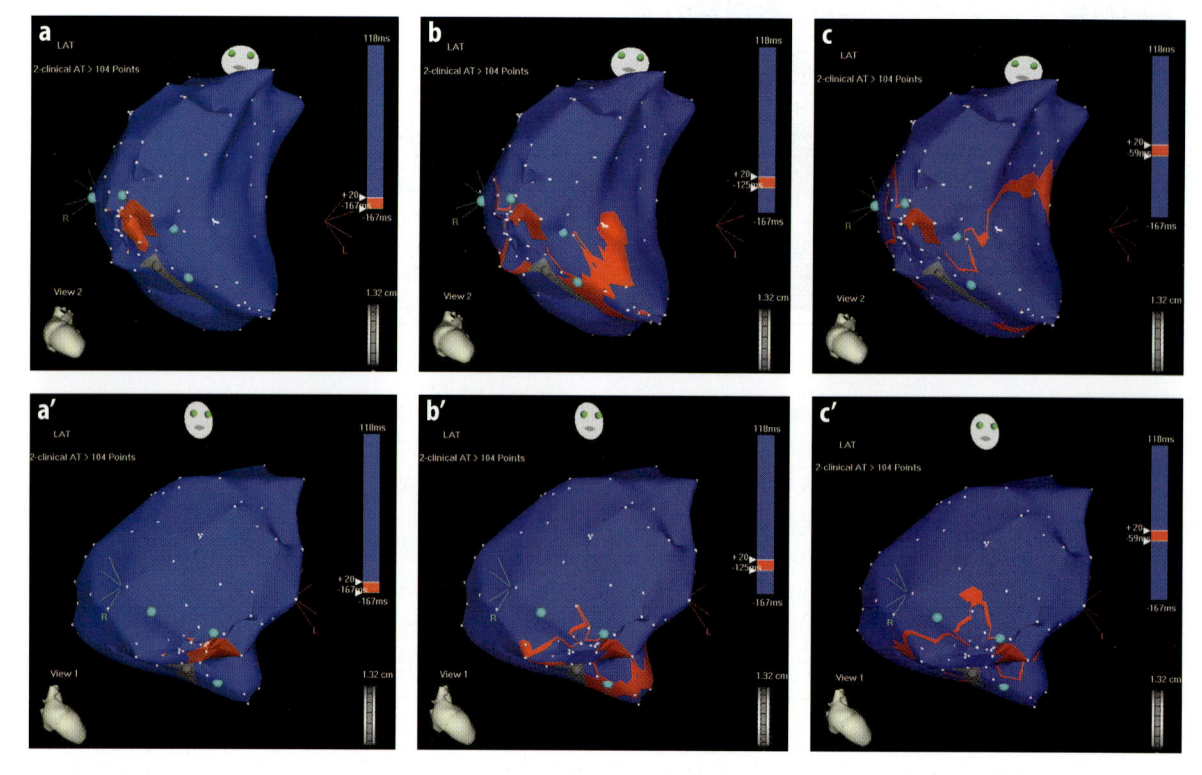

**Fig. 6a–f'.** Sequential frames of the propagation map of the right atrium during clinical atrial flutter in caudal anteroposterior (**a–f**) and RAO (**a'–f'**) views. The counter-clockwise single-loop reentry in the right atrium, similar to that of typical atrial flutter, is evident

mus showed conduction block (Fig. 6b', d') and did not participate in the circuit. A second wavefront originating from the main one (arrow in Fig. 6d) rotated clockwise around the inferior vena cava and terminated as a dead-end pathway at the wide area of block posterior to the mid-diastolic isthmus. The length of the reentrant circuit was 19.7 cm. The conduction velocity was lower in the mid-diastolic isthmus (48 cm/s) and higher in three evaluated tracts along the outer loop (76, 84, 70 cm/s). Stimulation at the mid-diastolic isthmus for entrainment was not possible because of the lack of capture even at maximum output. The ablation strategy was aimed at the mid-diastolic isthmus. Radiofrequency energy delivered by an irrigated-tip catheter (maximum output 40 W, cut-off temperature 43°C, maximum duration 60 s) to transect the mid-diastolic isthmus from posterior to anterior (Fig. 7) terminated the flutter after its cycle length had been prolonged and a line of double potentials was produced. Subsequently, the clinical flutter was no longer inducible even by burst atrial stimulation. Instead, this aggressive stimulation protocol induced a non-clinical atrial flutter with positive P waves in the inferior leads (Fig. 8) and a shorter cycle length (270 ms). After mapping of this new morphology, it was found that right atrial activation spanned 99% of the tachycardia cycle length (Fig. 9a, b). The mid-diastolically activated area was unusually wide (7.7 cm) and corresponded to the entire vertical length of the crista terminalis. It was bounded superiorly by the suture of the superior vena cava and inferiorly by the area of prior ablation, evident as double potentials. The reentrant circuit was again a single-loop reentry in the right atrium and measured 22.4 cm. As seen in the propagation map in Figure 10a–d, from the mid-diastolic area the wavefront moved posteriorly (Fig. 10a, b), rotated medially and then directed anteriorly (Fig. 10c) to re-enter the area of mid-diastolic activation (Fig. 10d). Analysis of the conduction velocities along the reentrant circuit showed higher values in the mid-diastolically activated area (67 cm/s) and in three tracts of the outer loop (106, 100 and 72 cm/s). Bipolar voltage mapping during this second morphol-

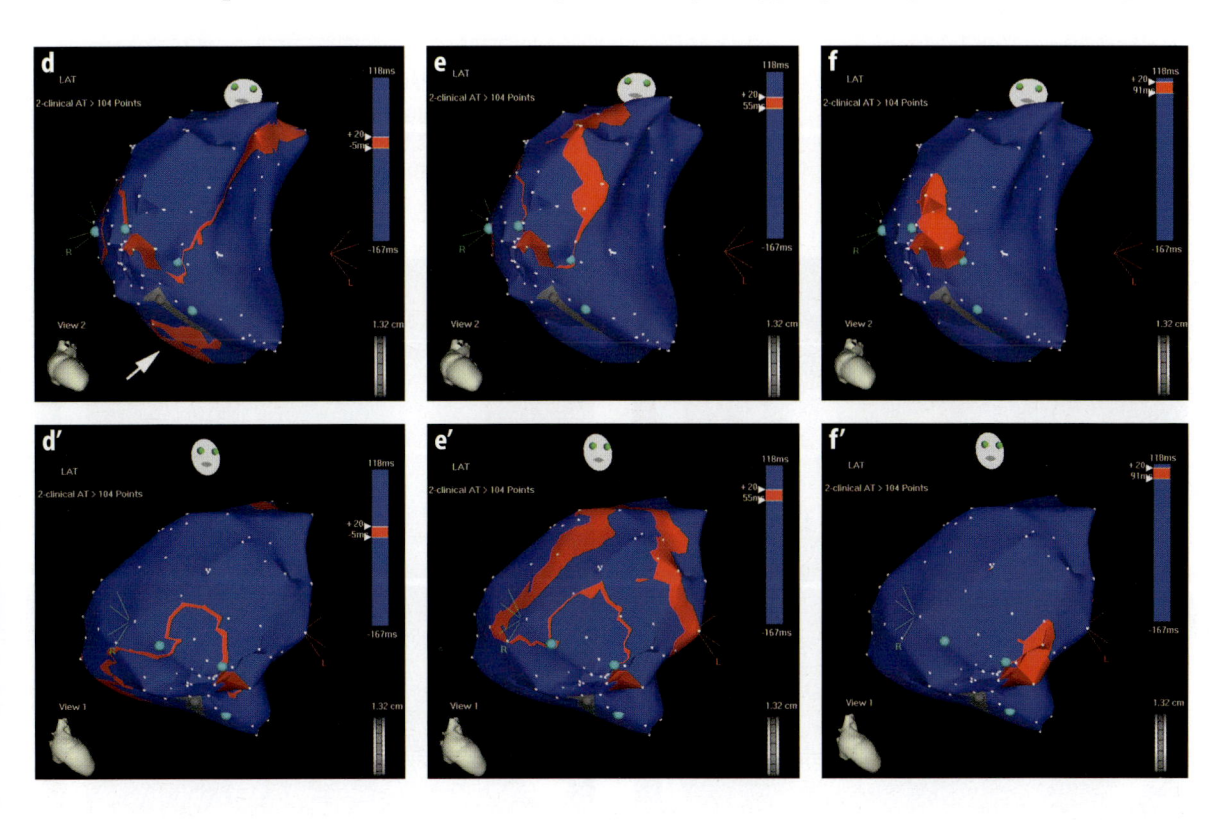

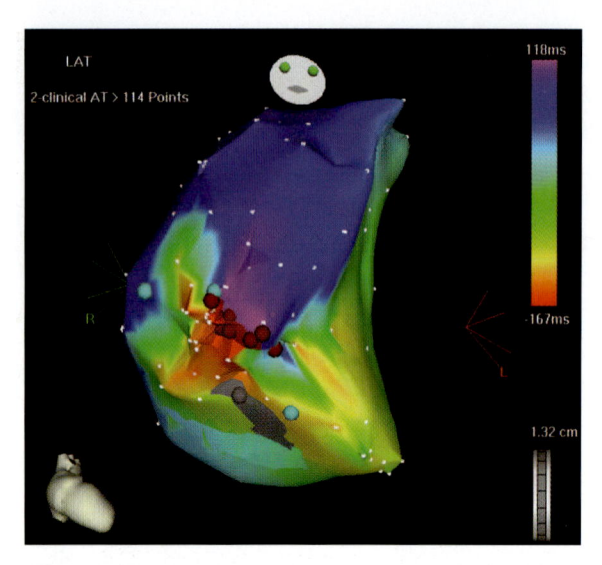

**Fig. 7.** Activation map of the right atrium during clinical atrial flutter in caudal right anterior view. *Red dots* indicate the ablation line

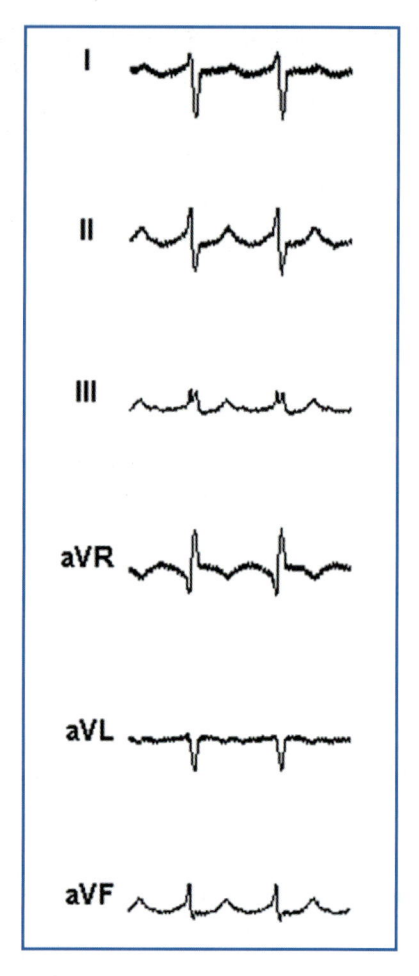

**Fig. 8.** Surface electrocardiogram of the atrial flutter with 2:1 atrioventricular conduction induced after ablation of the index morphology. Positive P waves in the inferior leads are superimposed on the T waves

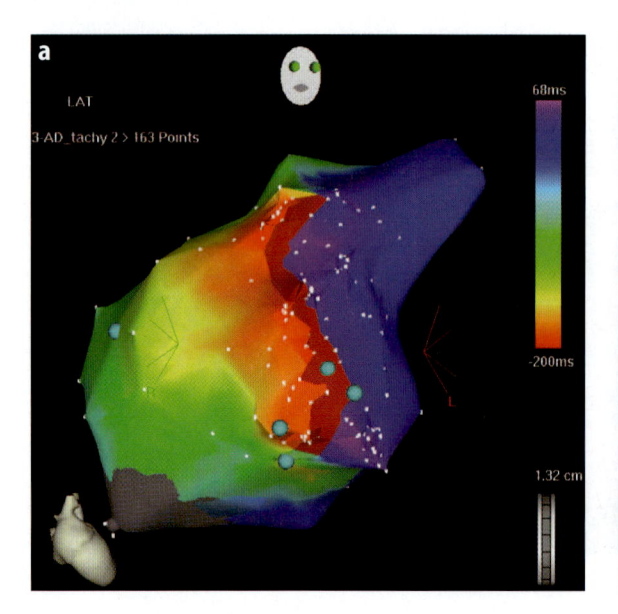

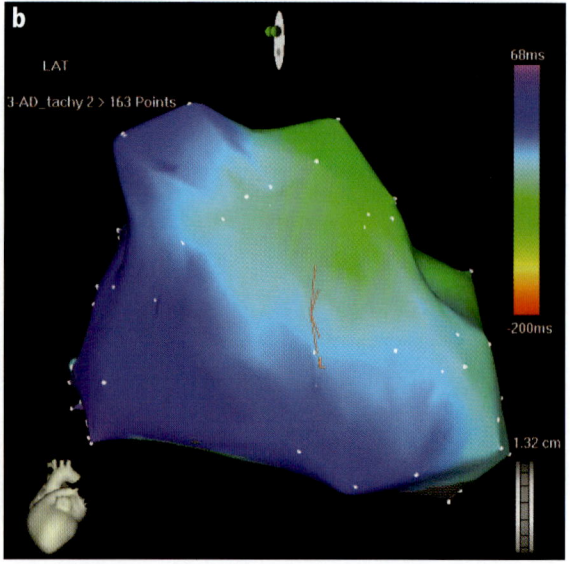

**Fig. 9a, b.** Activation map of the right atrium during the second atrial flutter morphology in RAO (**a**) and left lateral (**b**) views. The wide extension (7.7 cm) of the mid-diastolic isthmus, corresponding to the crista terminalis, is evident in this morphology

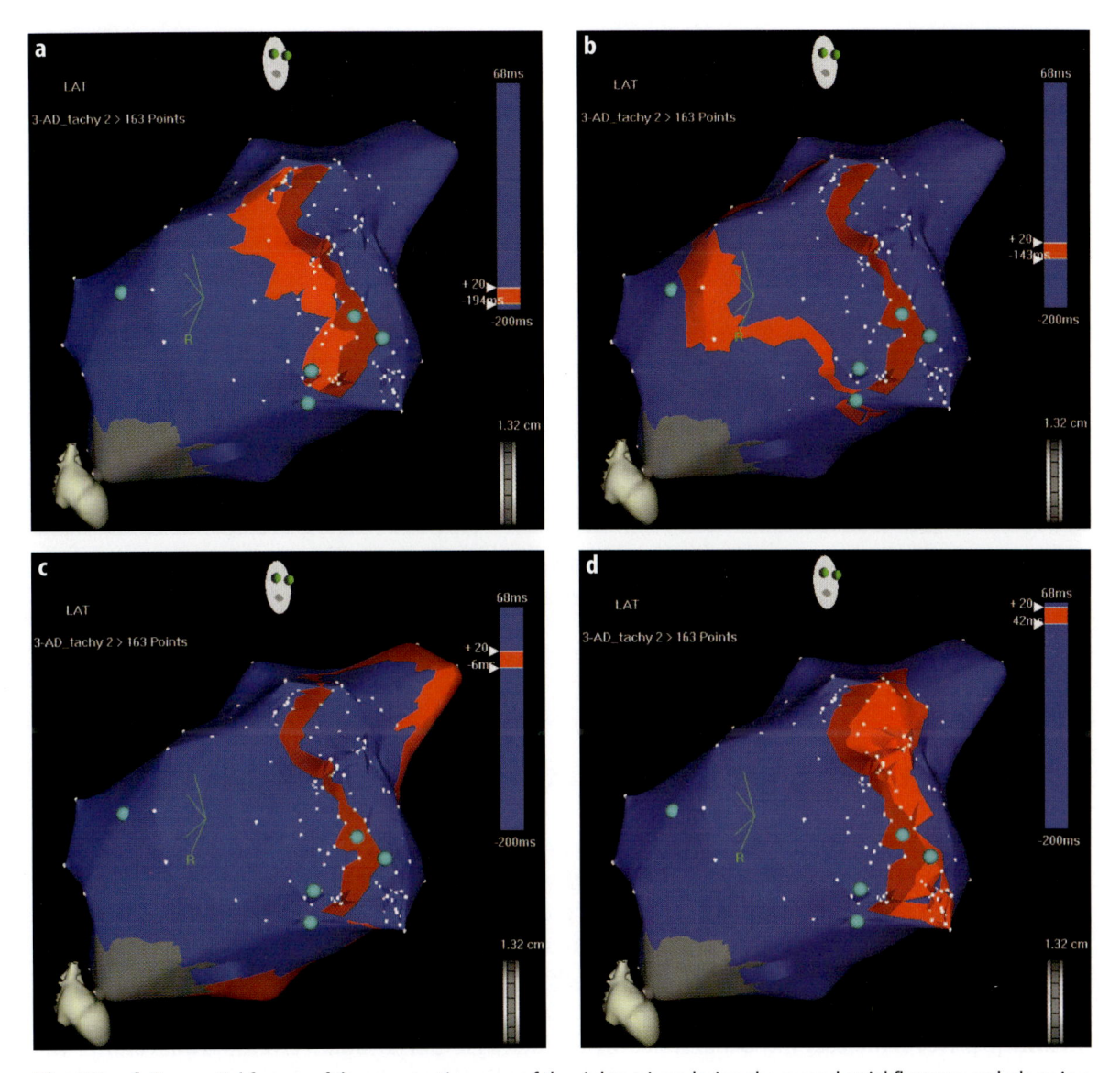

**Fig. 10a-d.** Sequential frames of the propagation map of the right atrium during the second atrial flutter morphology in a right lateral view. The reentrant circuit rotating around the right atrium is evident

ogy (Fig. 11a, b) confirmed, as observed before, low-amplitude potentials in the lateral wall and especially in the lower crista terminalis, where ablation had been previously performed. Relatively higher voltage signals were measured in the mid-diastolically activated area and ranged from 0.31 to 2.96 mV, with a wider area of higher amplitude being present in the central part of the crista terminalis (Fig. 11a). This second arrhythmia was not targeted for ablation and the procedure was terminated after electrical cardioversion for the following reasons: (1) the arrhythmia was not clinical, (2) the creation of complete line block along the isthmus appeared challenging for its extent and the presence of the areas of preserved voltage in the central crista terminalis, and (3) incomplete ablation resulting in flutter cycle prolongation could have been proarrhythmic, favoring 1:1 atrioventricular conduction (antegrade Wenckebach point at baseline 300 ms). On the same previously ineffective antiarrhythmic drug (amiodarone), the patient remained asymptomatic for 1 year. Subsequently, since he had recurrences of the non-targeted atrial flutter, he underwent surgical operation to create an extracardiac Fontan with positioning of a prosthetic conduit between the inferior vena cava and the right pulmonary artery, reduction of the right atrial volume, and maze procedure.

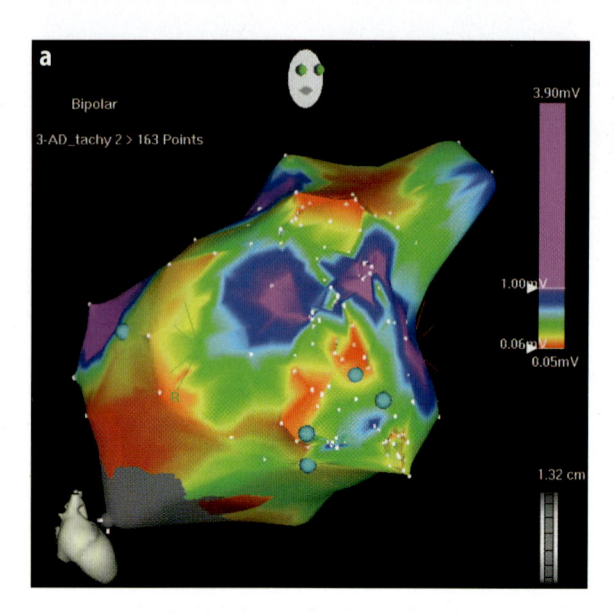

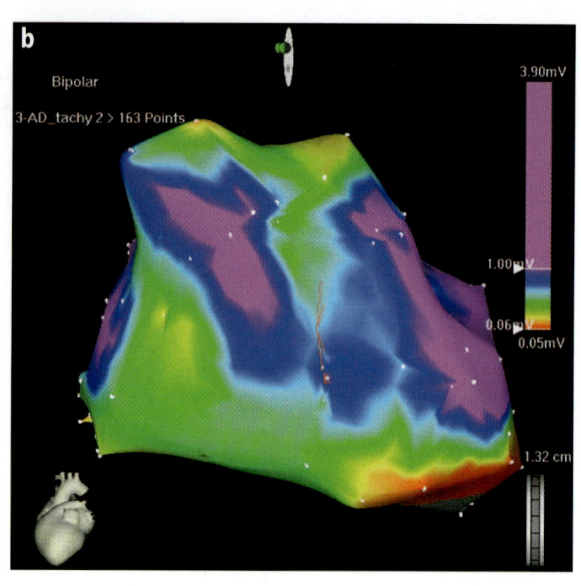

**Fig. 11a, b.** Bipolar voltage map of the right atrium during the induced flutter in right lateral (**a**) and left lateral (**b**) views. According to the setting of the colour-coded scale, areas with voltage > 1.0 mV are shown in *purple*

## Commentary

Atrial arrhythmias are a frequent finding in Fontan patients. In a recently published report on the long-term results of Fontan surgery for double-inlet left ventricle [1], 57% of the early survivors developed at least one episode of supraventricular arrhythmia. Overall freedom from these tachyarrhythmias at 5, 10, 15 and 20 years was 93, 66, 36 and 19%, respectively. In patients with intraatrial reentrant tachycardia after surgical repair of congenital heart disease, especially in Mustard and Senning patients, the cavotricuspid isthmus has been identified as the culprit isthmus in the majority of cases [2]. Conversely, in Fontan patients the reentrant circuits are usually remote from the cavotricuspid isthmus and are located in the lateral wall of the right atrium [3]. Nevertheless, the occurrence of a clockwise periannular circuit transversing the cavotricuspid isthmus or its anatomic equivalent in a Fontan right atrium has been reported [4]. In the present case, the surface P wave morphology and the reentrant circuit were attributable to counter-clockwise isthmus-dependent atrial flutter, with the only difference being in the location of the mid-diastolic isthmus–here, in the low lateral right atrium. Unlike in other cases, in which the critical isthmus was between anatomic or iatrogenic obstacles and/or electrically silent areas, the anterior and posterior boundaries of the mid-diastolic isthmus in this patient consisted of two poorly definable lines of double potentials that separated the isthmus with lower voltage from adjacent areas of preserved voltage. The occurrence of conduction block in coincidence with regions having a significant voltage gradient, such as observed in this patient, was also described in patients with left atrial flutter [5]. Despite this unusual electroanatomic pattern, ablation limited to the mid-diastolic isthmus, as defined by electroanatomic criteria, completely abolished the arrhythmia.

This case is paradigmatic of the possible coexistence in the same patient of two different types of macroreentrant circuit, which could be referred to as "isthmic" and "rotational". "Isthmic" macroreentrant tachycardia/flutter, which comprised the first arrhythmia morphology of this patient, has a reentrant circuit characterized by the presence of an isthmus of limited extension in a given part of the reentry course. In our experience, this isthmus corresponds, in the vast majority of patients (see exception in Case 19), to the area of mid-diastolic activation, where the conduction velocity is significantly slower than that in the outer loop and the voltage amplitude is usually < 0.5 mV and certainly < 1.0 mV. Conversely, in "rotational" forms the reentrant circuit is a wide wavefront of activation that rotates in an atrial chamber without entering an isthmus of limited extension, as observed in the second morphology in this patient. In our experience of electroanatomic mapping of macroreentrant atrial tachycardias [6], the far more common "isthmic" form exhibits a longer cycle length (308±68 ms, on average), possibly related to slow conduction in the isthmus (27±13 cm/s, on average), and the mid-diastolic isthmus can be successfully targeted by ablation (13.2±12.4 radiofrequency energy applications, on average). The difficulty of ablation is related to the isthmus extension (21.7±13.5 mm on average, range 5–45 mm in successfully treated patients). "Rotational" forms are very rare, exhibit a shorter cycle length even in an enlarged atrium and ablation may be very challenging, since any candidate ablation site is of wide extension with preserved voltage and normal conduction velocity. These characteristics in our patient contraindicated ablation, as it may have been proarrhythmic in case of incomplete success. The arrhythmia later recurred, suggesting that these forms, although rare, do occur clinically.

***Acknowledgement.*** *The images for this case were provided by Fabrizio Drago, MD, Department of Paediatric Cardiology, Bambino Gesù Hospital, Rome, Italy*

# References

1. Earing MG, Cetta F, Driscoll DJ et al. Long-term results of the Fontan operation for double-inlet left ventricle. Am J Cardiol 2005; 96: 291-298.
2. Chan DP, Van Hare GF, Mackall JA et al. Importance of atrial flutter isthmus in postoperative intraatrial reentrant tachycardia. Circulation 2000; 102: 1283-1289.
3. Collins KK, Love BA, Walsh EP et al. Location of acutely successful radiofrequency catheter ablation of intraatrial reentrant tachycardia in patients with congenital heart disease. Am J Cardiol 2000; 86: 969-974.
4. Abrams D, Schilling R. Mechanism and mapping of atrial arrhythmia in the modified Fontan circulation. Heart Rhythm 2005; 2: 1138-1144.
5. Jaïs P, Shah DC, Haïssaguerre M et al. Mapping and ablation of left atrial flutters. Circulation 2000; 101: 2928-2934.
6. De Ponti R, Verlato R, Bertaglia E et al. Treatment of macroreentrant atrial tachycardia based on electroanatomic mapping: identification and ablation of the mid-diastolic isthmus. Europace 2007; 9: 449-457.

# Case 15
## Organised Atrial Arrhythmias after Atrial Fibrillation Ablation in the Left Atrium (Example 1): an Arrhythmogenic Incomplete Linear Lesion with Modified Left-to-right Atrial Propagation

## Case Presentation

This is a 61-year-old male patient with hypertension and only mild dilatation of the left atrium. At the age of 54, he underwent ablation for typical atrial flutter with complete bidirectional block of cavotricuspid isthmus conduction. Three years later, in another hospital, he underwent electrophysiologically guided pulmonary-vein isolation for recurrent atrial fibrillation refractory to multiple antiarrhythmic drugs and, during the same hospital stay, three ablation procedures were performed. The ablation strategy included a linear lesion between the mitral annulus and the right superior pulmonary vein os. In the months following ablation, atrial fibrillation did not recur, but the patient did experience episodes of palpitation. ECG documented atrial tachycardia with a stable cycle length of 280 ms and flat P wave morphology in all leads, except V1, which showed a distinct positive P wave (Fig. 1). In the month before undergoing the

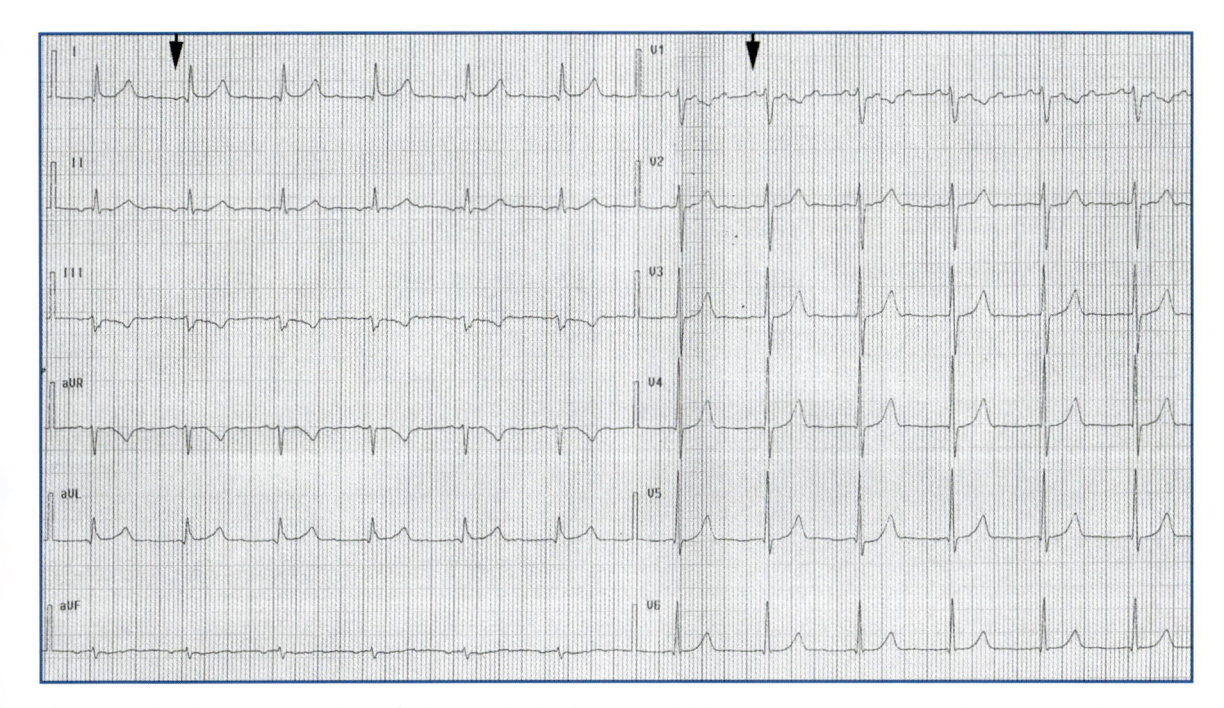

**Fig. 1.** Twelve-lead electrocardiogram of the clinical arrhythmia with 3:1 atrioventricular conduction; *arrows* indicate low-voltage P waves

procedure described below, the arrhythmia became persistent, was poorly tolerated and required electrical cardioversion. Upon arrhythmia recurrence, the patient was hospitalised to undergo an electrophysiologic procedure.

## Procedure

At baseline, the clinical arrhythmia, with a cycle length of 295 ms and variable atrioventricular conduction, was evident. Mapping was started in the right atrium; as a macroreentry arrhythmia was the most likely hypothesis, the window of interest was set accordingly. The peculiar aspects of activation mapping in the right atrium required the acquisition of 99 sites. Although right atrial activation spanned a considerable portion (76%) of the tachycardia cycle length, the activation pattern on the electroanatomic map did not show a clear "head-meets-tail pattern" with identification of a right-sided reentrant circuit. As shown in Figure 2a, b, the earliest activated area was a wide portion of the low posteromedial right atrium, from where the wavefront simultaneously propagated anteriorly and posteriorly to the os of the inferior vena cava. This excluded a lower-loop reentry around the inferior vena cava and instead suggested that conduction had resumed in the posterior area of the cavotricuspid isthmus. In fact, distinct double potentials were recorded in the anterior part of the cavotricuspid isthmus (blue dots in Fig. 2b), whereas there were single fragmented potentials (pink dots in Fig. 2b) in its posterior part. Moreover, right atrial activation was delayed (Fig. 3a–e) by an "independent" late wavefront in the anteromedial right atrium, which proceeded in a septal-to-lateral direction, in the region between the atrioventricular node and the line of cavotricuspid isthmus ablation. Although the origin of this late wavefront was unclear, it was apparently the result of left atrial propagation. A right atrial circuit was ruled out for the following reasons: (1) two different wavefronts collided in the right atrium, with 24% of the tachycardia cycle missing at high-density mapping, and (2) entrainment stimulation from different right atrial sites resulted in a return cycle markedly

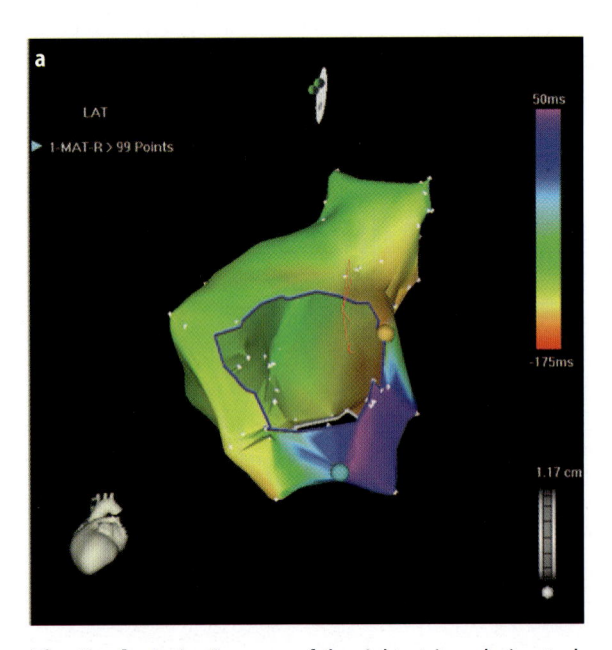

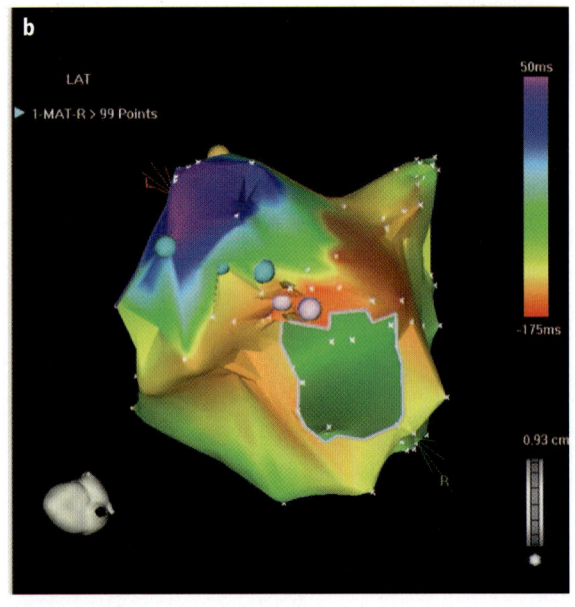

**Fig. 2a, b.** Activation map of the right atrium during tachycardia in caudal left anterior oblique (LAO) (**a**) and inferior (**b**) views. The *orange dot* indicates the site of His-bundle recording. *Blue dots* indicate sites of double potentials corresponding to the line of block in the cavotricuspid isthmus; the *pink dots* indicate the sites of fragmented but single potential, where a conduction gap in the isthmus line was present. Block of the cavotricuspid isthmus conduction was completed after ablation of the index arrhythmia, during coronary-sinus pacing

**Fig. 3a-e.** Sequential frames of the propagation map of the right atrium during tachycardia in an inferior view. The uniform propagation around the os of the inferior vena cava (**a**, **b**) and the delayed propagation in the anteromedial right atrium (**d**, **e**) are evident

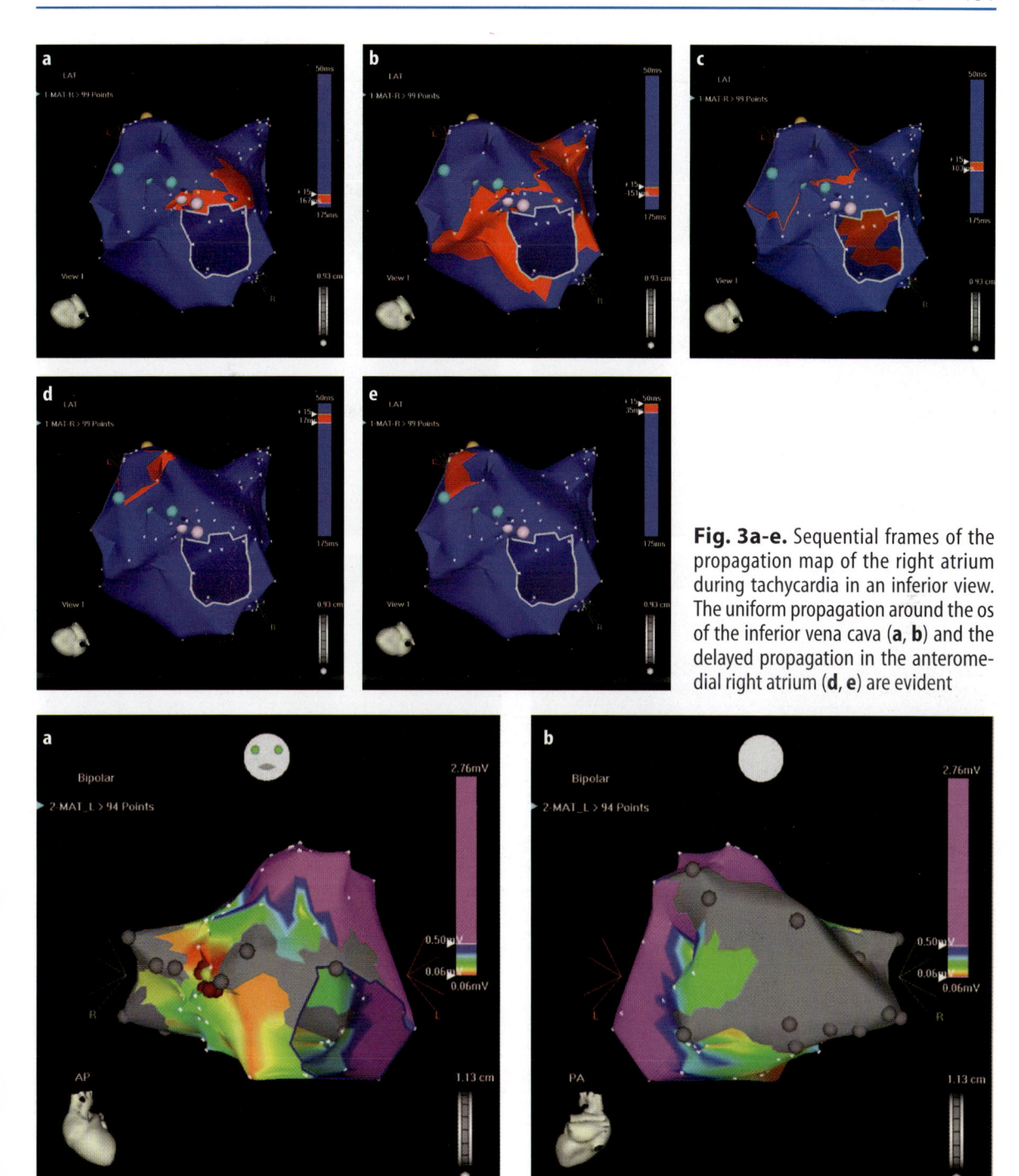

**Fig. 4a, b.** Bipolar voltage map of the left atrium during tachycardia in anteroposterior (**a**) and posteroanterior (**b**) views. According to the setting of the colour-coded scale, areas of preserved voltage are shown in *purple*. Electrically silent areas are tagged by *grey dots*. The *red dots* in the conducting gap in the electrically silent line indicate the site of ablation, while the *yellow dot* indicates the site where concealed entrainment with a post-pacing interval equalling the tachycardia cycle length was obtained

longer than the tachycardia cycle length. Therefore, after transseptal puncture, mapping was continued in the left atrium and cavotricuspid isthmus conduction block was completed later. The extensive map of the left atrium evidenced the absence of electrical activity in a large area around the oses of the four pulmonary veins and in the posterior left atrium, likely related to previous ablation (Fig. 4a, b). Low voltage was recorded in the medial left atrium, where a con-

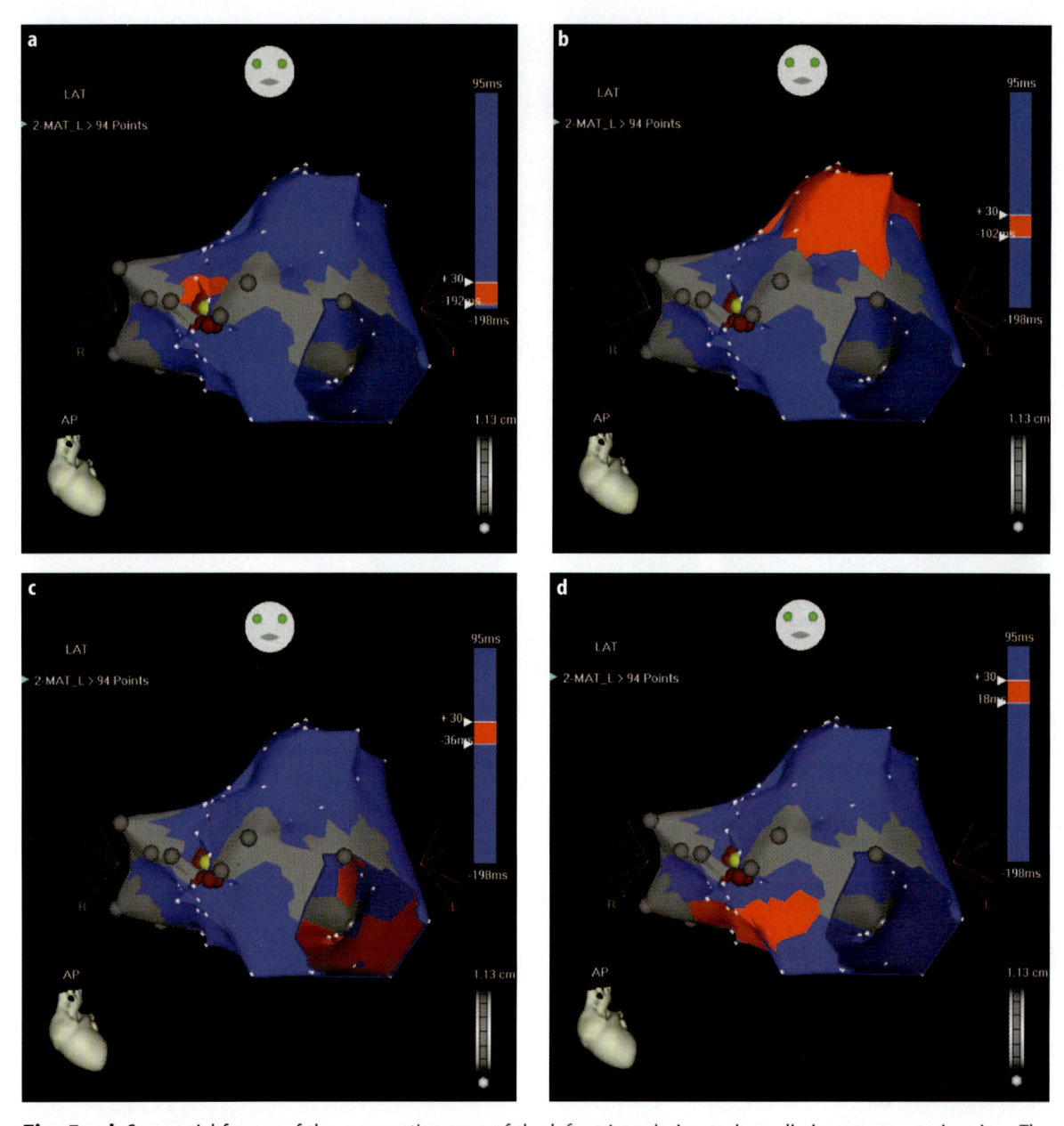

**Fig. 5a-d.** Sequential frames of the propagation map of the left atrium during tachycardia in anteroposterior view. The clockwise circuit in the left atrium is evident

ducting gap was observed in an electrically silent line extending from the mitral annulus at 11 o'clock to the right superior pulmonary vein os, probably the result of linear ablation performed in this area, as described in a previous procedure report. Low voltage was present also in the vicinity of scar tissue in the posterior left atrium, whereas voltage was preserved around the left atrial appendage. Left atrial activation spanned 99% of the tachycardia cycle length. As shown by the propagation map (Fig. 5a–d), the arrhythmia was sustained by a single-loop clockwise reentry in the left atrium. The mid-diastolic isthmus corresponded to the conducting gap in the electrically silent line in the medial left atrium (Fig. 6). Interestingly, analysis of the biatrial propagation map (Fig. 7) showed that the late wavefront propagating in the anteromedial right atrium derived from the left reentrant circuit, upon its arrival in the anteromedial left atrium. This confirmed the hypothesis that the late wavefront in the right atrium was the result of

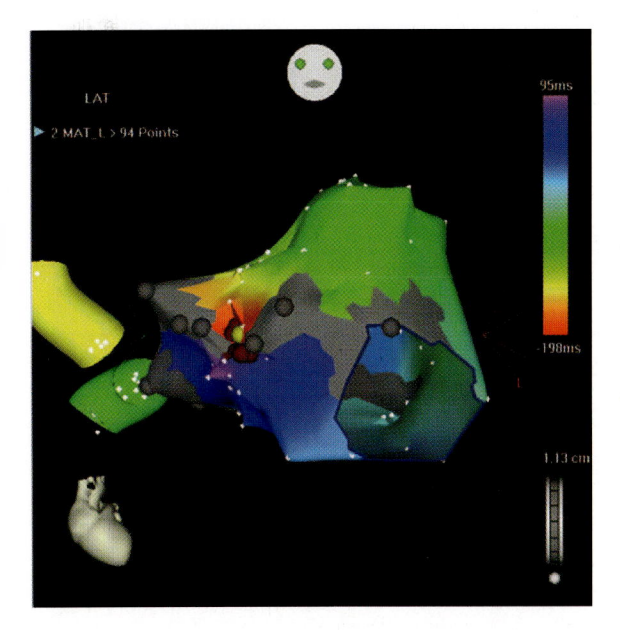

**Fig. 6.** Activation map of the left atrium during tachycardia in anteroposterior view. Tags as in Fig. 4. Right pulmonary veins are indicated by tubular icons

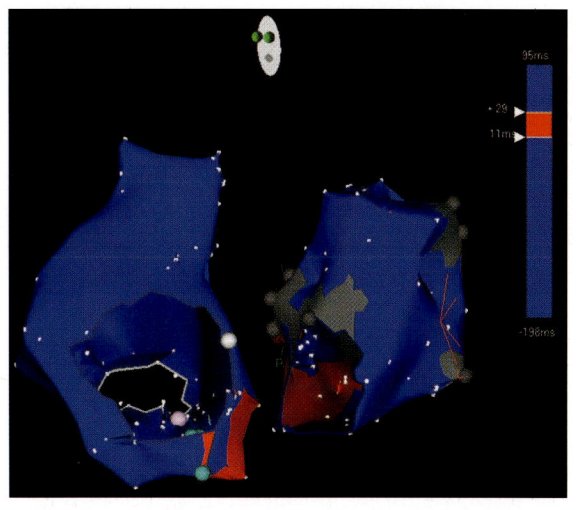

**Fig. 7.** Frame of the biatrial propagation map during tachycardia in LAO view, showing the peculiar interatrial propagation in this case. Due to the presence of the ablation line in the medial left atrium, the anteromedial right atrium is activated late by the left reentrant circuit, just before reentering the mid-diastolic isthmus. The two atrial chambers have been slightly separated at septal level to better evaluate propagation of each chamber

left-to-right bystander activation from a left atrial circuit. It also showed that the peculiar right atrial activation was due to an interatrial propagation altered by the linear lesion. In fact, the presence of the left "septal" linear lesion prevented uniform propagation of the wavefront from left to right. The posterior part of the medial right atrium, in electrical continuity with the area of the left atrium above the linear lesion, was activated early from the reentrant circuit just after exiting the mid-diastolic isthmus, whereas the anteromedial right atrium, below the linear lesion, was activated late by the reentrant circuit before reentering the mid-diastolic isthmus. Concealed entrainment with a post-pacing interval equalling the tachycardia cycle length was obtained in the mid-diastolic isthmus (yellow dot in Fig. 6). Very low bipolar voltage (<0.10 mV) was present in the mid-diastolic isthmus, suggesting that the substrate would be relatively easy to ablate. Radiofrequency energy delivery using a cool-tip catheter (maximum power 35 W, cut-off temperature 43°C, duration 60 s) in the mid-diastolic area resulted in early termination of the tachycardia (Fig. 8). Ablation was continued in the same area to produce complete disappearance of local electrical activity and to complete the linear lesion. At the end of the procedure, no arrhythmia was inducible by aggressive atrial pacing, and the patient was arrhythmia-free without antiarrhythmic drugs in a 30-month follow-up.

## Commentary

Regular, organised atrial tachyarrhythmias occurring in the months following left atrial ablation for atrial fibrillation have been described in multiple reports [1–7]. In some cases, the arrhythmia mechanism is predominantly focal, from reconnected pulmonary vein ostia [3, 6], while in others the arrhythmia is macroreentrant in nature and related to incomplete linear lesions around the pulmonary veins oses or in the left atrium [1, 2, 4, 6, 7].

The present case is paradigmatic of how a left atrial linear lesion, deployed to prevent the recurrence of atrial fibrillation, can result in an incomplete line of block with a residual gap of

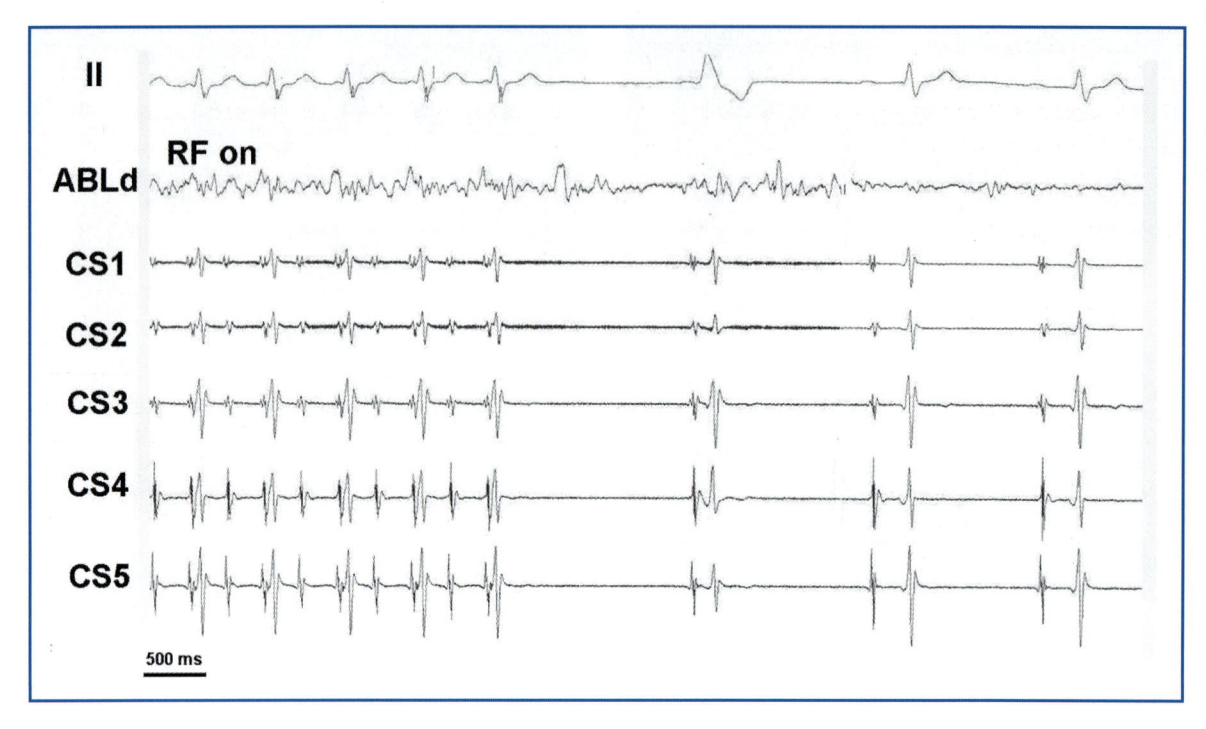

**Fig. 8.** Surface and intracavitary recordings upon tachycardia termination. From *top to bottom*, lead II, bipolar recordings from the distal electrode pair of the ablation catheter (ABLd) and from the coronary sinus catheter (CS1–CS5, from distal to proximal) are shown. Radiofrequency delivery is ongoing and tachycardia terminates with the restoration of sinus rhythm

conduction able to sustain left atrial macroreentry. The most difficult part of the procedure was not characterisation and ablation of the left atrial circuit, but interpretation of the unusual right atrial activation pattern. The typical pattern of by-stander activation of the right atrium during a macroreentrant left atrial tachycardia was shown in Case 10. Variants to this typical pattern due to cavotricuspid isthmus conduction block and delayed right atrial conduction for an atrial myopathy were presented in Case 11 and Case 7, respectively. Here, right atrial activation was unusually and unexpectedly delayed by the presence of a late septal wavefront, apparently independent if the right atrial activation was analysed alone. In fact, although both ablation lines had small conducting gaps, their concomitant presence in the medial cavotricuspid isthmus and in the left septum greatly modified the left-to-right propagation pattern, with the anteromedial area between these two lines being activated late by the "tail" of the reentrant left atrial circuit. This complex activation pattern could be understood only by analysing the biatrial propagation map, once mapping was completed also in the left atrium. This variant of the typical by-stander activation pattern should be kept in mind when right atrial activation is evaluated in patients with recurrent organised atrial arrhythmias after extensive left atrial ablation for atrial fibrillation, including linear lesions in the medial left atrium.

The lack of electrical activity in a wide area of the left atrium in this patient might have been the long-term result of an aggressive ablation strategy. The possible association with loss of left atrial haemodynamic function and its clinical implications should be carefully considered in the long-term management of these patients.

***Acknowledgement.*** *The images of this case were provided by Roberto Verlato, MD, Diagnostic and Interventional Electrophysiology Unit, Civile Hospital, Camposampiero, Padua, Italy.*

# References

1. Villacastin J, Perez-Castellano N, Moreno J, Gonzales R. Left atrial flutter after radiofrequency catheter ablation of focal atrial fibrillation. J Cardiovasc Electrophysiol 2003; 14: 417-421.
2. Mesas CE, Pappone C, Lang CCE et al. Left atrial tachycardia after circumferential pulmonary vein ablation for atrial fibrillation. J Am Coll Cardiol 2004; 44: 1071-1079.
3. Gerstenfeld EP, Callans DJ, Dixit S et al. Mechanism of organized left atrial tachycardias occurring after pulmonary vein isolation. Circulation 2004; 110: 1351-1357.
4. Jaïs P, Hocini M, Hsu LF et al. Technique and results of linear ablation at the mitral isthmus. Circulation 2004; 110: 2996-3002.
5. Kobza R, Hindricks G, Tanner H et al. Late recurrent arrhythmias after ablation of atrial fibrillation: incidence, mechanism, and treatment. Heart Rhythm 2004; 1: 676-683
6. Cummings JE, Schweikert R, Saliba W et al. Left atrial flutter following pulmonary vein antrum isolation with radiofrequency energy: linear lesions or repeat isolation. J Cardiovasc Electrocphysiol 2005; 16: 293-297.
7. Chugh A, Oral H, Lemola K et al. Prevalence, mechanism, and clinical significance of macroreentrant atrial tachycardia during and following left atrial ablation for atrial fibrillation. Heart Rhythm 2005; 2: 464-471.

# Case 16
## Organised Atrial Arrhythmias after Atrial Fibrillation Ablation in the Left Atrium (Example 2): Association of Multiple Potentially Pro-arrhythmogenic Factors Resulting in a Tachycardia with a Longer Cycle Length

## Case Presentation

This is a 66-year-old male patient with ischemic heart disease and prior inferior myocardial infarction with stenting of the left circumflex coronary artery. Three years before the current procedure, he underwent surgical mitral valvuloplasty for mitral regurgitation. For postoperative recurrent episodes of atrial fibrillation, amiodarone administration was initiated but was withdrawn after a few months due to hyperthyroidism. Then, two years before the current procedure, the patient underwent two procedures at another centre for catheter ablation of atrial fibrillation in the left atrium. Detailed descriptions of those procedures and of the surgical intervention could not be obtained. However, prior surgery did not imply any intraoperative ablation for atrial fibrillation. Subsequently, based on evidence of poor left ventricular function (ejection fraction 33%), a dual-chamber cardioverter-defibrillator was implanted by another centre. In the months before the procedure, the patient had episodes of atrial tachycardia causing congestive heart failure. This tachycardia had a 410 ms cycle length (with frequent 1:1 atrioventricular conduction periods) and a low-voltage P wave, negative in the inferior leads, positive in V1, flat in all the other leads (Fig. 1). For this reason, the patient was referred for catheter ablation of the arrhythmia.

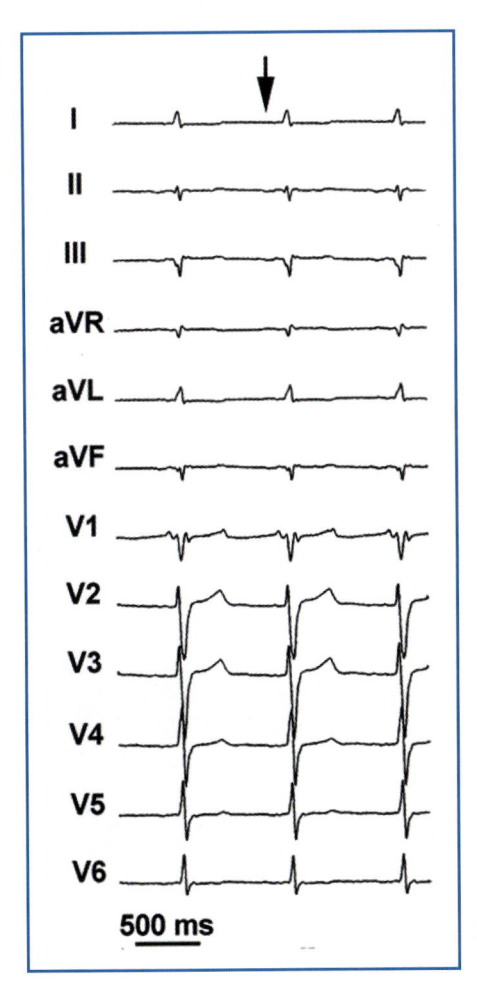

**Fig. 1.** Twelve-lead electrocardiogram of the atrial tachycardia with 2:1 atrioventricular conduction; the *arrow* indicates the low-voltage P wave

## Procedure

At the beginning of the procedure, the clinical arrhythmia was present with unchanged cycle length. A decapolar catheter was placed into the coronary sinus and a tetrapolar catheter was positioned in the His-bundle area. Bipolar atriograms from the coronary-sinus catheter showed presystolic activation with a proximal to distal activation sequence. The window of interest was set as for a macroreentrant arrhythmia and mapping in the right atrium was commenced. A right atrial activation pattern consistent with propagation from the left atrium of a left-sided arrhythmia was identified (Fig. 2a, b). Specifically, the area around the coronary sinus os showed early activation, and a homogeneous propagation pattern from the medial to the lateral right atrium was observed in the cavotricuspid isthmus, suggesting that isthmus ablation had not been performed in previous ablation procedures. Right atrial activation spanned only 40% of the tachycardia cycle length. The right atrial volume was increased (128 ml) and no area of double potentials suggesting prior right atriotomy was present. Therefore, mapping was continued in the left atrium after transseptal catheterisation was accomplished. Early during mapping, it was evident that a wide area of the posterior wall, as well as the four pulmonary veins (tagged by tubular icons), were electrically silent (Fig. 3a). Mapping was continued in this enlarged left atrium (volume 126 ml) until the reconstructed activation sequence spanned 95% of the tachycardia cycle length. Catheter manipulation in the posteromedial left atrium was difficult. A combination of catheter looping, rotational movements and withdrawal of the transseptal sheath allowed precise catheter positioning in this region, the electroanatomic characterisation of which was very critical in this case. Analysis of the activation map evidenced a mid-diastolic isthmus located in the posteromedial left atrium, inferior to the os of the right inferior pulmonary vein (Fig. 3b), bounded posteriorly by the electrically silent area and anteriorly by a continuous line of double potentials. This was likely related to a surgical posterior paraseptal left atriotomy between the two right pulmonary veins. Analysis of the propagation map (Fig. 4) evidenced that reentry was sustained by two synchronous loops sharing the same mid-diastolic isthmus. Upon exiting the mid-diastolic isthmus, the first loop rotated counter-clockwise in the left atrium (Fig. 4a–g), passing inferiorly (Fig. 4b, c), laterally (Fig. 4d, e) and then superiorly (Fig. 4f) to the

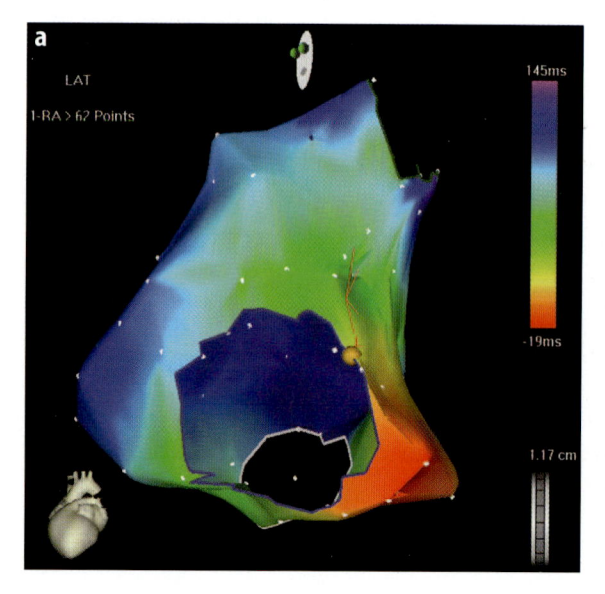

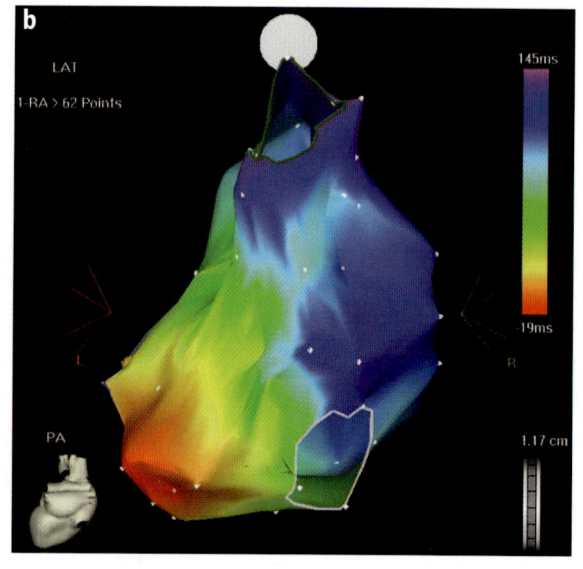

**Fig. 2a-b.** Activation map of the right atrium during tachycardia in caudal left anterior oblique (LAO) (**a**) and posteroanterior (**b**) views. The *orange dot* indicates the site of His-bundle recording

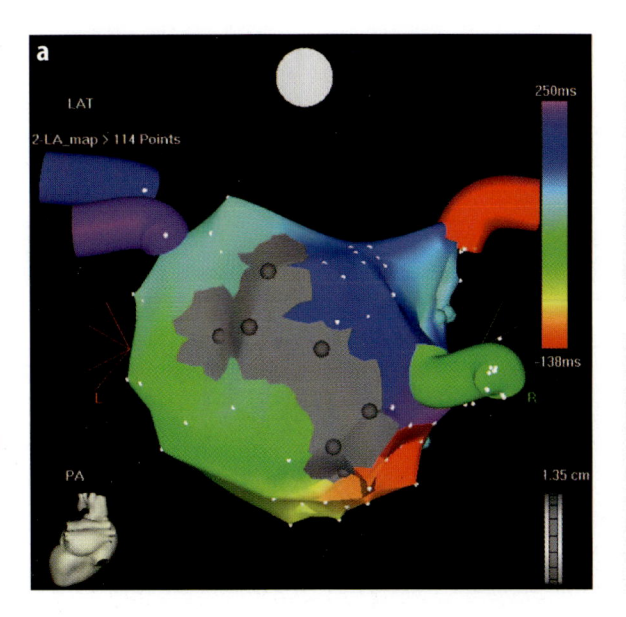

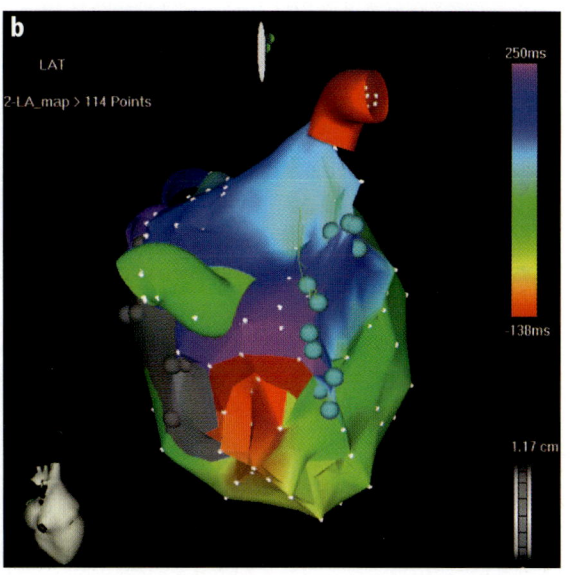

**Fig. 3a, b.** Activation map of the left atrium during tachycardia in posteroanterior (**a**) and caudal right lateral (**b**) views. The four pulmonary veins are tagged by tubular icons. The electrically silent area in the posterior wall is shown in *grey*, while the uninterrupted line of double potentials (*blue dots*) shown in (**b**) is likely related to prior surgical atriotomy to access the left atrium for mitral surgery

electrically silent area located in the posterior wall. The second loop rotated counter-clockwise around the line of double potentials (Fig. 4a'–g'). First, it passed inferior (Fig. 4b') and anterior (Fig. 4 c', d') to the line and then slowed down upon entering the gap between the line and the os of the right superior pulmonary vein (Fig. 4e, e'). Finally, it rejoined the other loop (Fig. 4f) and re-entered the mid-diastolic isthmus (Fig. 4g, g'). The length of the first loop was 22.5 cm, whereas the second loop was shorter (19.8 cm). Analysis of the conduction velocities showed a very low value in the mid-diastolic isthmus (21 cm/s). The average conduction velocity of the first loop was higher than that of the second loop. In the three segments of the outer part of the first and second loops, the values were 74, 79, 46 cm/s vs. 61, 54 and 55 cm/s, respectively. Analysis of the bipolar voltage map (Fig. 5a, b) showed very low voltage in the mid-diastolic isthmus, with values ranging from 0.09 to 0.22 mV, while the only area with preserved voltage amplitude was the anterolateral wall. The combination of a limited extension of the mid-diastolic isthmus (9 mm) with the very low voltage in this area suggested an easily ablatable substrate. Ablation was started from the posterior area of the isthmus using an irrigated-tip catheter (maximum power 35 W, cut-off temperature 43°C and maximum duration 60 s). As expected, the second application prolonged the tachycardia cycle length and terminated the arrhythmia (Fig. 6). Another six applications sequentially delivered during sinus rhythm along the isthmus led to complete disappearance of the electrical signal in this area (Fig. 7). Afterwards, electrical stimulation with an aggressive protocol (S2S3 at 600 and 400 ms cycle length drive and bursts up to 250 ms) did not induce any arrhythmia. Non-inducibility persisted at 30 min; therefore, the procedure was terminated. The patient had no arrhythmia recurrence without antiarrhythmic drugs during a 16-month follow-up.

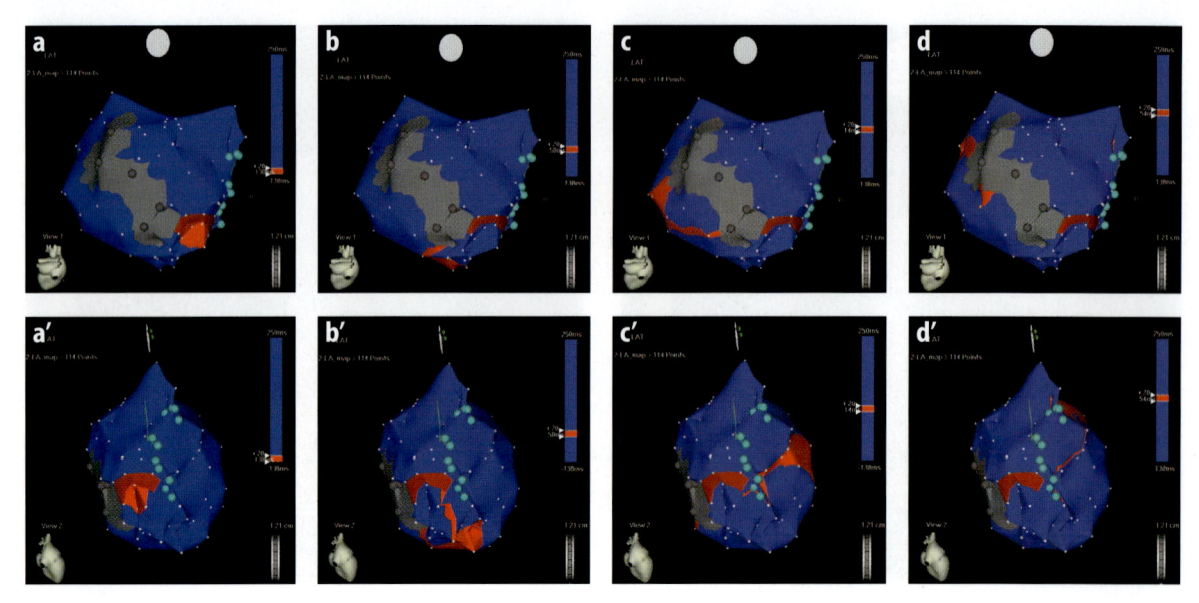

**Fig. 4a-g.** Sequential frames of the propagation map of the left atrium during tachycardia in posteroanterior (**a–g**) and caudal right lateral (**a'–g'**) views. The double-loop reentry with a shared mid-diastolic isthmus is evident

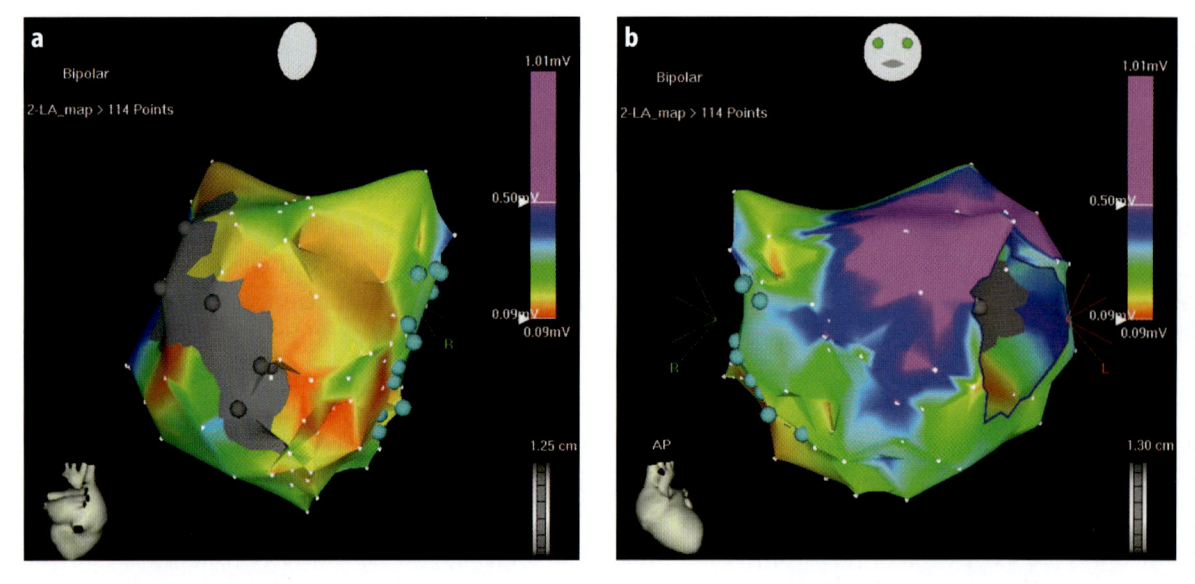

**Fig. 5a, b.** Bipolar voltage map of the left atrium during tachycardia in caudal right lateral (**a**) and anteroposterior (**b**) views. According to the colour-coded scale, areas with preserved voltage are shown in *purple* and are limited in this case to the anterolateral wall around the left appendage

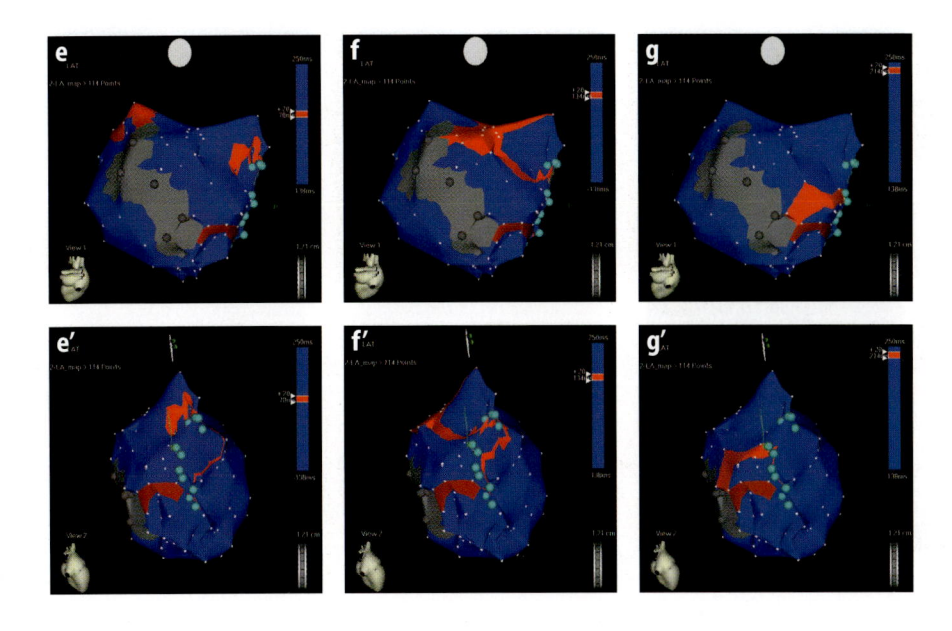

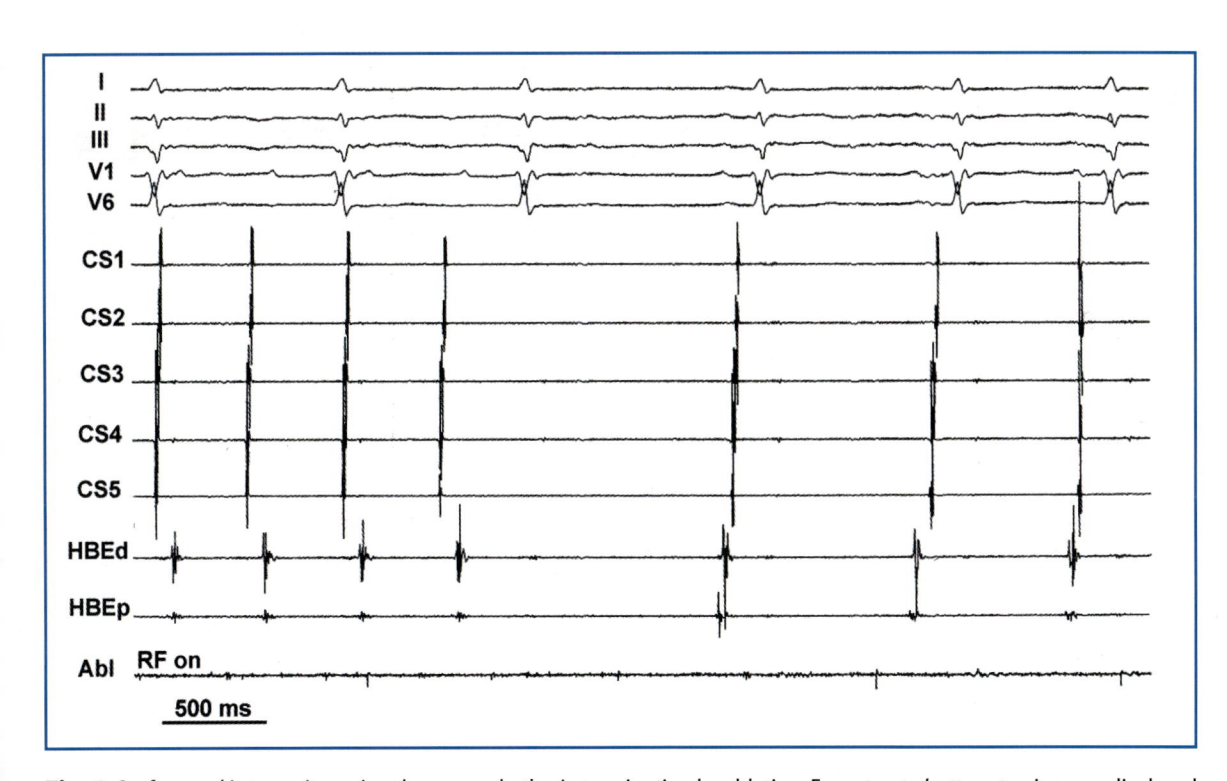

**Fig. 6.** Surface and intracavitary signals upon arrhythmia termination by ablation. From *top to bottom*, tracings are displayed as follows: leads I, II, III, V1, V6, bipolar recordings of the coronary sinus catheter from distal to proximal (CS1–5), bipolar recordings of the His-bundle catheter from distal to proximal (HBEd-p), bipolar recordings from the distal electrode pair of the ablation catheter (Abl). Tachycardia is early terminated by radiofrequency energy delivery with restoration of stable sinus rhythm

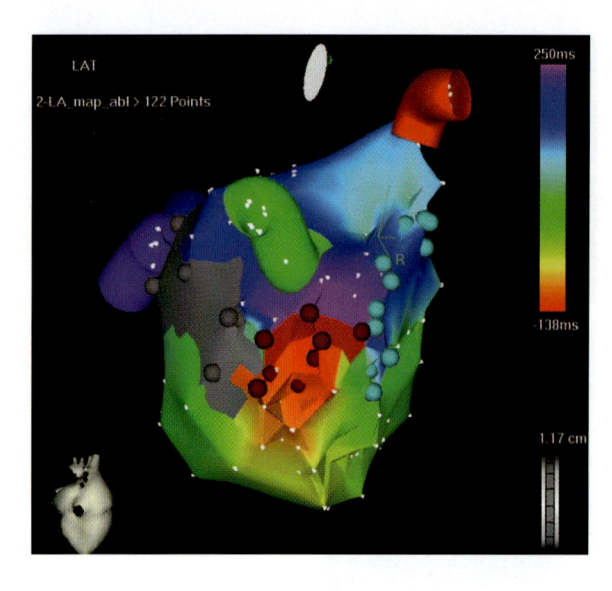

**Fig. 7.** Activation map of the left atrium during tachycardia in caudal right lateral view. Ablation sites are shown by the *red dots*

## Commentary

The occurrence of atrial flutter with a reentry circuit in the left septum in patients on amiodarone and without prior surgery or ablation was previously reported [1]. The peculiarity of this arrhythmia is the small reentrant circuit, confined to the left septum with a shorter cycle length (278±39 ms, range 230-340 ms). This circuit is responsible for a particular atrial activation pattern that results in prominent P waves only in lead V1, while limb leads show a flat P-wave morphology.

In spite of a similar P wave morphology, the case presented here is different from those of the above-mentioned study and from other organised arrhythmias after atrial fibrillation ablation. This macroreentrant tachycardia had a longer cycle length. Actually, the term "postablation" may not be appropriate here. If the time relationship between ablation and arrhythmia occurrence is excluded, the cause-effect relationship of ablation in determining this arrhythmia is not very evident. In fact, in this patient, the combination of multiple potentially pro-arrhythmogenic factors, namely valvular disease and prior surgery with atriotomy and pulmonary-vein encircling, may have led to the development of the macroreentrant arrhythmia. As discussed in Case 9, a variable pattern of electrically silent areas can be found in the left atrium of non-surgical patients, both in those with rheumatic and in those with non-rheumatic heart disease. In this case, mitral valve regurgitation could have been responsible for left atrial enlargement with scarring in the posterior wall. Moreover, the surgical atriotomy placed in the Waterstone groove for mitral surgery created the second artificial barrier in this patient and catheter pulmonary-vein encircling completed the pro-arrhythmogenic scenario, slowing down conduction around the right pulmonary veins. The lesson from this case may thus be that, in some patients, left atrial ablation for atrial fibrillation is not "per se" arrhythmogenic, but could contribute to the development of organised left atrial arrhythmias by: (1) eliminating the most disorganised arrhythmia, namely atrial fibrillation, and (2) combining with other pro-arrhythmogenic factors to favour left atrial macroreentry in patients with structural heart disease.

In such patients, the good news is that these organised arrhythmias can be successfully treated and permanently abolished by a further ablation procedure, especially when a short isthmus combines with low-amplitude potentials, as in this case. However, detailed reconstruction of the left atrium (114 sites acquired in this case) is required with the use of several "tricks" to map sites such as the inferoposteromedial region, which is not easily reachable.

One last peculiarity of this case is represented by the fact that, in spite of biatrial enlargement and the persistence of conduction over the cavotricuspid isthmus, the patient never experienced typical atrial flutter either before the procedure or during follow-up.

## References

1. Marrouche NF, Natale A, Wazni OM et al. Left septal atrial flutter: electrophysiology, anatomy and results of ablation. Circulation 2004; 109: 2440-2447.

# Case 17
## Organised Atrial Arrhythmias after Atrial Fibrillation Ablation in the Left Atrium (Example 3): do Lesions in the Left Atrium Have a Mid-term Evolution?

## Case Presentation

This is a 66-year-old male patient with persistent atrial fibrillation and hypertensive cardiomyopathy. In the two years prior to the procedure described here, he had suffered episodes of atrial fibrillation, which had become persistent and recurred within one week of DC-shock cardioversion, in spite of antiarrhythmic drug therapy. Echocardiography showed biatrial dilatation, with mild hypertrophy of the left ventricle and only mild impairment of left ventricular function (ejection fraction 53%). For this reason, the patient underwent atrial fibrillation ablation guided by CARTO_Merge, with complete electrical disconnection of the four pulmonary veins (Fig. 1). During the procedure, 63 sites were acquired in the left atrium and no electrically silent area was observed. Ablation was performed at the venoatrial junction using an irrigated-tip catheter with the following settings: maximum power 30 W, cut-off temperature 43°C and duration of 60 s. In the weeks following the procedure, sinus rhythm was stably restored. After ten weeks, the patient had atrial flutter that showed a surface P wave morphology not very dissimilar from typical atrial flutter (Fig. 2), except for the less-negative P waves in the inferior leads. The ablation procedure had not been aimed at cavotricuspid isthmus conduction. The arrhythmia recurred with the same cycle length and morphology and a prevalent 2:1 atrioventricular conduction after DC-shock cardioversion. Therefore, a second procedure was planned.

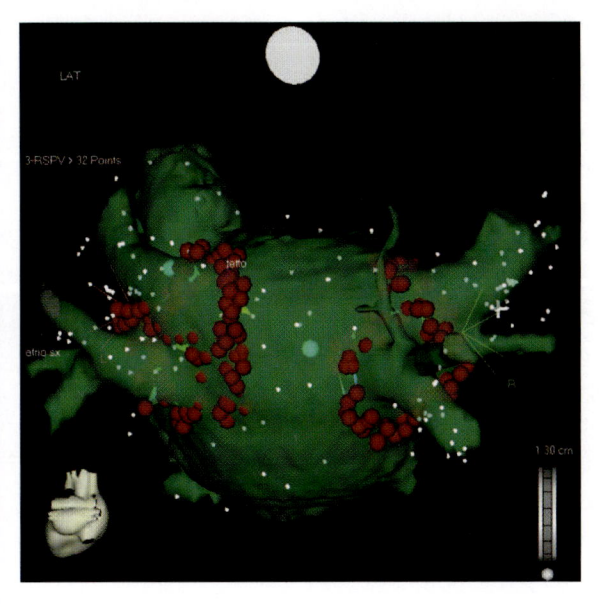

**Fig. 1.** Three-dimensional computed tomography image superimposed on the electroanatomic reconstruction of the left atrium and the pulmonary veins, in posteroanterior view. *Red dots* indicate the lesion pattern used in the first procedure for pulmonary vein ablation

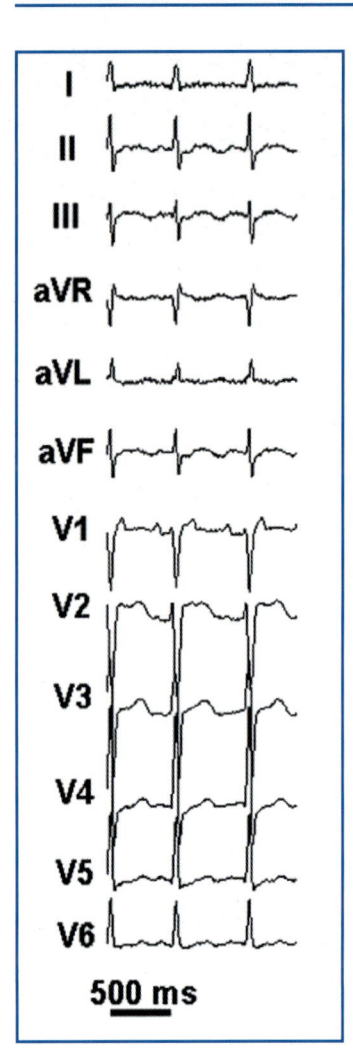

**Fig. 2.** Twelve-lead electrocardiogram of the recurrent atrial flutter after atrial fibrillation ablation, with 2:1 atrioventricular conduction

## Procedure

At the beginning of the procedure, the clinical flutter with a cycle length of 260 ms was present. A decapolar catheter was placed into the coronary sinus, where mid-diastolic atriograms were present; a bipolar recording with a single-component atrial deflection from the proximal coronary sinus was taken as the electrical reference. Right atrial volume was 109 ml. Very early during right atrial mapping, the hypothesis of a non-isthmus dependent right atrial flutter, suggested by the coronary sinus chronology, was confirmed by the activation sequence in the right atrium (Fig. 3a, b). From a wide area of early activation around the coronary sinus os, a concentric propagation pattern moved towards the latest activated area in the lateral right atrium. Although cavotricuspid isthmus conduction was not blocked, right atrial activation was relatively prolonged and corresponded to 56% of the flutter cycle length. However, this pattern was clearly indicative of propagation from a left atrial arrhythmia. Before transseptal puncture, a short tract of the coronary sinus, where mid-diastolic potentials were present, was mapped (Fig. 4). The mapping catheter could not be safely advanced further into the coronary sinus, due to the likely presence of a valve in the mid-coronary sinus. Although the mapped portion of the coronary sinus suggested an "early-meets-late" pattern, the entire reentry course could not be identified. For this reason, it was decided not to proceed to ablation into the conorary sinus, but to instead perform additional mapping in the left atrium. Left atrial mapping reconstructed 98%

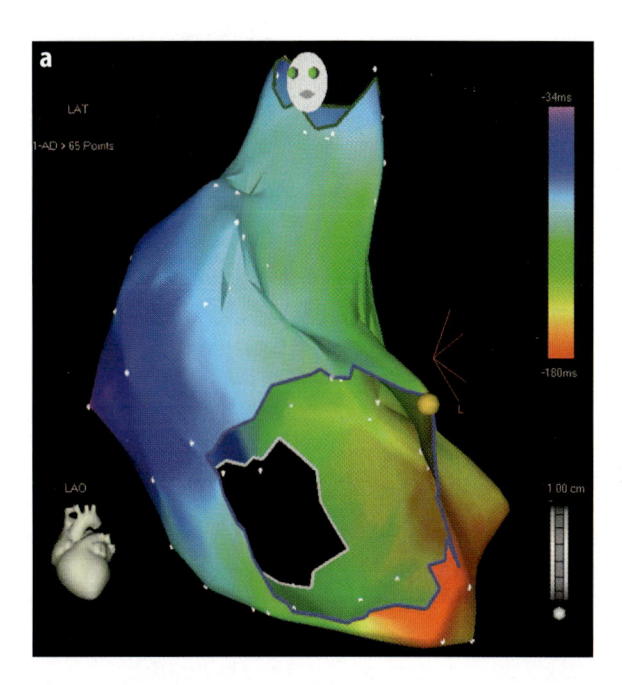

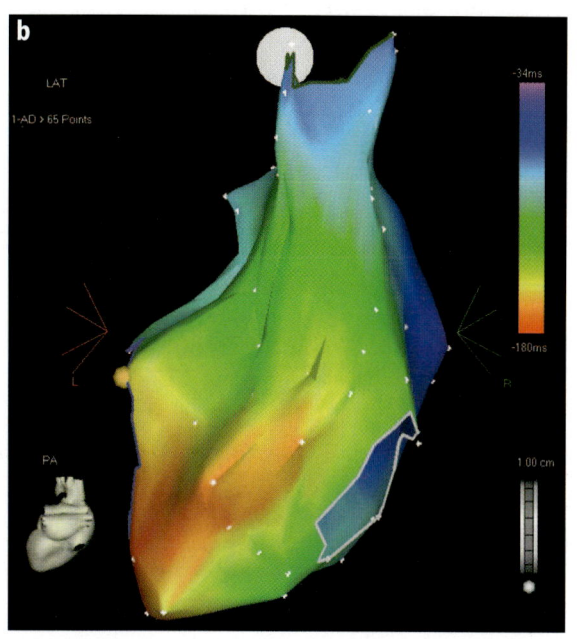

**Fig. 3a, b.** Activation map of the right atrium during atrial flutter in left anterior oblique (LAO) (**a**) and posteroanterior (**b**) views. *Orange dot* indicates the site of the His-bundle recording

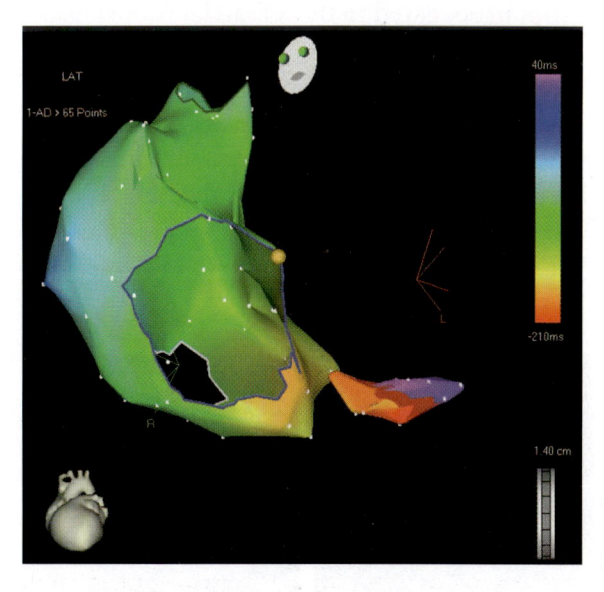

**Fig. 4.** Activation map of the right atrium and proximal part of the coronary sinus during flutter in caudal LAO view. The presence of mid-diastolic potentials in the coronary sinus is shown in *red and purple*

of the reentry course, which consisted of a single clockwise loop (Fig. 5a). The estimated left atrial volume was 136 ml. The mid-diastolic isthmus was identified in the posterior wall, between a wide electrically silent area and the mitral annulus at 6 o'clock (Fig. 5b), and involved coronary sinus fibres. No electrical activity was found in the four pulmonary veins. A comparison of the size and location of the electrically silent area (whose inferomedial limit was carefully defined by high-density mapping) with the line of lesion around the left pulmonary veins in the index procedure (Fig. 1) suggested that the extension of the electrically silent area in the current procedure exceeded the limit of the ablation lesion, extending linearly in the posterior left atrium. Analysis of the propagation map (Fig. 6a–h) confirmed a single-loop reentry in the left atrium. The propagation wavefront, upon exiting the mid-diastolic isthmus involving coronary sinus fibres (Fig. 6a), moved medially in the left atrium (Fig. 6b) and propagated over the coro-

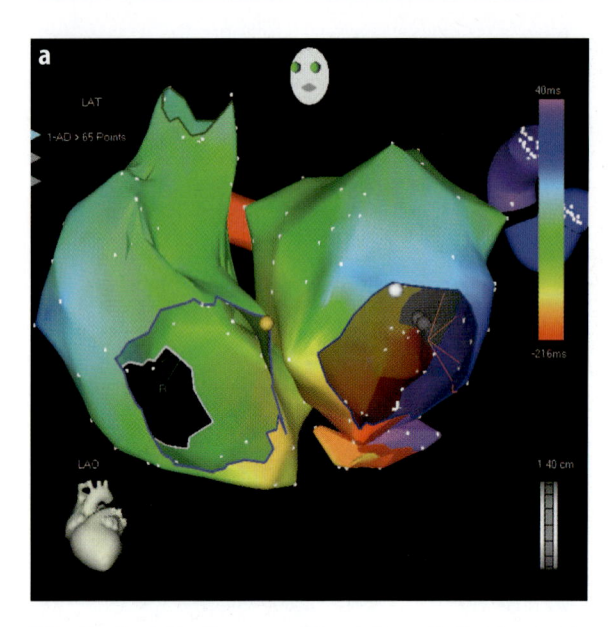

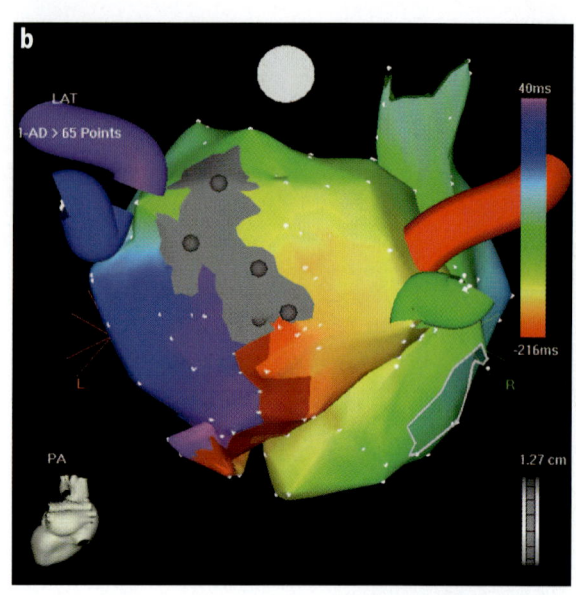

**Fig. 5a, b.** Activation map of the right and left atrium and proximal part of the coronary sinus during atrial flutter in LAO (**a**) and posteroanterior (**b**) views. Pulmonary veins are tagged by tubular icons and electrically silent area by *grey dots*

nary sinus os to the right atrium, whose by-stander activation was clearly demonstrated (Fig. 6c–e). From the medial left atrium, the main wavefront propagated to the left atrial roof (Fig. 6c, d) and then in a lateral (Fig. 6e) and posterior (Fig. 6f, g) direction to reenter the mid-diastolic isthmus, again involving the coronary sinus fibres (Fig. 6h). Analysis of the conduction velocities evidenced that the lowest value was found in the mid-diastolic isthmus (45 cm/s), whereas normal conduction velocities were recorded in the outer loop of the reentrant circuit: 67 cm/s in the posterior wall, 105 cm/s at the roof and 74 cm/s in the lateral wall. Analysis of the bipolar voltage map (Fig. 7) identified an amplitude of 0.63±0.20 (range 0.35–0.99) mV in the mid-diastolic isthmus, which extended for 4.1 cm. The anatomically shortest isthmus between the electrically

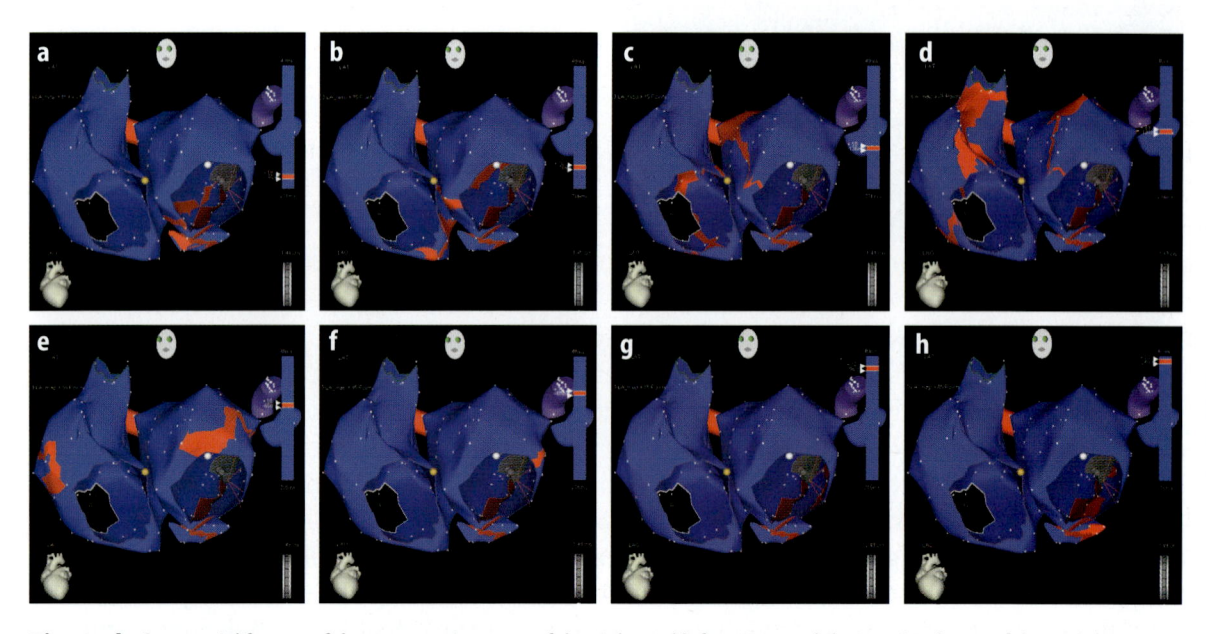

**Fig. 6a-h.** Sequential frames of the propagation map of the right and left atrium and the proximal part of the coronary sinus during atrial flutter in LAO view. The clockwise circuit in the left atrium with involvement of the coronary sinus fibres and by-stander activation of the right atrium are evident

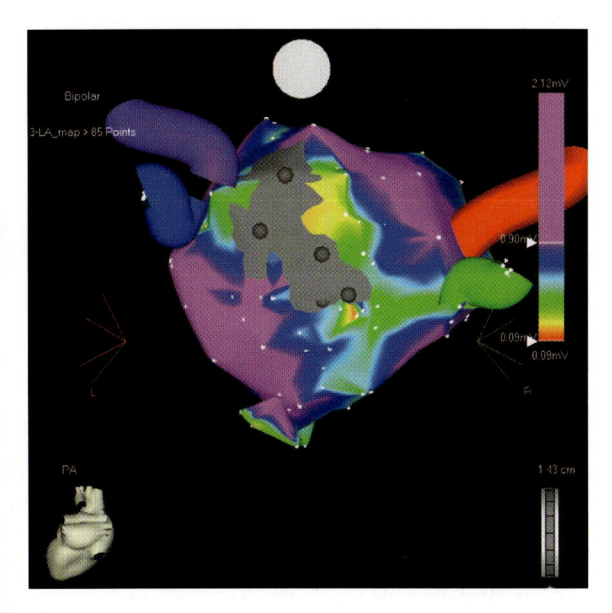

**Fig. 7.** Bipolar voltage mapping of the left atrium during atrial flutter in posteroanterior view. According to the colour-coded scale, areas with voltage > 0.9 mV are shown in *purple*

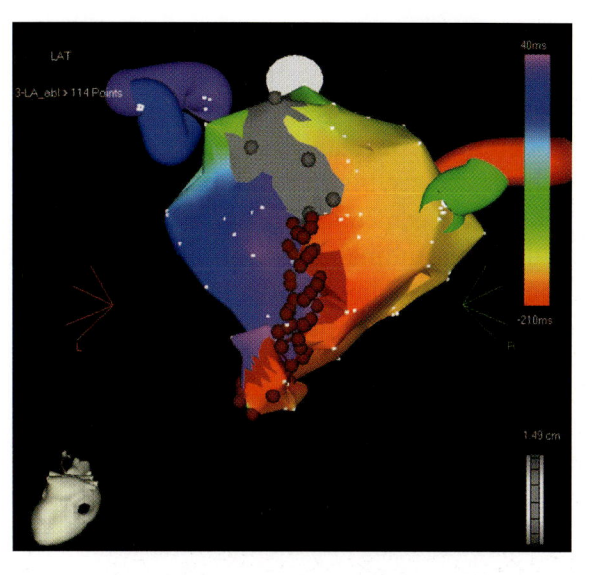

**Fig. 8.** Activation map of the left atrium and proximal part of the coronary sinus during atrial flutter in caudal posteroanterior view. The *red dots* indicate the ablation line in the mid-diastolic isthmus

silent area/left inferior pulmonary vein and the mitral annulus in the lateral position ("mitral isthmus") measured 3.6 cm, but the bipolar signal amplitude was higher (1.04±0.58, range 0.46–1.71 mV). Ablation was aimed at the mid-diastolic isthmus instead of at the more lateral and more commonly ablated "mitral isthmus" based on the following considerations: (1) lower amplitude potentials and slower conduction velocity in the mid-diastolic isthmus than in the "mitral isthmus" were considered indicative of easier ablation; (2) ablation in the coronary sinus was highly probable due to evidence of its involvement in the circuit and its distal part was impossible to reach safely, but it was required if the shortest anatomical "mitral isthmus" was to be targeted; (3) a more proximal ablation into the coronary sinus was considered safer, both during the procedure and in the long-term, thus avoiding possible postablation stenosis; (4) ablation aimed at the "mitral isthmus" would not have prevented the possible development of another flutter circuit rotating around the right pulmonary veins and using slow conduction of the non-ablated mid-diastolic isthmus. Twenty-nine sequential applications in the mid-diastolic isthmus, from the upper to the lower part, with an irrigated-tip catheter (maximum power 40 W, cut-off temperature 43°C, duration 60 s) abolished the electrical signal in this area and prolonged the arrhythmia cycle length to 300 ms. Therefore, ablation continued in a corresponding area of the coronary sinus, where another six applications terminated the arrhythmia and restored sinus rhythm. Afterwards, no other arrhythmia was inducible by programmed atrial stimulation. The patient was arrhythmia free at a 12-month follow-up.

## Commentary

In this patient, the P wave pattern of the atrial flutter that recurred after atrial fibrillation ablation resembled that of the typical counter-clockwise isthmus-dependent atrial flutter; therefore, a simple ablation procedure was expected. However, a more difficult arrhythmogenic substrate was found, requiring extensive mapping and ablation in the left atrium and in the coronary sinus. Therefore, caution should be used both in the evaluation of atrial flutter morphology after atrial fibrillation ablation and during the preprocedure evaluation regarding the predicted dependence on the cavotricuspid isthmus. Even cavotricuspid-isthmus-dependent atrial flutter may exhibit a P wave pattern very different from the typical one after atrial fibrillation ablation in the left atrium [1]. In fact, left atrial activation may be altered by prior left atrial ablation by a debulking effect and marked reduction in left atrial voltage.

Interestingly, the electrically silent area found in the posterior left atrium during the second procedure seemed larger than the lesion around the left pulmonary veins, exceeding the latter with a longitudinal extension towards the posterior left atrium. During the index procedure, a double ablation line was deployed in this area for a particularly resistant posterior breakthrough of the left superior pulmonary vein. One might speculate as to whether the larger lesion found during the second procedure was related to indirect ischaemic injury, possibly of an atrial coronary branch, in the course of prior ablation with an irrigated-tip catheter, although the power was limited to 30 W. In any case, in this patient the formation of a larger electrically silent area in the posterior left atrium seemed crucial to the development of a left macroreentrant arrhythmia a few weeks after ablation.

This case brings up the dilemma whether prophylactic ablation of the "mitral isthmus" is appropriate in every patient undergoing pulmonary-vein ablation, to prevent this type of reentry circuit. The efficacy of associated "mitral isthmus" ablation was previously discussed in detail [2]. However, epicardial ablation through the distal coronary sinus is required in 68% of patients, in whom complete left isthmus block is achieved in 84%. Moreover, postablation recurrences deriving from incomplete block or recovered conduction over the "mitral isthmus" account for 5% of cases [3]. The lesson from the anatomy is that the "left atrial isthmus" is not an anatomic entity, since individual anatomic variants are present that vary widely in extent (17–51 mm from the left pulmonary vein to the mitral annulus) and wall thickness (1.4–7.7 mm), with the possibility that the left atrial myocardium continues onto the atrial aspect of the mitral valve leaflet [4]. These anatomic characteristics would sufficiently justify the difficulties encountered in permanent and complete "mitral isthmus" ablation. In our experience [5], the arrhythmia observed in this patient is rare, even if the "mitral isthmus" is not systematically targeted during left atrial ablation for atrial fibrillation. In a series of 65 patients with 81 morphologies of atypical atrial flutter, this isthmus represented the critical slow conduction pathway only in a few patients]. Moreover, in this case, a more medial pathway was the better ablation target, based on electroanatomic and procedural considerations. Taken together, these observations lead to the conclusion that the systematic use of prophylactic ablation of the "mitral isthmus" to prevent left macroreentry is questionable.

## References

1. Chugh A, Latchamsetty R, Oral H et al. Characteristics of cavotricuspid isthmus-dependent atrial flutter after left atrial ablation of atrial fibrillation. Circulation 2006; 113: 609-615.
2. Jaïs P, Hsu LF, Hocini M et al. The left atrial isthmus: from dissection bench to ablation lab. J Cardiovasc Electrophysiol 2004; 15: 813-814.
3. Jaïs P, Hocini M, Hsu LF et al. Technique and results of linear ablation at the mitral sthmus. Circulation 2004; 110: 2996-3002.
4. Becker AE. Left atrial isthmus: anatomic aspects relevant for linear catheter ablation procedures in humans. J Cardiovasc Electrophysiol 2004; 15: 809-812.
5. De Ponti R, Verlato R, Bertaglia E et al. Treatment of macroreentrant atrial tachycardia based on electroanatomic mapping: identification and ablation of the mid-diastolic isthmus. Europace 2007; 9: 449-457.

# Case 18
# A Non-clinical Macroreentrant Right Atrial Tachycardia with Two Independent Loops: the Exception to the Rule of a Shared Mid-diastolic Isthmus in Double-loop Reentry

## Case Presentation

This is a 34-year-old male patient with congenital ventricular septal defect and subvalvular aortic stenosis. At the age of 1, he underwent surgical closure of the ventricular septal defect, which involved surgical incision of the right atrium. At the age of 11, the subvalvular aortic stenosis was surgically corrected. Before this intervention, at the age of 8, he underwent right pneumectomy for hemoptisis due to congenital absence of the right pulmonary artery. Six months before the procedure he complained of two episodes of palpitations. These were documented by surface ECG as counter-clockwise typical atrial flutter, requiring DC-shock cardioversion to restore sinus rhythm. Subsequently, he was referred for an electrophysiology procedure while on sinus rhythm and in wash-out from antiarrhythmic drug therapy. Echocardiography showed neither residual shunts nor significant gradient in the left outflow tract; left ventricular function was preserved.

## Procedure

At the beginning of the procedure, the patient was in sinus rhythm with right bundle branch block. A decapolar catheter was positioned along the crista terminalis and two tetrapolar catheters were placed in the His-bundle area and coronary sinus. Since the heart was clockwise rotated and rightward displaced as a consequence of right pneumectomy, the coronary sinus was difficult to cannulate; therefore, a tetrapolar steerable catheter was used and positioned distally in the coronary sinus to avoid displacement. Since the patient had previously undergone surgery with right atrial atriotomy, it was felt that it was incorrect to directly proceed to ablation of cavotricuspid isthmus conduction on the assumption, based on the surface P wave pattern, that the clinical arrhythmia was necessarily dependent on isthmus conduction. Therefore, attempts to induce clinical flutter were made. Programmed electrical stimulation from the right atrium and the coronary sinus consisting of up to three extrastimuli failed to induce arrhythmia. Burst stimulation from the coronary sinus induced atrial flutter with a stable cycle length of 225 ms and 2:1 atrioventricular conduction. Since the atrioventricular conduction ratio and the presence of a wide QRS due to right bundle branch block prevented complete evaluation of the P wave morphology, an intravenous bolus of adenosine was administered and transient atrioventricular block was obtained. As shown in Figure 1, the P wave morphology was positive in leads I, II, III, aVF, V2–V6, flat in aVL and V1 and negative in aVR. Nonetheless, the intracav-

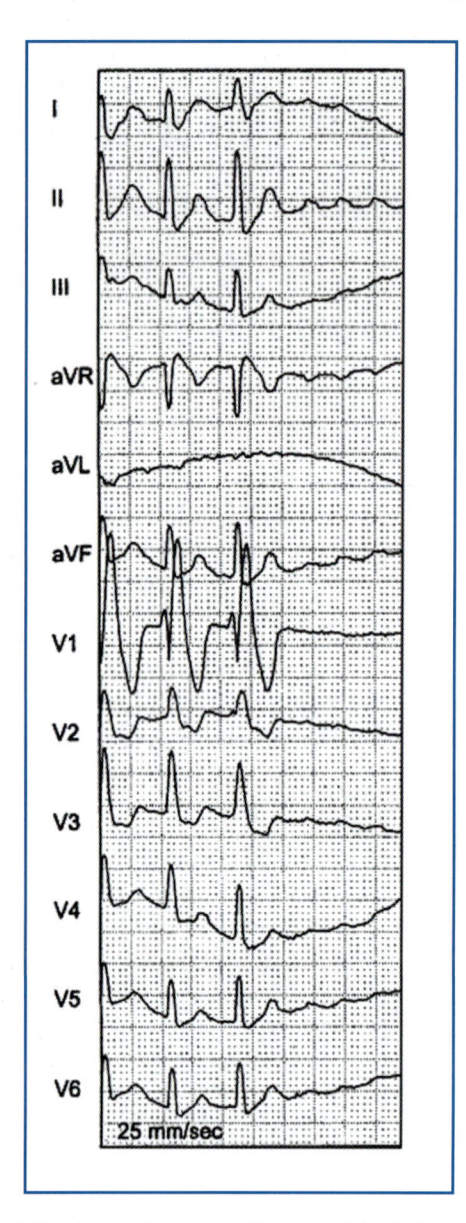

**Fig. 2.** Surface and intracavitary signals during the induced atrial flutter. From *top to bottom*, tracings are displayed as follows: limb leads and precordial leads V1 and V6, bipolar recordings of the catheter positioned along the crista terminalis, from the upper to the lower part (CT5–1), bipolar signals from the coronary sinus (CS2) and from the distal (CTI1) and proximal (CTI2) electrode pairs of the catheter positioned in the cavotricuspid isthmus. The activation sequence is similar to that of isthmus-dependent atrial flutter, with the difference that the upper crista terminalis is almost synchronous with the coronary sinus

**Fig. 1.** Twelve-lead electrocardiogram of the induced atrial flutter. On the right hand side, the P wave morphology is unmasked by intravenous adenosine injection

itary activation sequence, recorded on a conventional system (Fig. 2), was not very dissimilar from that of typical counter-clockwise atrial flutter with superior to inferior activation of the crista terminalis, which preceded activation of the medial cavotricuspid isthmus. Activation of the coronary sinus followed and was inscribed at the beginning of the P wave; this was difficult to identify during 2:1 atrioventricular conduction due to superimposition of the QRS complex and the T wave. Although the arrhythmia was different from the one documented clinically, its cycle length and intracavitary activation sequence were very stable. Accordingly, it was decided to proceed with electroanatomic mapping, with a coronary sinus atriogram as reference and the window of interest set as for macroreentry. Early during mapping, an electrically silent area was found in the lower portion of the posterolateral wall, likely related to prior atriotomy. Quite unusually, diastolic activation was observed both just above this area and in the cavotricuspid isthmus. For this reason, high-density mapping of the right atrium with the acquisition of more

Case 18   153

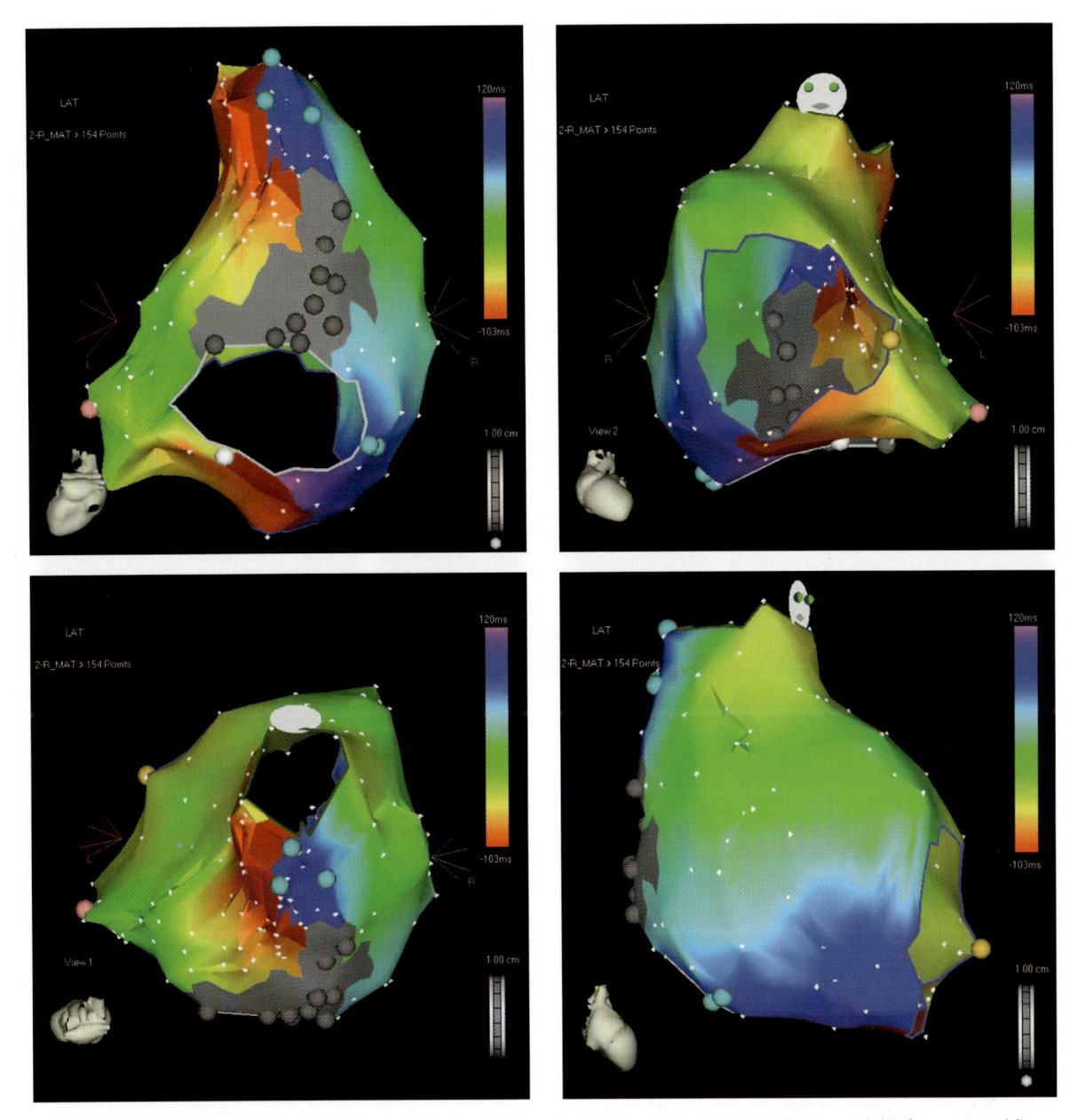

**Fig. 3a-d.** Activation map of the right atrium during induced atrial flutter in right lateral (**a**), caudal left anterior oblique (LAO) (**b**), cranial posteroanterior (**c**) and right anterior oblique (**d**) views. The *orange dot* indicates the site of His-bundle recording; the *pink dot* indicates the os of the coronary sinus. Sites of double potentials are tagged by *blue dots* and the electrically silent area by *grey dots*

than 150 sites was carried out until 99% of the tachycardia cycle length was reconstructed. Right atrial volume was 126 ml. As shown in Figure 3a, the presence of two mid-diastolic isthmi in the right atrium was confirmed, the first located in the cavotricuspid isthmus and the second in the posterior high right atrium, between the electrically silent area and the superior vena cava os. From these mid-diastolic isthmi, two symbiotic but independent loops originated, both fulfilling the definition of a reentrant circuit, i.e. unidirectional activation of a wavefront spanning at least 90% of the tachycardia cycle length with return of the activation wavefront to the site of earliest activation. The first loop was not dissimilar from the peritricuspid loop of a typical counter-clockwise atrial flutter, as shown by the sequence of colours around the tricuspid annulus in Fig-

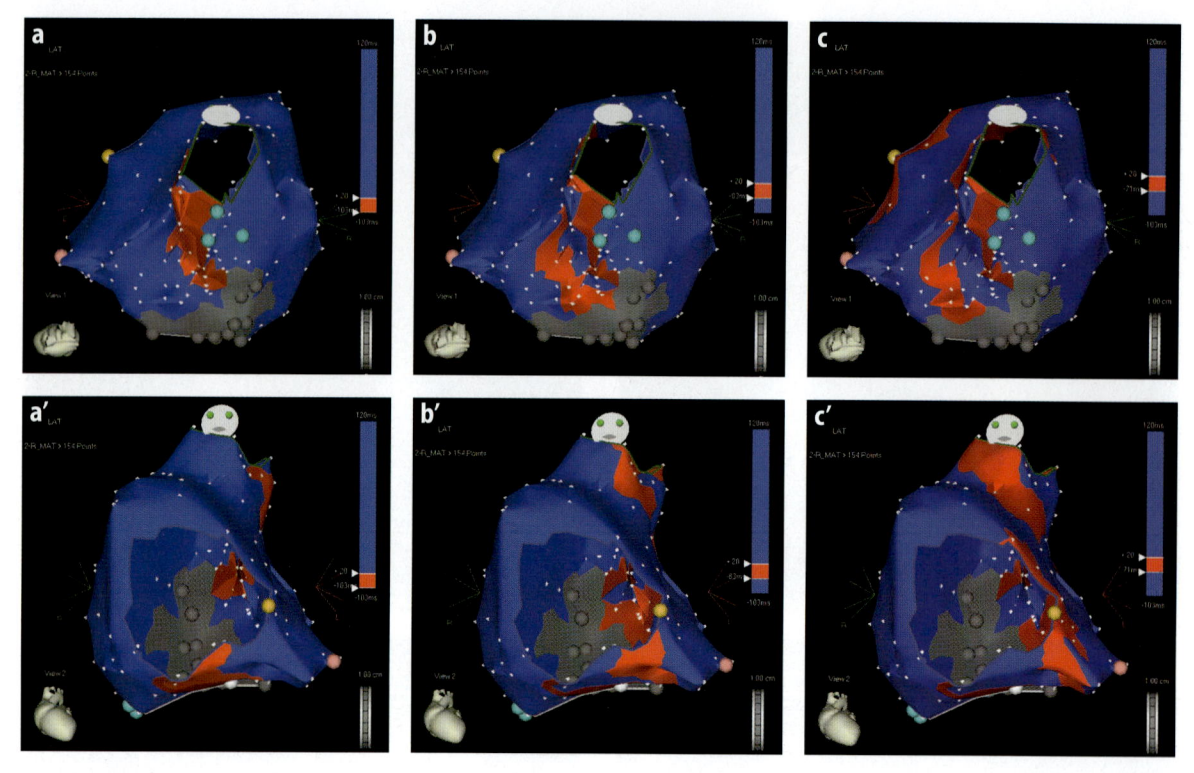

**Fig. 4a–f'.** Frames of the propagation map of the right atrium during induced atrial flutter in cranial posteroanterior (**a–f**) and caudal LAO (**a'–f'**) views

▶

ure 3b. The estimated length of this loop was 14.7 cm and conduction velocities in the mid-diastolic isthmus and in three segments along the outer loop were 23, 75, 89 and 81 cm/s. As shown in Figure 3c, the second loop rotated counter-clockwise around the superior vena cava os. Its estimated length (11.2 cm) was shorter than that of the first loop, but longer than expected in a loop around the superior vena cava, since the presence of an area of double potentials close to the superior vena cava os (Fig. 3a, c, d) forced the wavefront to follow a zig-zag course in this part of the circuit. The estimated conduction velocities in this loop were significantly slower: 13 cm/s in the mid-diastolic isthmus and 65, 57 and 60 cm/s in three segments of the outer loop. Sequential frames of the propagation map of the upper and peritricuspid loop are shown in Fig. 4a–f and 4a'–f', respectively. As evident in Figure 4d, d' the two loops shared a limited tract of the outer loop, in the area between the tricuspid annulus at 12–11 o'clock and the superior vena cava os. Also of interest in Figure 4d, d' is the presence of a third delayed wavefront in the medial right atrium and atrial septum (indicated in the figures by the arrow), which came from the upper loop and slowly proceeded anteroinferiorly towards the coronary sinus os (pink dot). This delayed wavefront contributed to separating the two loops by preventing activation of the medial cavotricuspid isthmus by the second loop. A fourth, dead-end wavefront was also present (arrow in Fig. 4e, e'), fed by both loops and colliding against the lateral side of the electrically silent area. At this point it was decided to further evaluate this unusual finding by entrainment mapping; unfortunately, stimulation at 200 ms cycle length produced, not unexpectedly, degeneration into sustained atrial fibrillation, which required DC-shock to restore sinus rhythm. No arrhythmia could be induced afterwards, even by very aggressive stimulation during isoprenaline infusion. Evaluation of the bipolar voltage map during flutter evidenced a distinct channel of very-low-amplitude potentials in the mid-diastolic isthmus of the upper loop, between the electrically silent area and the superior vena cava os (Fig. 5a), while an almost preserved voltage pattern was present in the cavotricuspid isthmus (Fig. 5b). Although the two isthmi could have been ablated during sinus rhythm, ablation was limited to cavotricuspid isthmus conduction. Electrical stimulation and test applications at reduced power output in the upper isthmus resulted in very evident phrenic nerve stimulation. Based on this evidence, the fact that the clinical arrhythmia had the P wave morphology of typical atrial flutter and the patient's important comorbidity, it was decided that limiting ablation to the cavotricuspid isthmus was a safer strategy. In the subsequent 18-month follow-up, the patient remained arrhythmia-free in the absence of antiarrhythmic drug therapy.

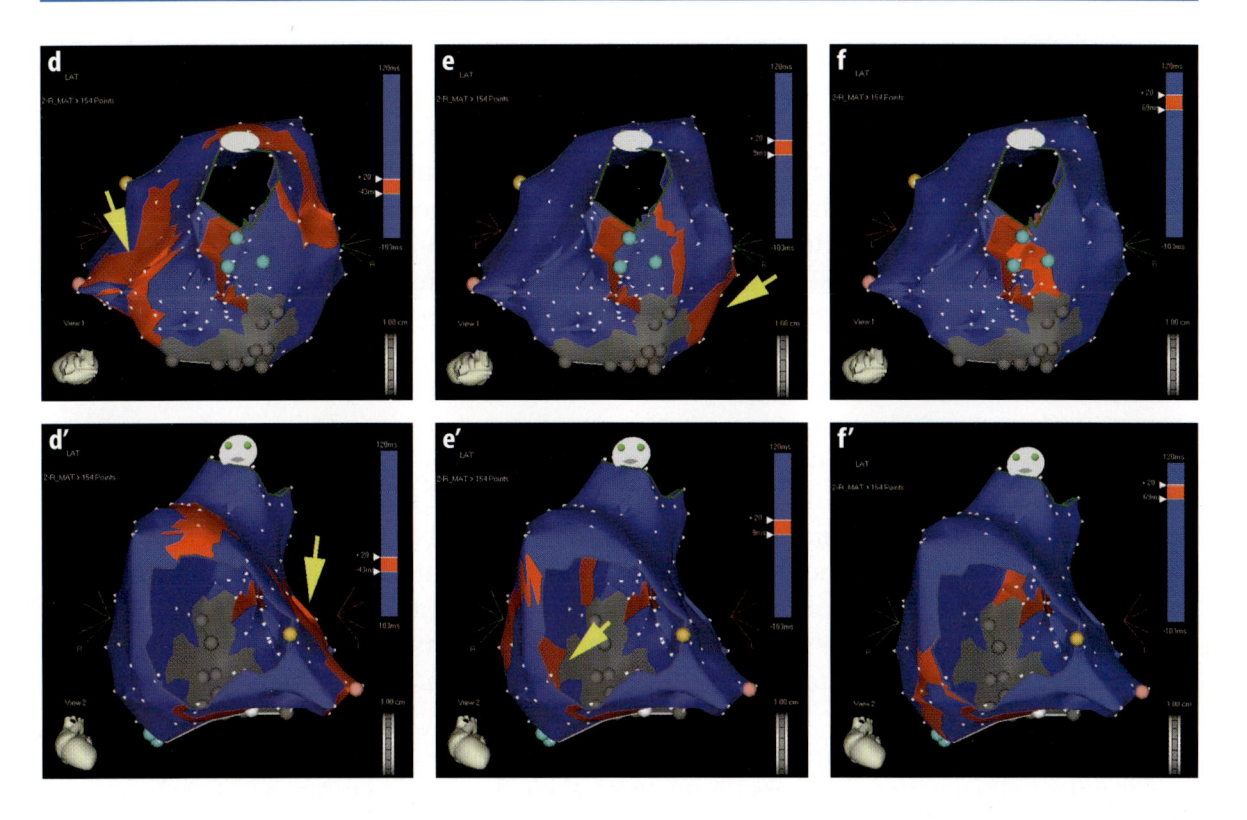

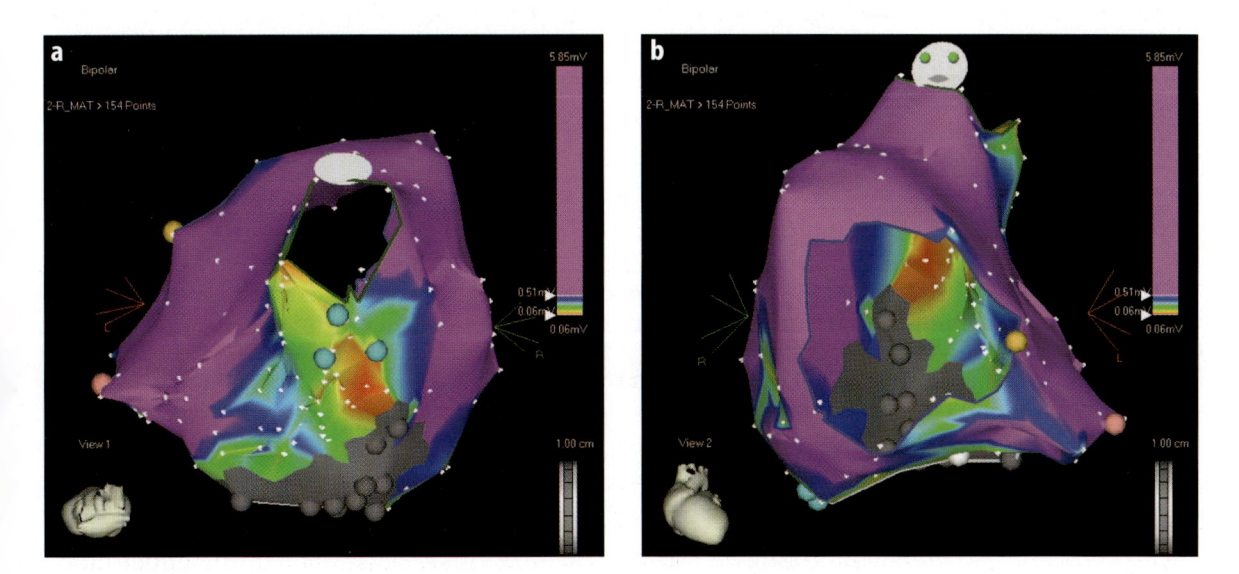

**Fig. 5a, b.** Bipolar voltage map of the right atrium during the induced atrial flutter in cranial posteroanterior (**a**) and caudal LAO (**b**) views. According to the setting of the colour-coded scale, areas of preserved voltage are shown in *purple*

## Commentary

Although incomplete, this case is presented because of the peculiar coexistence of two independent loops not sharing the mid-diastolic isthmus. In fact, the presence of two loops with a shared mid-diastolic isthmus is relatively common in our experience, accounting for roughly one third of the morphologies in macroreentrant atrial tachycardia/flutter [1]. The description of the typical "figure-of-eight" reentrant circuit, with two loops rotating around two different areas of block with a common channel of slow conduction, dates back to the experimental evidence produced by El Sherif [2]. Examples of the "figure-of-eight" double-loop reentry are provided in Cases 3, 8, 9, 11, 13, 16, 22. The present case is the only example in our experience of a reentry involving two independent loops in the same heart chamber colliding at the outer loop, while each loop has its own mid-diastolic isthmus. Although the true prevalence of this type of double-loop reentry is still unknown, its occurrence is expected to be rare. In fact, slow conduction, usually observed in the mid-diastolic isthmus, is expected to be the major determinant of the average speed of the reentrant wavefront (and therefore of the cycle length of each loop) in anatomically fixed reentry, since variations of conduction velocity over the outer loop are more limited. Therefore, it should be quite rare that two loops with two different areas of slow conduction synchronize to originate a reentry with two independent loops of the same cycle length. In this case: (1) the shortest loop (the upper loop around the superior vena cava) showed slower conduction velocities, both in the mid-diastolic isthmus and in the outer loop; (2) an area of double potentials (functional or possibly anatomical block related to prior surgery) close to the posterior area of the superior vena cava os forced this reentrant wavefront in a zig-zag pathway and rendered the upper loop longer than expected; (3) a third wavefront of delayed conduction, moving from the upper medial right atrium down to the atrial septum and coronary sinus os, helped keep the two loops separated upon exiting from the mid-diastolic isthmus. It is likely that all these elements significantly contributed to prevent invasion of the peritricuspid loop by the upper loop.

It is also interesting that the P wave morphology was mainly determined by the upper loop, which initiated a propagation wavefront from cranial to caudal both in the right and, probably, in the left atrium, with the second loop confined to around the tricuspid ring.

It should also be noted that this was an induced non-clinical arrhythmia. Although the arrhythmia was very stable during the entire mapping time, it degenerated into atrial fibrillation during entrainment stimulation and never recurred during mid-term follow-up. It is unknown whether this arrhythmia could have existed and how much could have persisted in this form in a clinical setting.

## References

1. De Ponti R, Verlato R, Bertaglia E et al. Treatment of macroreentrant atrial tachycardia based on electroanatomic mapping: identification and ablation of the mid-diastolic isthmus. Europace 2007; 9: 449-457.
2. El Sherif N, Mehra R, Gough WB et al. Reentrant ventricular arrhythmias in the late myocardial infarction period: interruption of reentrant circuits by cryothermal techniques. Circulation 1983; 8: 644-656.

# Case 19
# A Peculiar Clockwise Peritricuspid Atrial Flutter: the Exception to the Rule of Aiming at the Mid-diastolic Isthmus

## Case Presentation

This is a 51-year-old male patient with a history of idiopathic paroxysmal atrial fibrillation. Five years prior to the procedure described here, he underwent catheter ablation of atrial fibrillation in our centre, with electrical disconnection of the pulmonary veins. Subsequently, he was arrhythmia-free, until six months before the second procedure, when he began complaining of palpitation recurrence. This was documented on electrocardiogram as typical reverse atrial flutter (Fig. 1), with a cycle length of 250 ms, a prolonged surface P wave (160 ms) and predominantly 2:1 atrioventricular conduction. During a persistent episode, the patient was again referred to our institution for the second electrophysiology procedure.

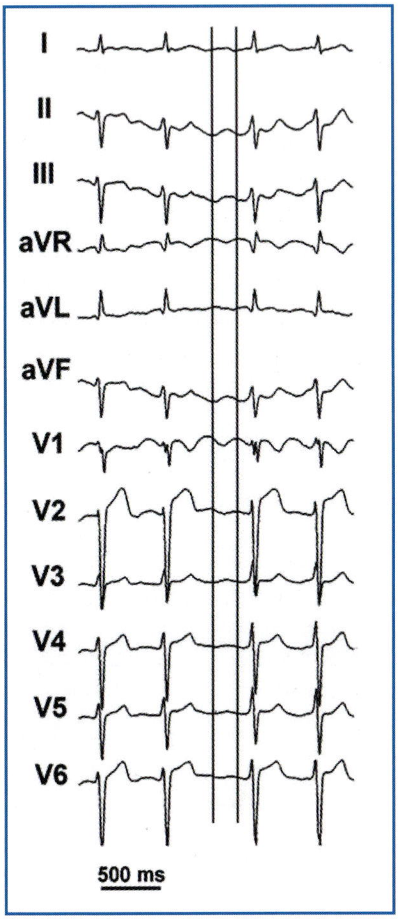

## Procedure

At the beginning of the procedure, the clinical arrhythmia persisted. A decapolar catheter was positioned in the coronary sinus and a tetrapolar catheter in the His-bundle area. With a coronary sinus atriogram as the electrical reference, mapping was started in the right atrium. The window of interest was set as for a macroreentrant arrhythmia. High-density mapping was easily performed and a clear clockwise peritricuspid reentry circuit was identified (Fig. 2a, b). Both from conventional recordings and the activation map, it was clear that the lateral right atrium showed diastolic activation, while the cavotricuspid isthmus showed an end-systolic chronology (pale blue and blue colours). The mid-diastolically activated area was located in the lateral wall and ex-

**Fig. 1.** Twelve-lead electrocardiogram of the clinical atrial flutter, with a cycle length of 250 ms. The duration of the P wave is indicated by the two *vertical lines*

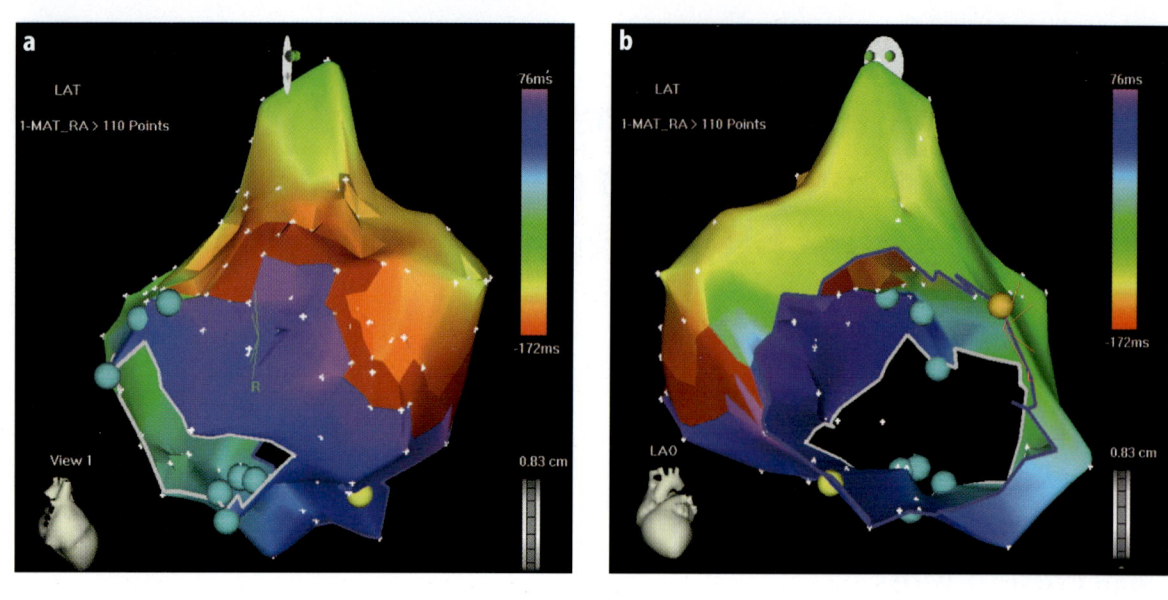

**Fig. 2a, b.** Activation map of the right atrium during atrial flutter in right lateral (**a**) and left anterior oblique (LAO) (**b**) views. The *orange dot* indicates the site of His-bundle recording and the *blue dots* the sites of double potentials, recorded both in the posterior wall and in the posterior part of the cavotricuspid isthmus. The *yellow dot* is the pacing site for entrainment

tended from an area of double potentials in the posterior wall, close to the inferior vena cava os, and the tricuspid annulus at 9 o'clock (Fig. 2a). A second short line of double potentials was observed in the posterior cavotricuspid isthmus, likely in the area of the Eustachian ridge. The

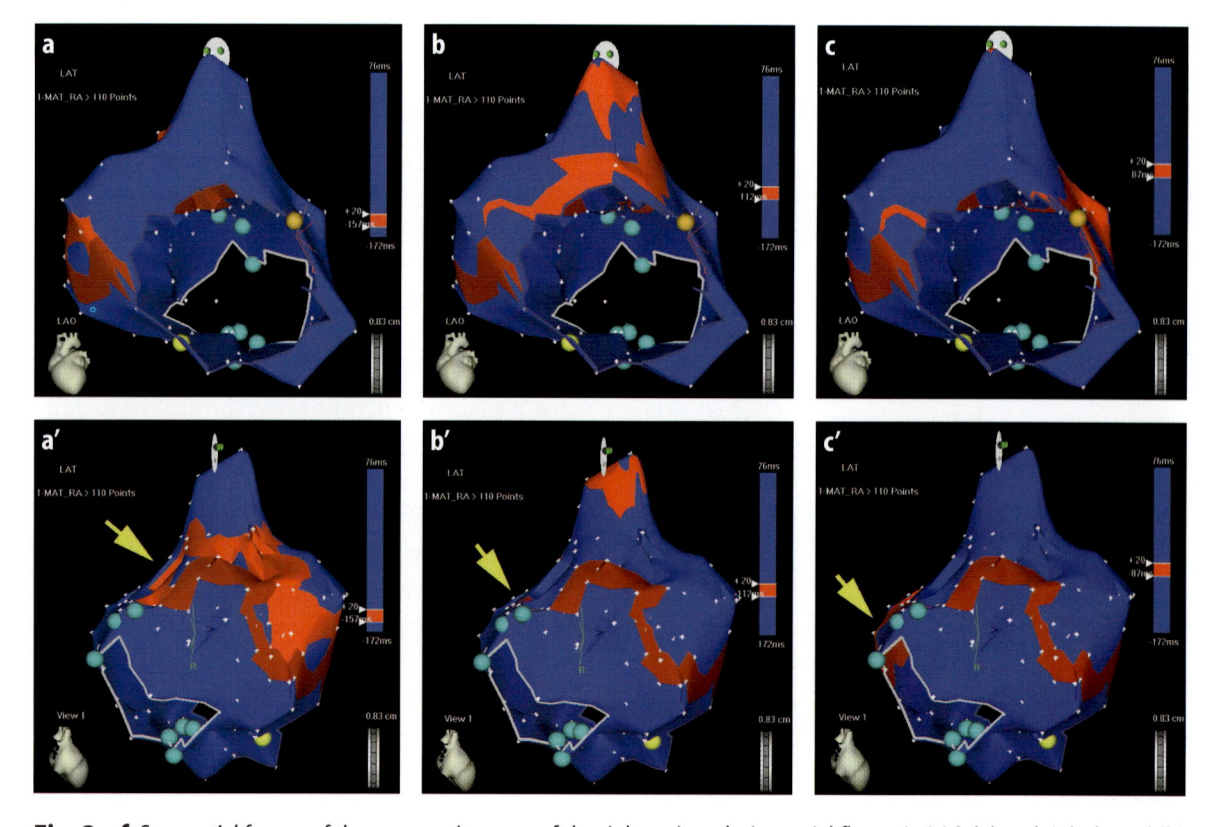

**Fig. 3a-f.** Sequential frames of the propagation map of the right atrium during atrial flutter in LAO (**a**) and right lateral (**b**) views. The complete peritricuspid loop, the incomplete posterior loop (*yellow arrows*) and the dead-end activation of the superior vena cava are evident

propagation map clearly showed a peritricuspid clockwise circuit (Fig. 3a–f and a'–f'). Dead-end activation of the superior vena cava (Fig. 3b, b') was also evident, as was the presence of a second incomplete loop (indicated by the arrow in Fig. 3a'–d'). This loop moved from the posterior part of the mid-diastolic area in a superoposterior direction, passing above the posterior line of double potentials and directing towards the medial right atrium, where it rejoined the dominant loop. The length of the peritricuspid reentry was 17.4 cm. Conduction velocity showed a lower value in the mid-diastolically activated area (40 cm/s) than in the three analysed segments in the outer loop (76, 72 and 67, respectively). Analysis of the bipolar voltage map (Fig. 4a, b) showed generally preserved voltage in the right atrium, with small areas of low voltage in the posterolateral wall, from the superior vena cava to the posterior area of double potentials, and in the lateral wall at the level of the mid-diastolic activation area. The extension of the mid-diastolic area from anterior to posterior measured 7.5 cm, with lower voltage in the anterior and posterior limits of this area (ranging from 0.16 to 0.24 mV) and preserved voltage in the central part of the mid-diastolic area (ranging from 1.74 to 4.11 mV). The anteroposterior extension of the cavotricuspid isthmus was 2.3 cm and was rendered even shorter by the presence of the line of block in its posterior aspect. The voltage in the cavotricuspid isthmus ranged from 1.19 to 1.72 mV. Electrical stimulation at 90% of the tachycardia cycle length in the central cavotricuspid isthmus (yellow dot in the previous figures) resulted in entrainment, with fusion of the intracavitary activation sequence and a post-pacing interval equalling the length of the tachycardia cycle (Fig. 5), which classified this site as being in the outer loop of the reentrant pathway. Unlike the other cases discussed in this book, an ablation strategy aimed at the narrowest anatomic isthmus instead of the mid-diastolic isthmus was by far more convenient in this case, considering the electroanatomic data of isthmus extension and voltage amplitude. Moreover,

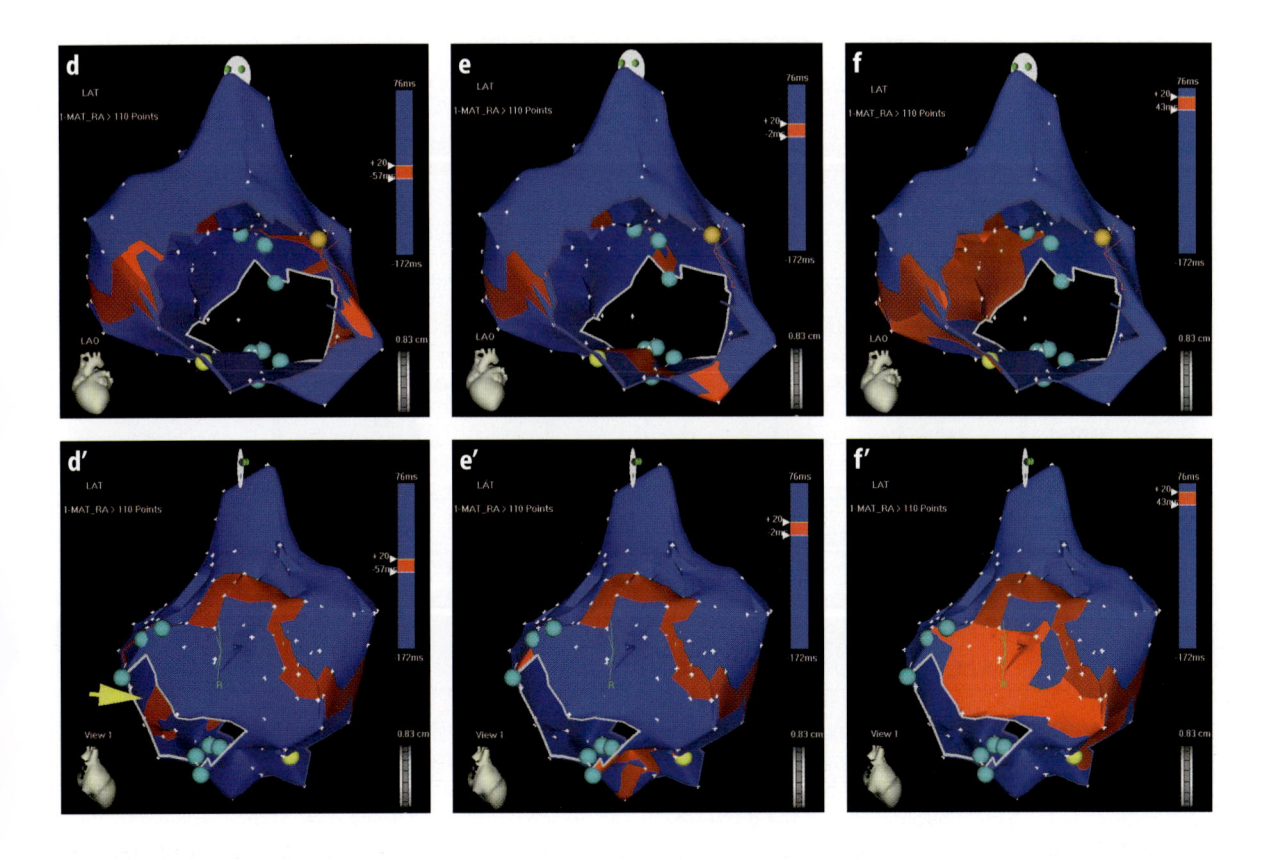

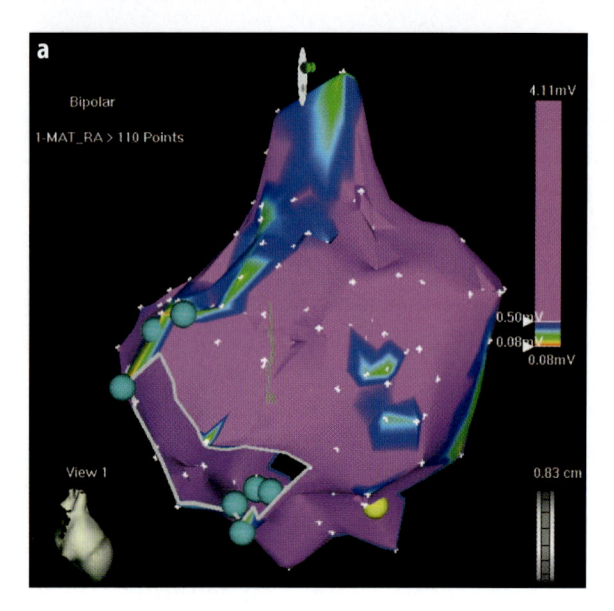

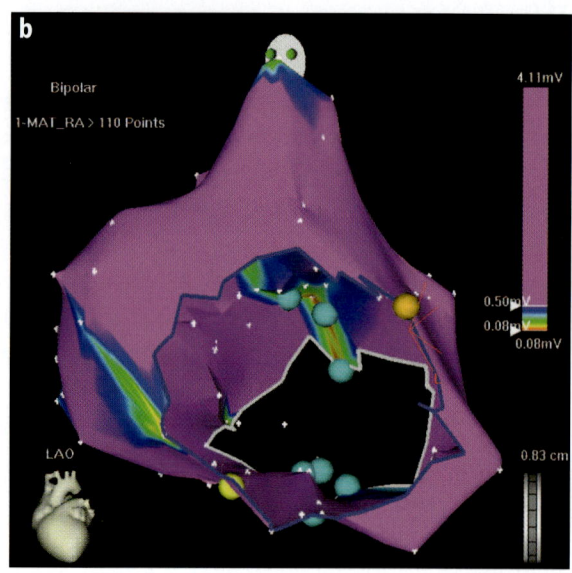

**Fig. 4a, b.** Bipolar voltage map of the right atrium during atrial flutter in right lateral (**a**) and LAO (**b**) views. According to the setting of the colour-coded scale, areas of preserved voltage are shown in *purple*

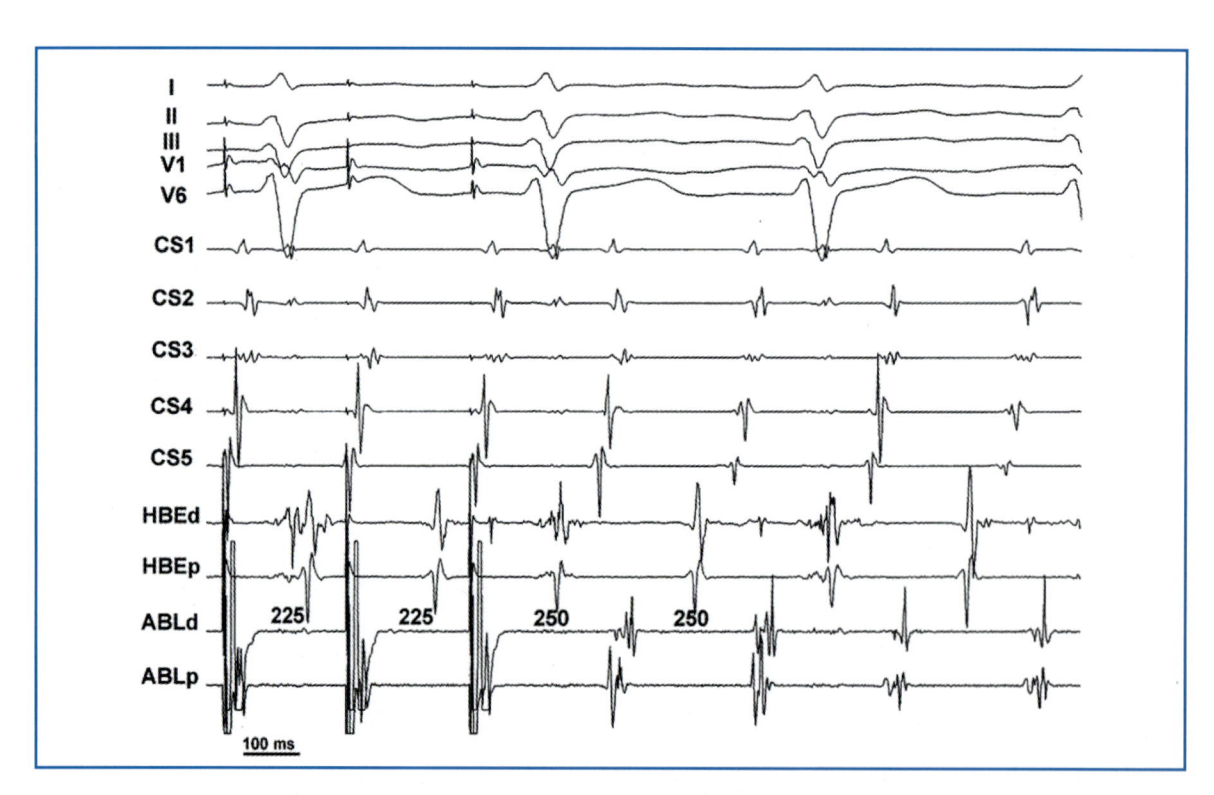

**Fig. 5.** Surface and intracavitary recordings during entrainment stimulation at the site indicated by the *yellow dot* in the previous figures. From *top to bottom*, tracings are displayed as follows: leads I, II, III, V1, V6, bipolar recordings of the coronary sinus catheter from distal to proximal (CS1–5), bipolar recordings from the distal (HBEd) and proximal (HBEp) electrode pairs of the His-bundle catheter, bipolar recordings from the distal (ABLd) and proximal (ABLp) electrode pairs of the mapping/ablation catheter, positioned in the central cavotricuspid isthmus. Atrial flutter was entrained at 225 ms, with modification of the intracavitary activation sequence (anticipation of the entrained site, compared to the atrial deflection in the coronary sinus and His-bundle area). The return cycle equalled the cycle length of the flutter. Values are in milliseconds and refer to tracing ABLd

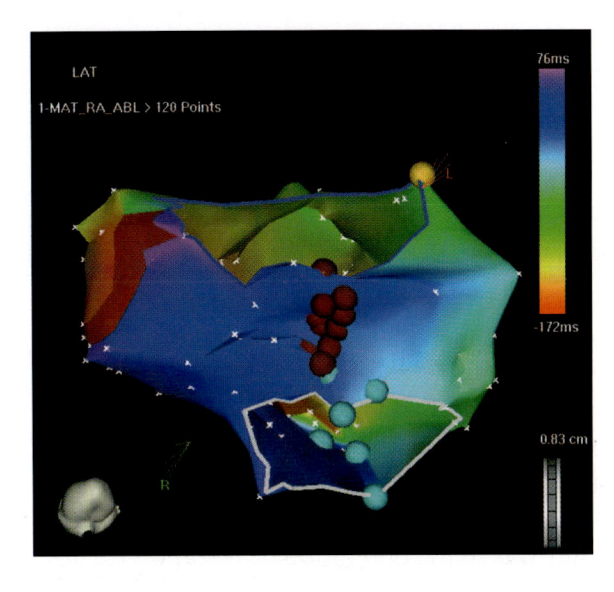

**Fig. 6.** Ativation map of the right atrium during atrial flutter in an inferior view. *Red dots* indicate the ablation line in the cavotricuspid isthmus

ablation of the cavotricuspid isthmus was safer than ablation in the lateral wall, where the line of ablation could have involved a perisinus area and/or an area close to the course of the right phrenic nerve. Therefore, ablation was started by delivering radiofrequency energy using an irrigated-tip catheter (maximum power 40 W, cut-off temperature 43°C, duration 45 s) from the tricuspid annulus to the os of the inferior vena cava (Fig. 6). When the ablation line approached the site of double potentials, radiofrequency energy delivery interrupted the arrhythmia (Fig. 7) and produced bidirectional complete cavotricuspid isthmus conduction block, as demonstrated by paging of the coronary sinus and low lateral right atrium. Afterwards, no other arrhythmia was inducible, even using a very aggressive stimulation protocol during isoprenaline infu-

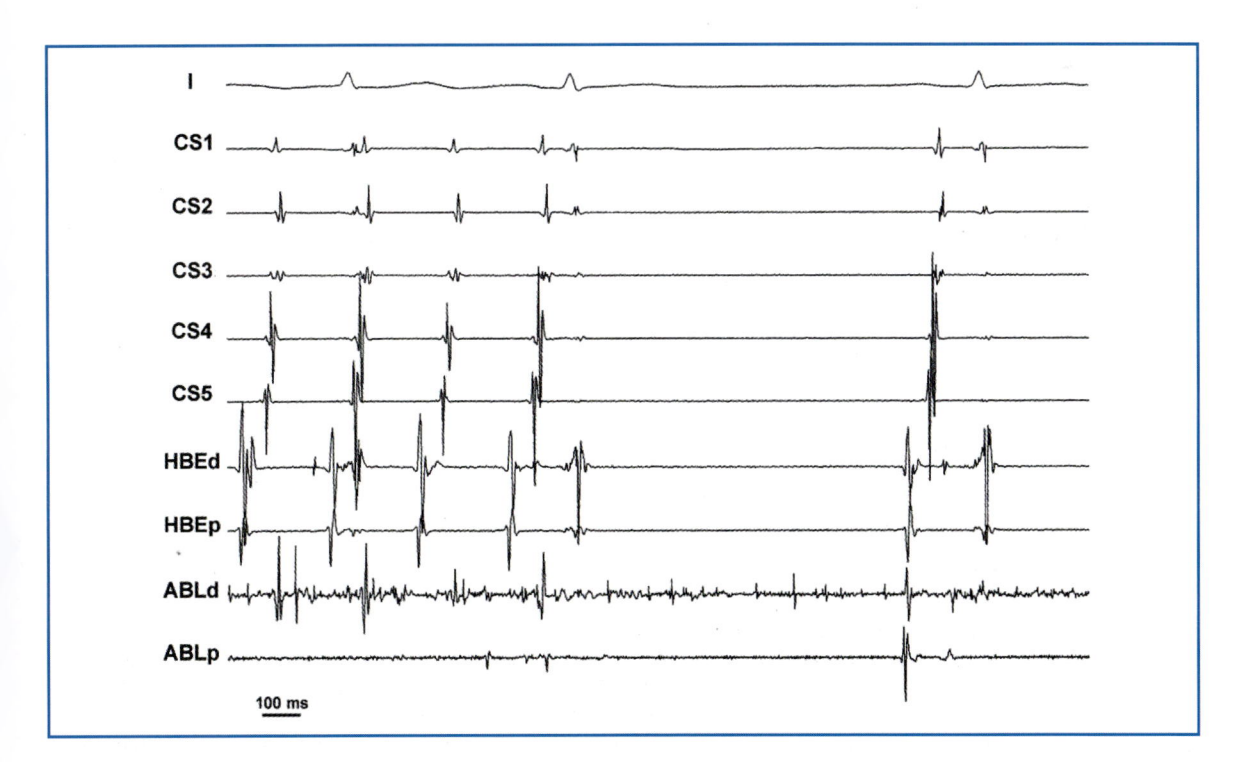

**Fig. 7.** Surface and intracavitary recordings upon flutter termination during radiofrequency energy delivery. Tracings are displayed as in Fig. 5, with the exception that only surface lead I is shown

sion. The result persisted after 30 min; therefore, the procedure was concluded. The patient was arrhythmia-free without antiarrhythmic drugs at a 6-month follow-up.

## Commentary

In patients with counter-clockwise typical atrial flutter, pacing from the central cavotricuspid isthmus results in concealed entrainment, with a post-pacing interval exceeding the flutter cycle by no more than 7 ms [1]. This finding confirms that this area is the protected isthmus of slow conduction of the reentrant circuit. Well-conducted studies using non-contact [2] and electroanatomic [3] mapping have provided evidence that, in the clockwise form of atrial flutter, the circuit is basically the same as in the counter-clockwise form, with a reverse direction of rotation and the cavotricuspid isthmus still serving as the slow conduction pathway.

One peculiar aspect of this case was mid-diastolic activation with slow conduction located in the right lateral wall, while the cavotricuspid isthmus was in the outer loop of reentry with normal conduction velocity, as confirmed by electroanatomic mapping, with a specific setting of the window of interest, and by entrainment. The reason why the slow conduction area "migrated" to the lateral wall in this case is unknown. The presence of small areas of low voltage in the right lateral wall may have been indicative of an initial degenerative process, which might have favoured slow conduction, whereas preserved voltage was found in the cavotricuspid isthmus. Consequently, in this patient, the reentrant circuit may have been rendered possible only by the presence of delayed conduction in the lateral wall, while the cavotricuspid isthmus had preserved conduction velocity.

However, the focus of this case is the ablation strategy, which was very different from the one adopted in the other cases presented in this book. The advantages of targeting the mid-diastolic isthmus in macroreentrant atrial tachycardia/flutter were pointed out both in our study [4] and in other reports [5, 6]. This is the only case in our experience in which ablation of an anatomically defined isthmus was far more convenient than ablation of the mid-diastolic isthmus. This case confirms the need for treatment tailored to each patient, with exceptions to the general rules in particular cases.

## References

1. Olgin JE, Kalman JM, Fitzpatrick AP, Lesh MD. Role of right atrial endocardial structures as barriers to conduction during human type I atrial flutter. Circulation 1995; 92: 1839-1848.
2. Schilling RJ, Peters NS, Goldberger J et al. Characterization of the anatomy and conduction velocities of the human right atrium flutter circuit determined by noncontact mapping. J Am Coll Cardiol 2001; 38: 385-393.
3. Rodriguez LM, Timmermans C, Nabar A et al. Biatrial activation in isthmus-dependent atrial flutter. Circulation 2001; 104: 2545-2550.
4. De Ponti R, Verlato R, Bertaglia E et al. Treatment of macroreentrant atrial tachycardia based on electroanatomic mapping: identification and ablation of the mid-diastolic isthmus. Europace 2007. 9: 449-457.
5. Jaïs P, Sanders P, Hsu L et al. Flutter localized to the anterior left atrium after catheter ablation of the atrial fibrillation. J Cardiovasc Electrophysiol 2006; 17: 279-285.
6. Kaltman JR, Schultz JR, Wieand TS et al. Mapping the critical diastolic pathway in intra-atrial reentrant tachycardia using an automated voltage mapping program. J Cardiovasc Electrophysiol 2006; 17: 786-788.

# Part III

# Atrial Ablation Based on Substrate Mapping in Sinus Rhythm

# Case 20
## Non-inducible Atrial Flutter in a Patient with Prior Surgery for Congenital Heart Disease (Example 1): Ablation Based on Substrate Mapping in Sinus Rhythm

## Case Presentation

This is a 27-year-old male patient who at the age of 5 underwent surgical closure of an ostium secundum atrial septal defect using a Dacron patch. One year before the procedure described here, he began complaining of palpitations, with the ECG equivalent of atrial flutter (Fig. 1) of 240 ms cycle length. The P wave morphology was very similar to that of typical atrial flutter, although symmetric negative P waves were present in the inferior leads, instead of the classic "saw-tooth" morphology. Moreover, unlike typical atrial flutter, the P wave morphology in V1 was biphasic, with a predominant negative late component. Initially, the patient refused the procedure and was cardioverted, but the arrhythmia recurred with the same morphology in the following months. Consequently, the patient accepted the procedure and was referred for ablation while on a persistent episode of atrial flutter. The day before the procedure, probably as a result of its prolonged duration, the arrhythmia degenerated into atrial fibrillation. A previous transthoracic echocardiography in sinus rhythm showed no marked dilation of the heart cham-

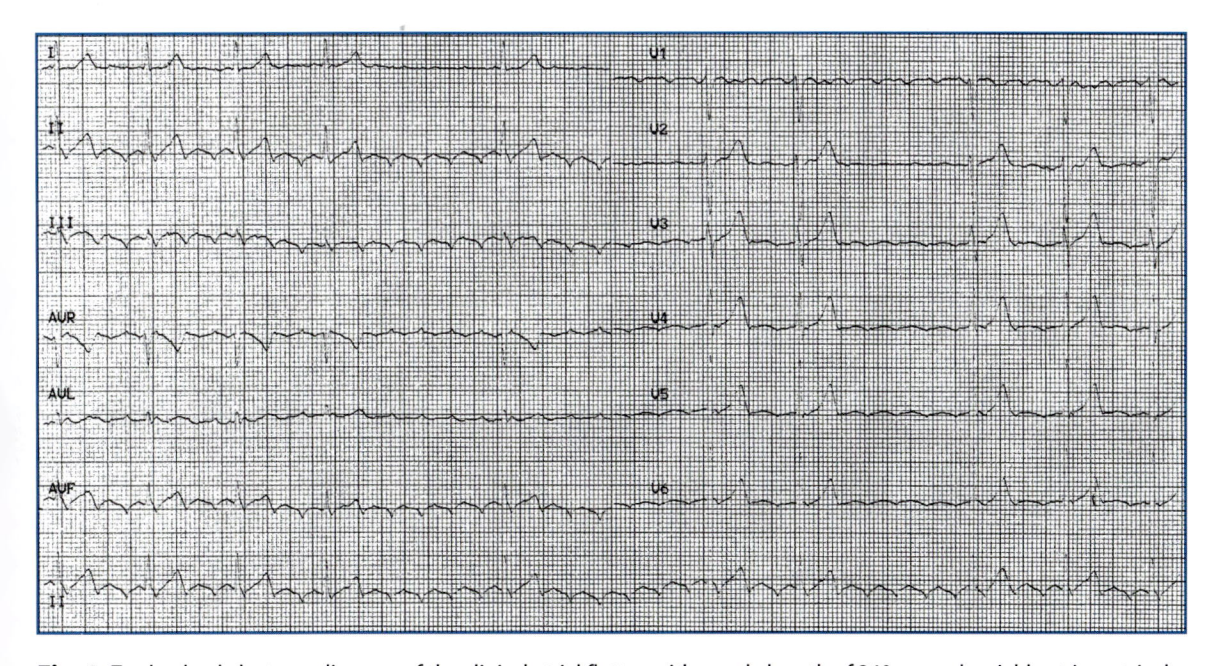

**Fig. 1.** Twelve-lead electrocardiogram of the clinical atrial flutter, with a cycle length of 240 ms and variable atrioventricular conduction

bers and normal ventricular function. Preprocedure transoesophageal echocardiogram excluded intracavitary thrombi.

## Procedure

At the beginning of the procedure, the patient was still in atrial fibrillation with completely disorganised atrial electrical activity. Two decapolar catheters were placed, one into the coronary sinus and the other along the crista terminalis, while a tetrapolar catheter was placed in the His-bundle area. Afterwards, under sedation, the patient was cardioverted and sinus rhythm was stably restored. Induction attempts using a very aggressive protocol (programmed stimulation up to multiple extrastimuli from different sites of the right atrium and coronary sinus, and burst stimulation up to 180 ms cycle length, also during isoprenaline infusion) failed to induce arrhythmia. Therefore, mapping of the right atrium in sinus rhythm was carried out, with a coronary sinus atriogram as the reference signal. High-density mapping with the acquisition of 168 sites was performed (Fig. 2a–d), while 12-lead electrocardiographic monitoring showed a constant sinus P wave morphology. Interestingly, a Y-shaped line of double potentials separated by > 70 ms was easily identified in the posterolateral wall (Fig. 2a), corresponding to surgical atriotomy, which was likely performed in this way to gain greater access to the right atrium/atrial septum while sparing the sinus node area. The latter was of normal size and position (Fig. 2a, b). The line of block, which surrounded the lower part of the sinus node area and extended inferiorly along the posterolateral wall, had two effects on right atrial activation: (1) it prolonged right atrial activation up to 144 ms, and (2) it moved the latest activated area (normally located in the lower medial right atrium) to the lower area of the lateral wall (Fig. 2a, c, d). Analysis of the propagation map (Fig. 3) revealed the consequence of the presence of this line of block in greater detail. In fact, the impulse originating in the sinus node area (Fig. 3a) split early into four wavefronts (Fig. 3b, c and b', c'): (1) a dead-end wavefront directed towards the superior vena cava; (2) an anterior wavefront, slowly activating the anterior wall superior to the line of block; (3) a medial wavefront directed towards the medial upper right atrium and then the atrial septum and the coronary sinus os; (4) a wavefront posterior to the line of block, which moved from superior to inferior along the posterior wall. In the lower area of the posterior wall, this latter wavefront split in two components (Fig. 3d, e and d', e'). The first moved medially and joined the medial wavefront moving towards the atrial septum and the medial cavotricuspid isthmus. The second engaged the conducting gap between the line of block and the inferior vena cava. Finally (Fig. 3f, f'), the three still-active wavefronts (namely, the anterior, the medial and the one coming from the lower conducting gap) collided in the latest activated areas, located anteroinferiorly to the posterolateral atriotomy. Right atrial volume was 130 ml. The bipolar voltage map (Fig. 4a, b) showed generally preserved voltage amplitude, with the exception of the area of prior atriotomy and a small area at the superior vena cava os. Peculiarly, no evidence of either a large area of reduced voltage or of delayed conduction (as assessed by the quick movement of the medial wavefront) was present in the atrial septum, as the result of surgical repair of the atrial septal defect. Based on this analysis, three possibly critical isthmi were identified. The first isthmus was located between prior atriotomy and the inferior vena cava os. Its length was 15 mm, the voltage was between 0.26 and 0.87 mV (0.55±0.32 mV, on average) and the conduction velocity measured during sinus rhythm propagation was low (21 cm/s), as evidenced also by crowding of the isochronal line on the activation map (Fig. 2a) and by narrowing of the propagation band shown in Fig. 3e. The second isthmus was the cavotricuspid isthmus, which was 1.7 mm long and had normal conduction velocity (83 cm/s) and preserved voltage (2.73±2.13). The third isthmus was the 2.6 mm channel between the upper part of the line of double potentials

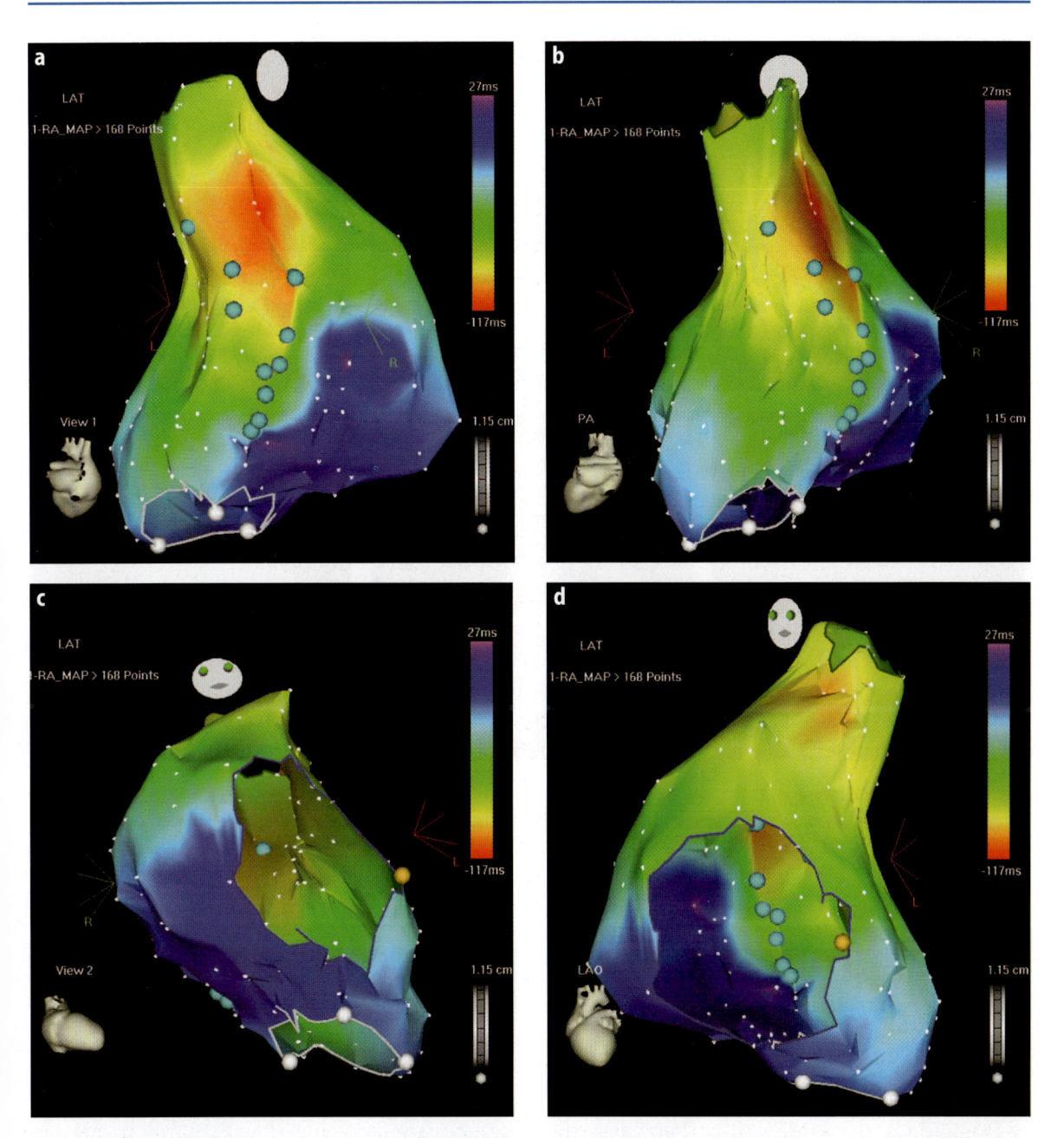

**Fig. 2a-d.** Activation map of the right atrium during sinus rhythm in posterolateral (**a**), posteroanterior (**b**), caudal anteroposterior (**c**) and left anterior oblique (LAO) (**d**) views. The *orange* and *blue dots* indicate the sites of His-bundle recording and of double potentials, respectively. To better define the inferior vena cava os, which was of crucial importance in this case for reconstruction of the caudal part of the right atrium, three ostial points with no electrical signal were acquired and tagged as "location only" (*white dots*).

and the superior vena cava os, where the voltage was preserved (1.32±0.85 mV, on average). However, the conduction velocity of transverse propagation across the isthmus could not be calculated in sinus rhythm, since propagation activated this area from inferior to superior and not transversally across the isthmus. In this patient, the area between prior atriotomy and the tricuspid annulus could not be considered an isthmus due to its extension and voltage values. Based on the morphology of the clinical arrhythmia (suggesting a lower-loop reentry in the right atrium) and the substrate mapping data, it was decided to ablate the cavotricuspid isthmus, to avoid peritricuspid and lower-loop reentry, and the inferolateral isthmus (between atriotomy and inferior vena cava os), to avoid clockwise and counter-clockwise reentry in the lat-

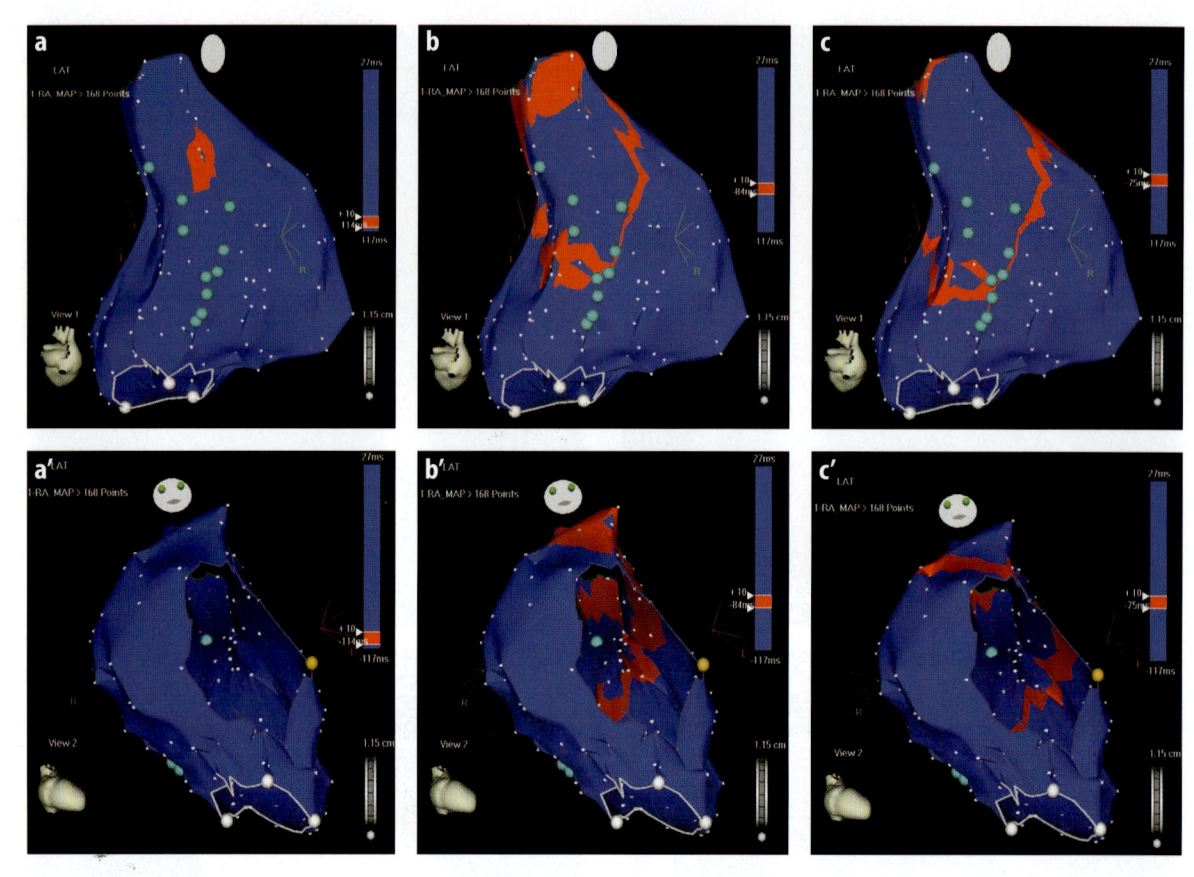

**Fig. 3a-f'.** Sequential frames of the propagation map of the right atrium in sinus rhythm in posterolateral (**a–f**) and caudal anteroposterior (**a'–f'**) views. Modification of the normal right atrial propagation pattern in sinus rhythm induced by the lateral line of block is evident

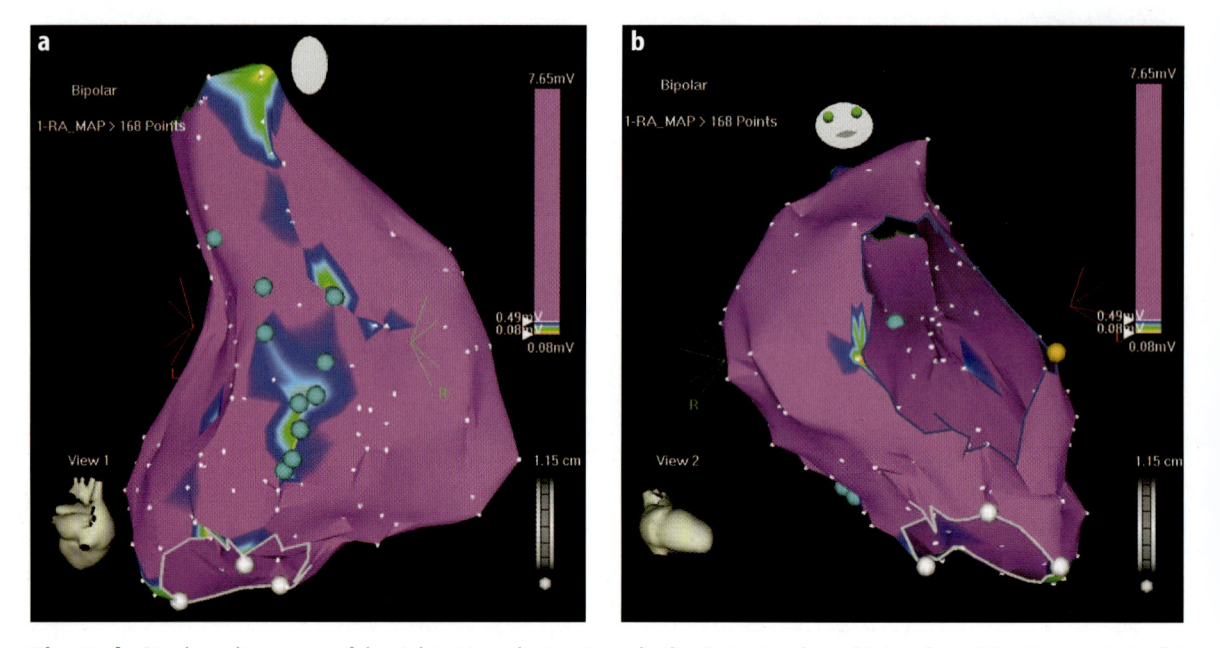

**Fig. 4a,b.** Bipolar voltage map of the right atrium during sinus rhythm in posterolateral (**a**) and caudal anteroposterior (**b**) views. According to the setting of the colour-coded scale, areas with preserved voltage are shown in *purple*

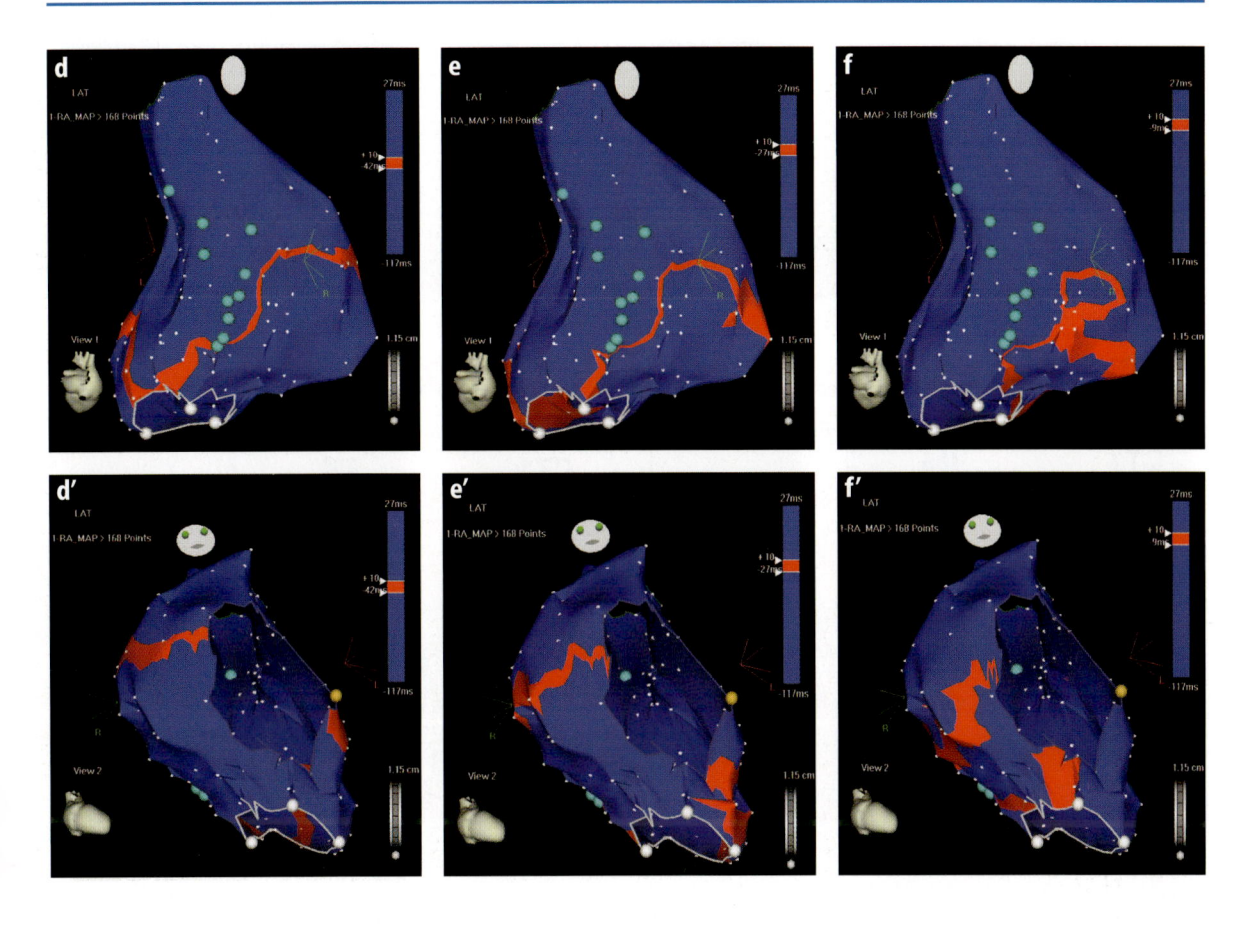

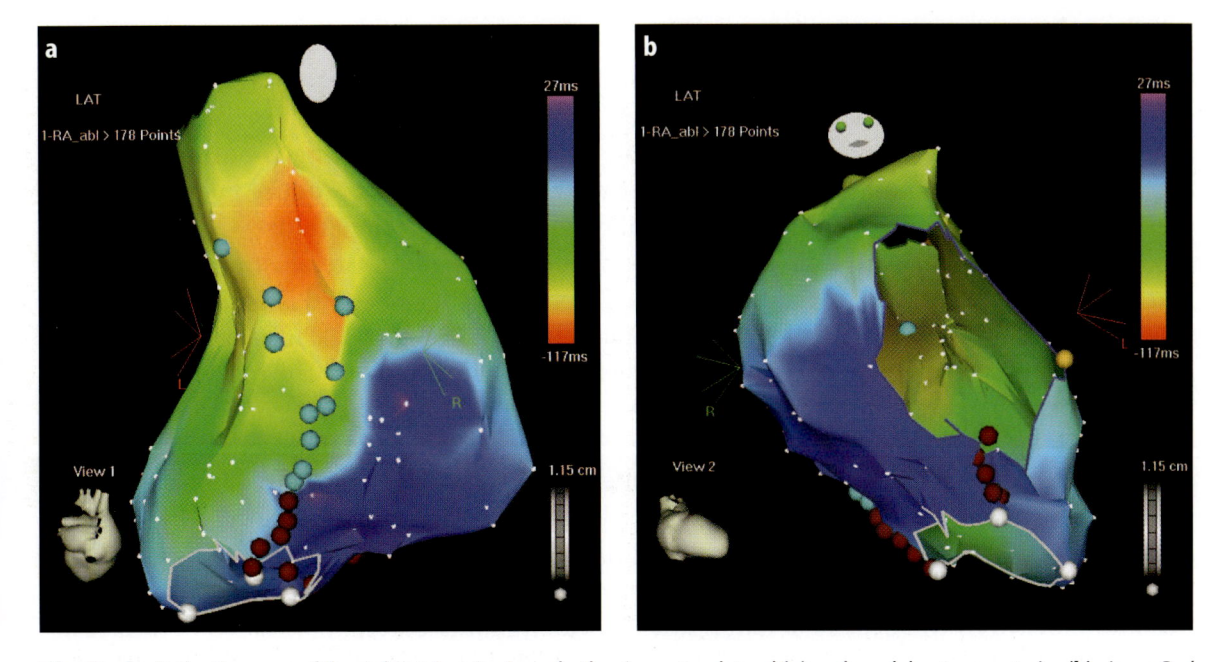

**Fig. 5a, b.** Activation map of the right atrium in sinus rhythm in posterolateral (**a**) and caudal anteroposterior (**b**) views. *Red dots* indicate the ablation line in the cavotricuspid and inferolateral isthmus

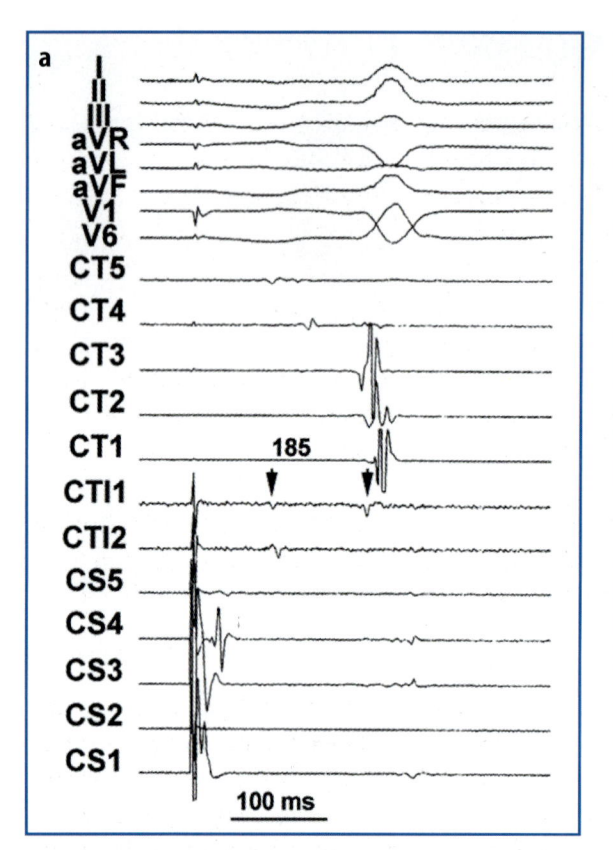

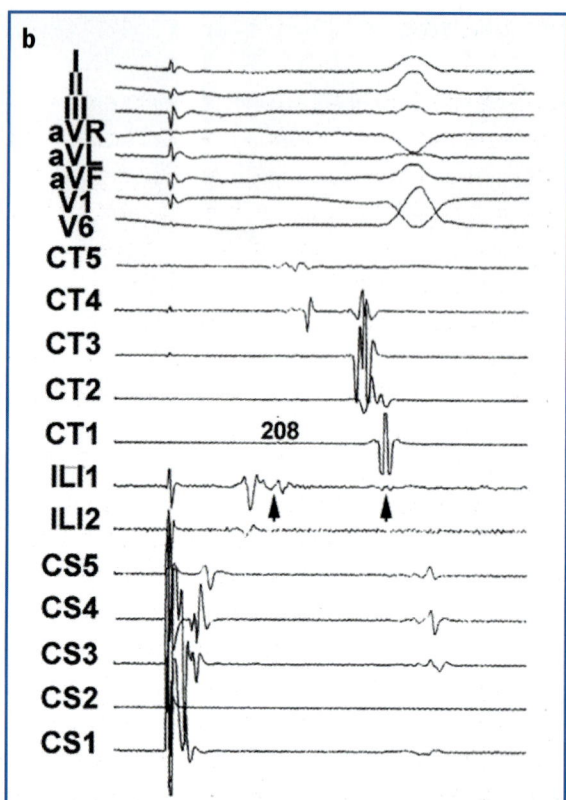

**Fig. 6a, b.** Surface and intracavitary recordings during coronary sinus pacing after ablation of the cavotricuspid isthmus (**a**) and inferolateral isthmus (**b**). From *top to bottom*, tracings are displayed as follows: limb and V1, V6 leads, bipolar recordings of the crista terminalis catheter from the upper to the lower part (CT5–1); in **a**, bipolar recordings from the distal (CTI1) and proximal (CTI2) electrode pairs of the ablation catheter positioned in the posterior cavotricuspid isthmus; in **b**, bipolar recordings from the distal (ILI1) and proximal (ILI2) electrode pairs of the same catheter now positioned in the inferolateral isthmus; bipolar recordings of the coronary sinus catheter, from proximal to distal (CS5–1). *Arrows* indicate double potentials. Numbers are in milliseconds and refer to the interval between coronary sinus activation and lower crista terminalis activation in CT1

eral wall around the line of block. Apart from its extension and voltage amplitude, the superior isthmus was not ablated for phrenic-nerve capture in this area during electrical stimulation. Five radiofrequency energy applications with an irrigated-tip catheter (maximum power 50 W, cut-off temperature 43°C, duration 60 s) in the cavotricuspid isthmus produced persistent bidirectional conduction block. Another five applications (cut-off temperature 43°C, maximum power 35 W, duration 60 s) produced conduction block of the inferolateral isthmus (Fig. 5a, b). During coronary sinus pacing, conduction block across the cavotricuspid isthmus (Fig. 6a) was assessed by an uninterrupted line of double potentials separated by > 100 ms along the ablation line, with the crista terminalis activated from the upper to the lower part. During coronary sinus pacing, the second potential in the posterior part of the cavotricuspid isthmus (second arrow in tracing CTI1 in Fig. 6a) preceded activation of the lower crista terminalis, suggesting the presence of a fast clockwise wavefront around the inferior vena cava os. Conduction block across the inferolateral isthmus (Fig. 6b) locally produced a line of double potentials separated by > 100 ms during coronary sinus pacing. Moreover, activation of the lower crista terminalis was delayed by 23 ms, confirming the presence of a previous wavefront around the inferior vena cava os, which was now blocked by this second ablation line. Repeated induction attempts failed to induce arrhythmia. Conduction block in the cavotricuspid and inferolateral isthmus persisted after 30 min; hence, the procedure was terminated. In an 18-month follow-up, the patient was arrhythmia-free without antiarrhythmic drugs.

## Commentary

In our experience, a minority of patients with atrial arrhythmias have been treated based on substrate mapping in sinus rhythm, since both the macroreentrant and the focal forms are persistent or easily inducible during the procedure. When a macroreentrant atrial tachycardia/flutter is not present nor inducible, high-density electroanatomic mapping may provide detailed information on how surgical intervention has modified normal activation in sinus rhythm; at the same time, it provides essential data for a rational ablative strategy. In patients with postsurgical macroreentrant forms, pace-mapping, as an alternative or complement to electroanatomic mapping in sinus rhythm, may not provide the type of data needed to plan the ablation strategy. In fact, electrical stimulation in these situations does not necessarily produce a surface P wave morphology similar to the one originated by the unidirectional course of the macroreentrant circuit.

As previously reported [1, 2], in normal human right atria there are three different activation wavefronts originating from the sinus node: (1) one dead-end wavefront towards the superior vena cava; (2) one lateral wavefront that activates the lateral wall/crista terminalis and (3) one medial wavefront that activates the medial right atrium and the atrial septum towards the coronary sinus os. The last two wavefronts rejoin in the lower medial right atrium, below the slow pathway, where in all normal cases right atrial activation ends. Normally, right atrial propagation lasts 92±10 ms, on average. However, there is clear evidence of individual modification of this normal pattern, even in a limited series of observations [1]. The case presented here is paradigmatic of how even a single atriotomy related to prior surgery may relevantly modify the normal activation pattern, by splitting the lateral wavefront into two components travelling superoanteriorly and inferiorly, respectively, to the atriotomy. A more complex activation pattern as a result of prior surgical atriotomy is given in Case 21. In the present case and in the next one, the line of conduction block produced by surgical atriotomy was well-evident during sinus rhythm, probably in relation to the atriotomy location and its proximity to the sinus node. Certainly, this facilitated the mapping procedure. Nonetheless, it cannot be excluded that, in the setting of a more complex surgical intervention for congenital heart disease, (1) sinus rhythm is not stable enough to allow high-density mapping, and/or (2) not all the atriotomy/lines of block can be identified in sinus rhythm. As already reported [3], this would require additional mapping during another rhythm (e.g. coronary sinus pacing), which will prolong the procedure and render it even more complex.

In this case, the ablation strategy was based on integration of the clinical evidence (morphology of the clinical atrial flutter) and all the data provided by electroanatomic mapping that were useful to identify candidate isthmi, such as isthmus extension and location, conduction velocity and voltage amplitude. To avoid overtreatment, the isthmus between the atriotomy and the superior vena cava os was not ablated, mainly because the clinical flutter morphology was unlikely to be related to this superior isthmus. Moreover, the proximity to the sinus node, the phrenic nerve capture during pacing in this area, and the extension and higher voltage of this isthmus could have rendered its ablation unsafe in addition to difficult. This relatively parsimonious strategy was very successful in this case, as determined in the mid-term follow-up.

Finally, of interest in this case and in Case 21, was the finding that no sign in terms of delayed conduction/reduced voltage was present at the site of atrial septal closure with a prosthetic patch.

## References

1. De Ponti R, Ho SY, Salerno-Uriarte JA et al. Electroanatomic analysis of sinus impulse propagation in the normal human atria. J Cardiovasc Electrophysiol 2002; 13: 1-10.
2. Lemery R, Soucie L, Martin B et al. Human study of biatrial electrical coupling: determinants of endocardial septal activation and conduction over interatrial connections. Circulation 2004; 110: 2083-2089.
3. Love BA, Collins KK, Walsh EP, Triedman JK. Electroanatomic characterization of conduction barriers in sinus/atrially paced rhythm and association with intra-atrial reentrant tachycardia circuits following congenital heart disease surgery. J Cardiovasc Electrophysiol 2001; 12: 17-25.

# Case 21
## Non-inducible Atrial Flutter in a Patient with Prior Surgery for Congenital Heart Disease (Example 2): Substrate Mapping in Sinus Rhythm with the Help of Imaging Integration

## Case Presentation

This a 49-year-old male patient who at the age of 24 underwent surgical closure of an ostium secundum atrial septal defect with a prosthetic patch. One year before the procedure, he began complaining of recurrent palpitations, documented at 12-lead ECG as atrial flutter with 240 ms cycle length. The morphology was consistent with a typical reverse form with negative P waves in V1–V2 and positive P waves in the inferior and lateral leads (Fig. 1). Most of the time, the arrhythmia was very symptomatic and required the patient's hospitalisation and treatment by DC-cardioversion. For this reason, he was referred for an electrophysiologic procedure while on sinus rhythm.

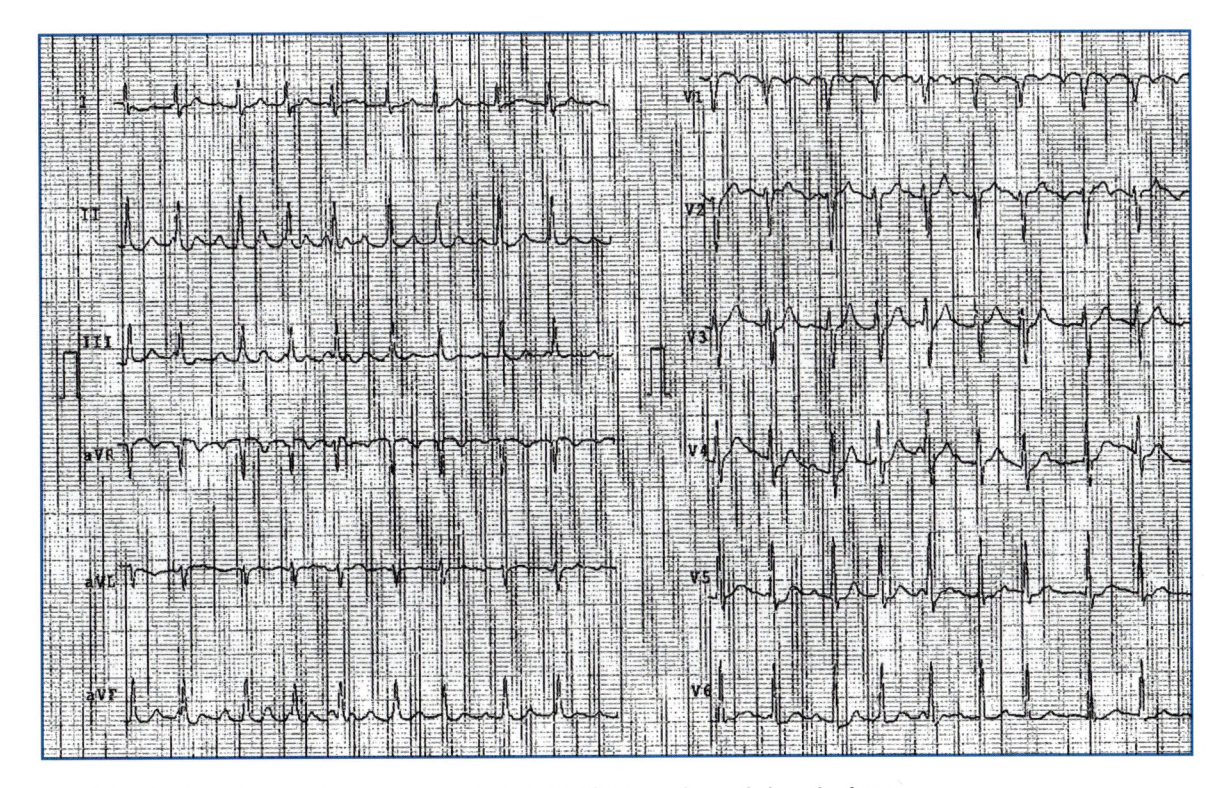

**Fig. 1.** Twelve-lead electrocardiogram of the clinical atrial flutter with a cycle length of 240 ms

## Procedure

At the beginning of the procedure, a decapolar catheter and two tetrapolar catheters were placed along the crista terminalis, in the coronary sinus and in the His-bundle area, respectively. Atrioventricular conduction was normal. As in the previous case, stimulation attempts by very aggressive protocols, also during isoprenaline infusion, did not induce arrhythmias. Since the patient had prior surgery involving right atrial atriotomy, it was felt that it was incorrect to empirically proceed to ablation of cavotricuspid isthmus conduction based on the assumption, from the P wave pattern, that the clinical arrhythmia was necessarily dependent only on isthmus conduction. Therefore, electroanatomic mapping of the right atrium in sinus rhythm was commenced, using a coronary sinus atriogram as the reference signal. After 80 sites were acquired, a pre-acquired three-dimensional image of a 16-slice computed tomography scan of the right atrium was superimposed on electroanatomic mapping using a single point at the coronary sinus os and the visual alignment/surface registration options. Superimposition, in the early phase of electroanatomic mapping, of the computed tomography image helped to better and more quickly identify the limits of the superior and inferior vena cava, tricuspid annulus, coronary sinus os and the extension of the cavotricuspid isthmus. Complete mapping was subsequently obtained, with the acquisition of 130 points (Fig. 2a, b). As for the left atrium, point acquisition in the right appendage was avoided, since placement of the mapping catheter in this structure may deform it. During pre-procedural segmentation, the right coronary artery was easy to isolate from its origin to the origin of the posterior interventricular branch. Integration of also the right coronary artery showed its zig-zag course along the cavotricuspid isthmus and the very close anatomic relationship of these two structures, although "penetration" of the right coronary artery in the paraseptal isthmus was clearly an artefact likely due to the different phases of the cardiac cycle in which the two images (computed tomography scan and electroanatomic mapping) were acquired. The activation map (Fig. 3a, b) clearly showed that the sinus node area was of normal size and position. The presence of two lines of block, identified by double potentials in the anterolateral wall (Fig. 3a), prolonged right atrial propagation to 130 ms

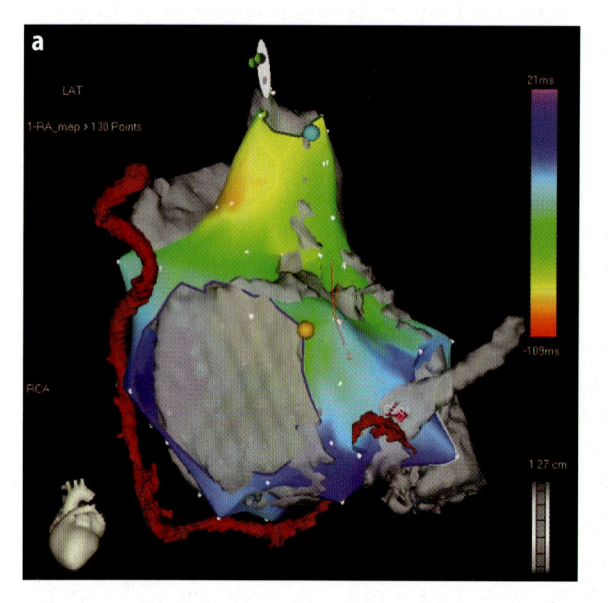

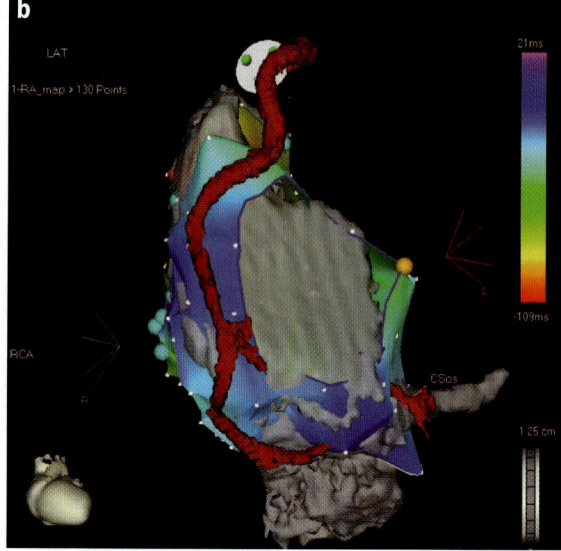

**Fig. 2a, b.** Activation map of the right atrium in sinus rhythm in caudal left lateral (**a**) and caudal anteroposterior (**b**) views. In *grey*, the three-dimensional image of the computed tomography scan is superimposed. The *red flag* labelled "CS os" indicates the site used for initial registration of the imported image. The *red tubular structure* is the right coronary artery, from its origin to the origin of the posterior interventricular branch

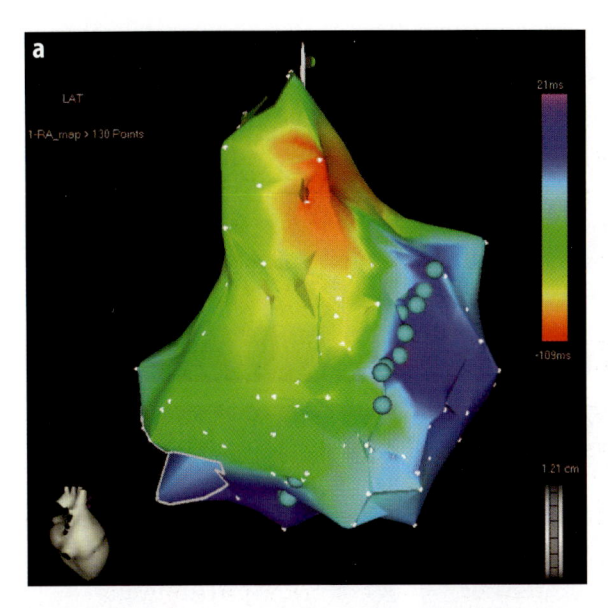

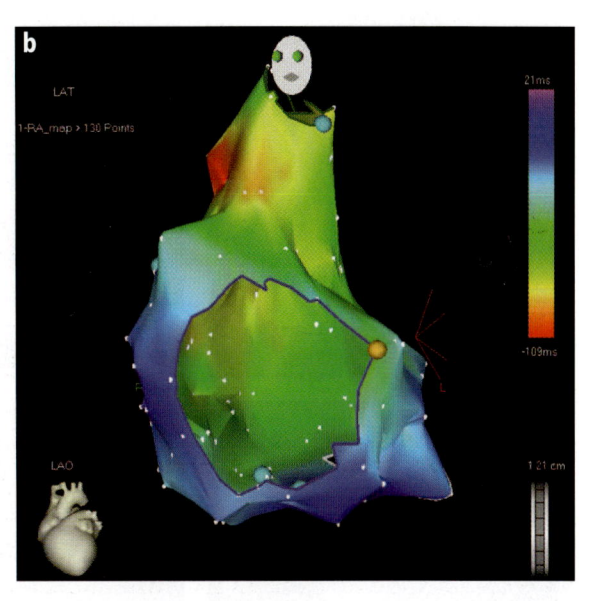

**Fig. 3a, b.** Activation map of the right atrium in sinus rhythm in right lateral (**a**) and left anterior oblique (LAO) (**b**) views. The *orange dot* indicates the site of His-bundle recording, and the *blue dots* the site of double potentials

and produced two different areas of latest activation in the lateral wall, anterior to the longer line of block (Fig. 3a) and in the central cavotricuspid isthmus (Fig. 3b). Analysis of the propagation map (Fig. 4) showed a complex pattern of wavefront fragmentation related to these two lines of conduction block, which can be described as follows: (1) as in the normal pattern, a dead-end activation of the superior vena cava was observed (Fig. 4a, b); (2) as expected, from the sinus node area, a medial wavefront originated and was directed towards the medial right atrium, the atrial septum, the coronary sinus os and the medial cavotricuspid isthmus (Fig. 4a'–e'); (3) the lateral wavefront, originating from the sinus node, directed anteroinferiorly and partly collided against the longer line of block (Fig. 4b), while partly continuing as (4) a superior wavefront that traveled superior to the line of block and activated from superior to inferior (Fig. 4d, e) the area between the line of block and the tricuspid annulus and as (5) an inferior wavefront, whose posteroinferior component passed in the very narrow posteroinferior channel between the shortest line of block and the inferior vena cava os (Fig. 4c–f), while its less inferior component, just after having activated the channel between the two lines of block (Fig. 4c), split into (6) a superior component that activated from inferior to superior the area between the longer line of block and the tricuspid annulus and collided with the superior wavefront (Fig. 4d–f) and (7) an anteroinferior component that directed medially along the cavotricuspid isthmus (Fig. 4d'–e') and finally collided in its central part with the medial wavefront (Fig. 4f'). Right atrial volume was 110 ml. The bipolar voltage map (Fig. 5a, b) showed generally preserved voltage, with low voltage only along the longer line of block, in small areas of the sinus node and of the cavotricuspid isthmus. As in Case 20, the site of closure of the atrial septal defect could not be identified by voltage mapping. Based on the electroanatomic data, three candidate isthmi were identified: (1) the isthmus between the two lines of block, which measured 10 mm, had a conduction velocity of 38 cm/s and bipolar voltage amplitude of 1.19±0.65 mV, on average; (2) the isthmus between the lower line of block and the inferior vena cava os, which measured 12 mm, with a conduction velocity of 37 cm/s and bipolar voltage amplitude between 0.27 and 4.9 mV; (3) the cavotricuspid isthmus, which had an extension from anterior to posterior of 19 mm and a bipolar voltage amplitude of 0.56±0.34 mV, with a conduction velocity (calculated during coronary sinus pacing, since collision of the two wavefronts in this isthmus did not allowed cor-

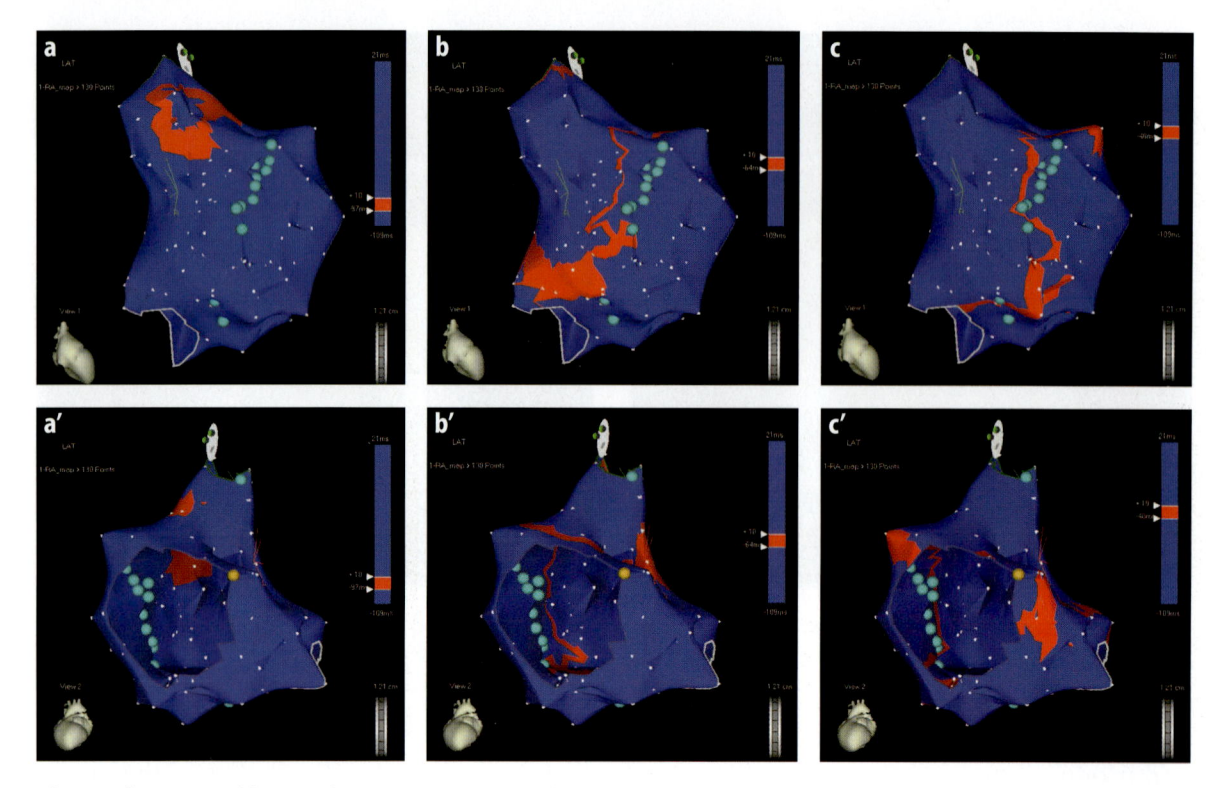

**Fig. 4a-f'.** Sequential frames of the propagation map of the right atrium during sinus rhythm in caudal right anterior oblique (RAO) (**a–f**) and caudal left lateral (**a'–f'**) views. Fragmentation of the propagation pattern due to the presence of the two atriotomies in the lateral wall is evident ▶

rect evaluation during sinus rhythm) of 65 cm/s. The first two isthmi could have sustained both lower-loop reentry around the os of the inferior vena cava and clockwise or counter-clockwise reentry in the lateral wall around the atriotomies, whereas the cavotricuspid isthmus may have been responsible for the peritricuspid loop, which could have combined with the right free wall loops to originate a double-loop reentry. The clinical morphology might have been sustained by one or by a combination of multiple loops; the most likely possibility being a clockwise peritri-

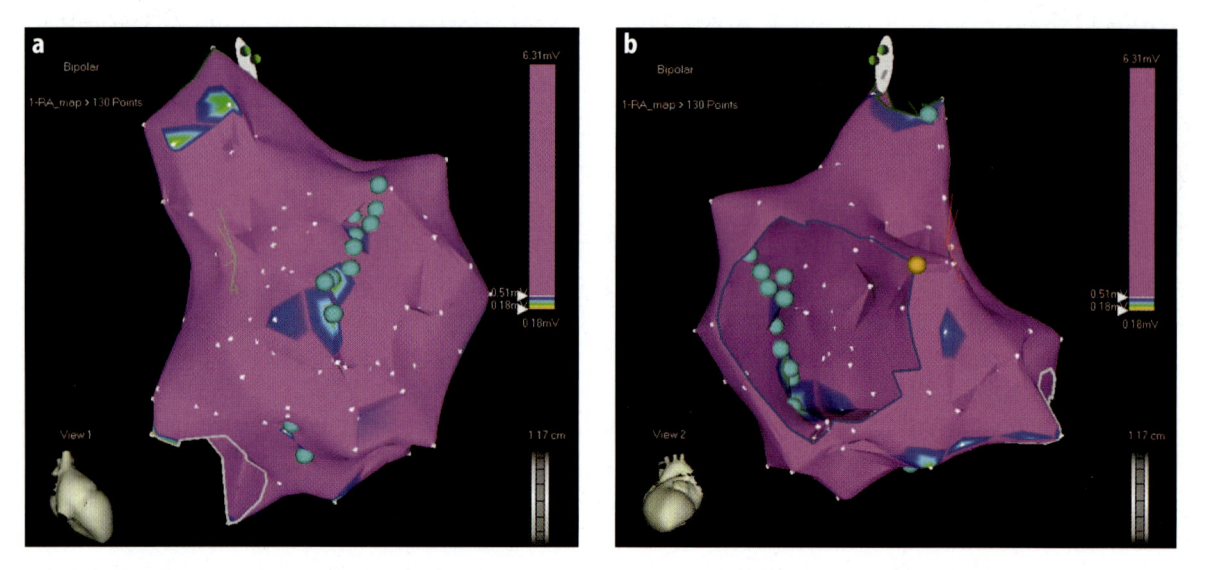

**Fig. 5a, b.** Bipolar voltage map of the right atrium during sinus rhythm in caudal RAO (**a**) and caudal left lateral (**b**) views. According to the setting of the colour-coded scale, areas with preserved voltage are shown in *purple*

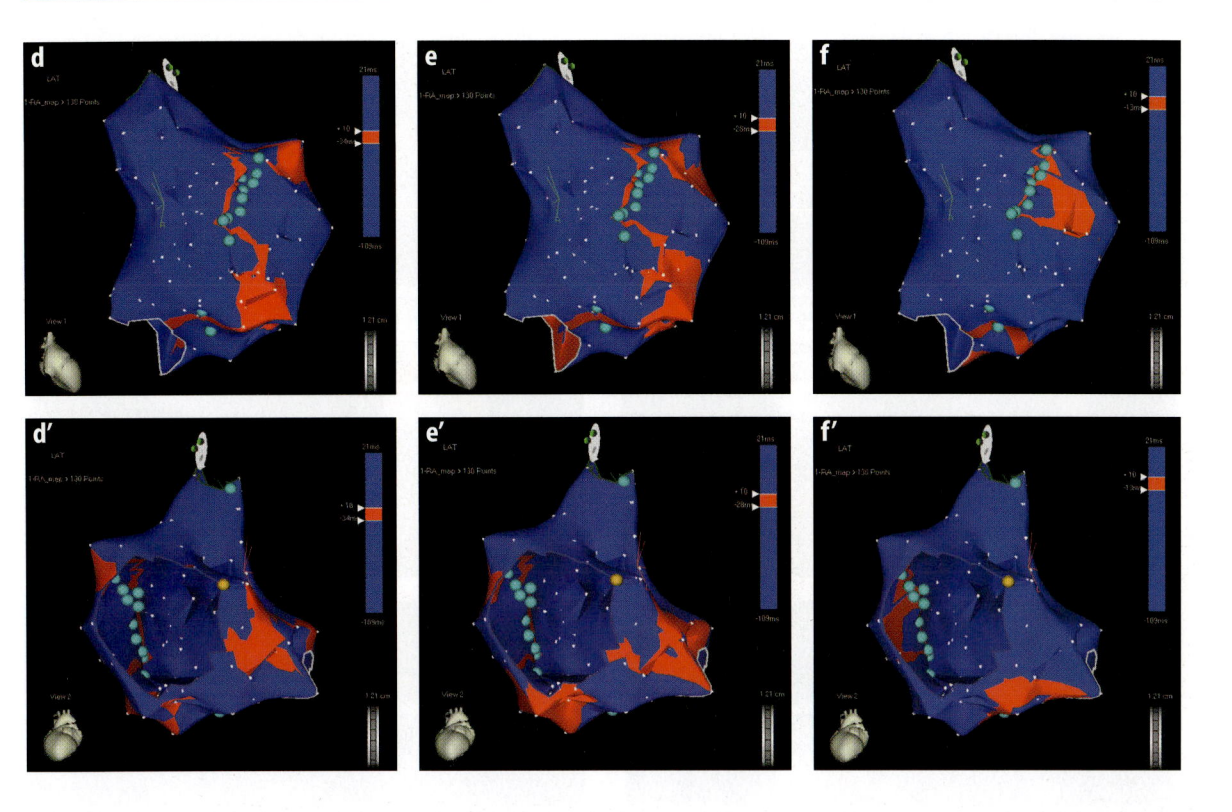

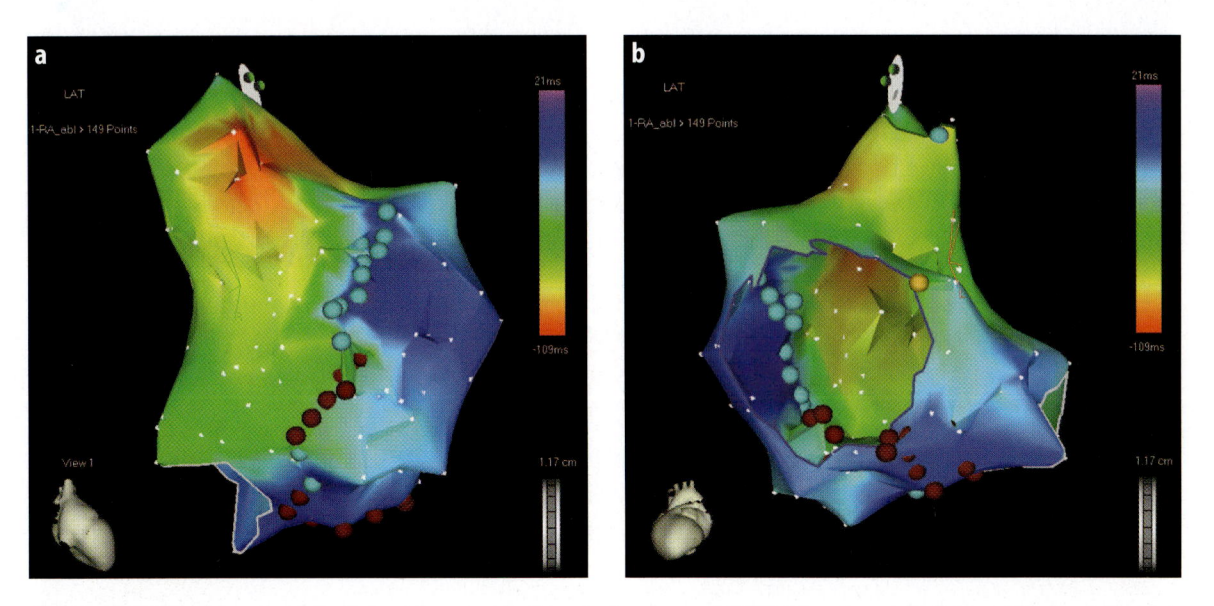

**Fig. 6a, b.** Activation map of the right atrium during sinus rhythm in caudal RAO (**a**) and caudal left lateral (**b**) views. *Red dots* indicate the ablation lines

cuspid reentry associated with a counter-clockwise reentry around one or both atriotomies in the right lateral wall. Neither the isthmus between the upper part of the line of block and the superior vena cava nor the one between the line of block and the tricuspid isthmus were considered as critical isthmi due to their extension, conduction velocity and voltage. The ablation line of the cavotricuspid isthmus was traced such that also the gap between the lower line of block and the inferior vena cava os was eliminated (Fig. 6a, b). Ten radiofrequency energy applications

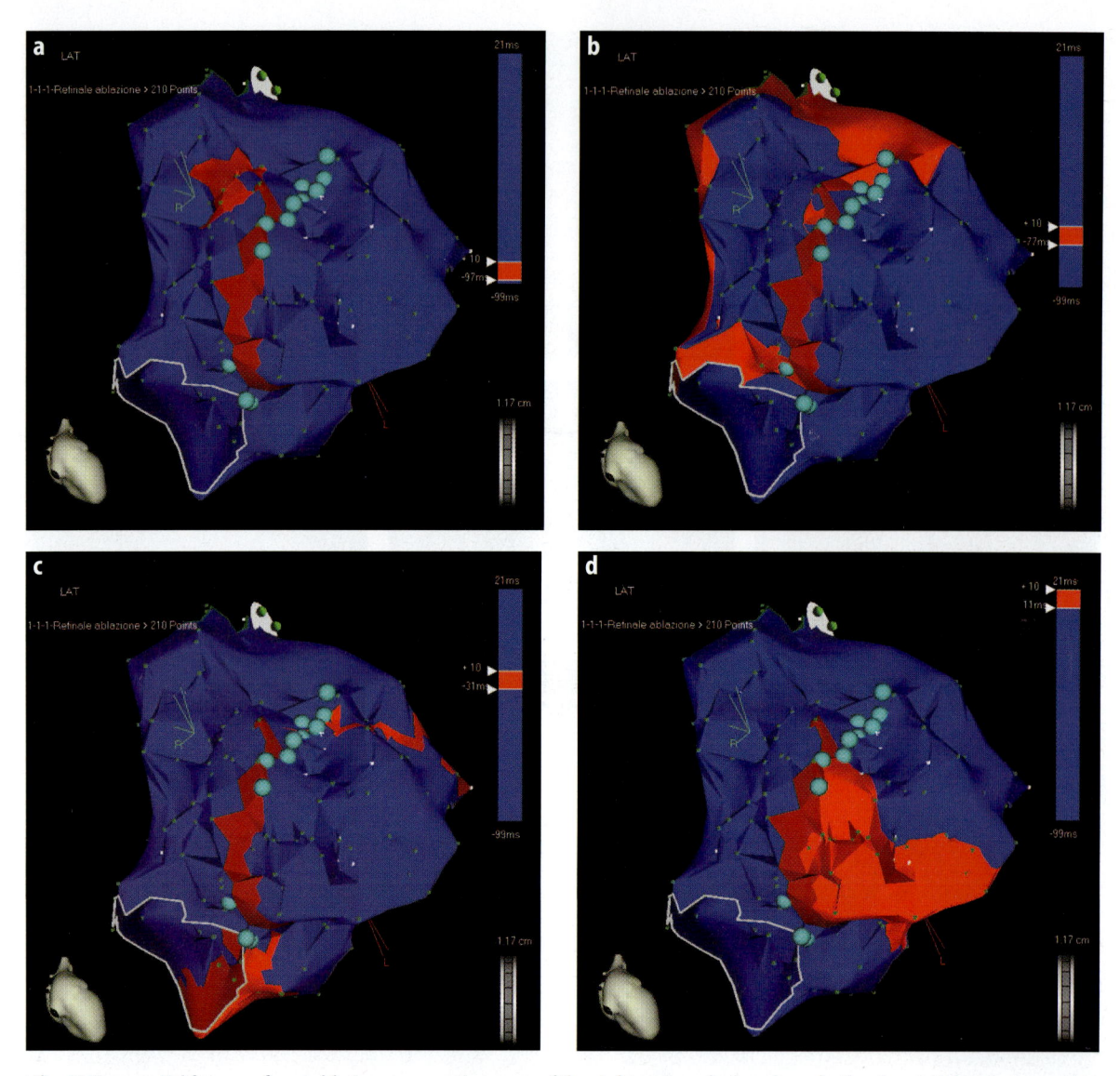

**Fig. 7.** Sequential frames of postablation propagation map of the right atrium during sinus rhythm in caudal RAO view, using the re-map option. After ablation of the conduction in the cavotricuspid isthmus and of the two gaps related to atriotomies, simplification of the propagation pattern is evident

using an irrigated-tip catheter (maximum power 45 W, temperature cut-off 43°C, duration 60 s) produced bidirectional conduction block over the cavotricuspid isthmus, as demonstrated by conventional methods. After the absence of phrenic-nerve capture was established by high output electrical stimulation, conduction over the remaining isthmus was abolished by further ablation, in which another nine applications were delivered with the same catheter and settings, with creation in this area of a continuous line of double potentials, separated by 70 ms. Remapping during sinus rhythm of the right atrium showed "simplification" of the activation pattern (Fig. 7). Four wavefronts originated from the sinus node area (Fig. 7a). The first two extinguished early in the superior vena cava and against the continuous line of block along the crista terminalis (Fig. 7b). The third was directed medially, activating the medial right atrium, the atrial septum and the medial cavotricuspid isthmus (Fig. 7c) and terminated against the line of cavotricuspid isthmus ablation. The fourth, from the sinus node area, moved anteriorly and activated from superior to inferior the dead-end channel between the lateral line of block, the ablation line in the cavotricuspid isthmus and the tricuspid annulus (Fig. 7d). Since the conduction block persisted along the lines of ablation 30 min after ablation was terminated, the procedure was terminated. The patient was arrhythmia-free without antiarrhythmic drug during a 16-month follow-up.

## Commentary

This case is both similar and different from the previous one. The two patients had similar surgical interventions for the same congenital defect and in both cases the complexity arose mainly from the fact that no arrhythmia was present or inducible at the time of the procedure. However, the same surgical procedure resulted in a different pattern of modified sinus propagation in the right atrium, with fragmentation into multiple wavefronts more evident in the present case. This difference may be explained by the difference, although minimal, in the surgical technique, which implied in the present case a different position and extension of the longer surgical incision and a second smaller atriotomy close to the inferior vena cava os.

In this case, mapping of the right atrium was integrated with the three-dimensional image obtained by computed tomography scan. Registration using a single point (coronary sinus os) and visual alignment/surface registration options resulted in imaging integration that contributed to a better and quicker localisation of the anatomic landmark in the right atrium and with the acquisition of a limited number of points, both crucial issues in an electroanatomic-based procedure. Certainly, a preprocedural computed tomography scan increases radiation exposure, although optimisation of the acquisition parameters minimises the dose delivered to the patient.

Last but not least, this case brings up the not negligible issue of the strict anatomic relationship between the right coronary artery and the cavotricuspid isthmus. In an interesting anatomic study [1], it was found that the right coronary artery runs epicardially in the right atrioventricular groove at a distance from the endocardium of 4.2±2.1 mm, on average, in the central isthmus (6 o'clock of the clock quadrant). Moreover, in 47% of the specimens, at the inferolateral isthmus, the right coronary artery is less than 4 mm from the endocardium. Based on these data and our imaging integration, the very low incidence of ischemic complications [2] resulting from ablation of the cavotricuspid isthmus, often offered as first-line treatment of typical atrial flutter, is perhaps surprising. This apparent discrepancy may be explained by the presence of a fat pad in the atrioventricular groove, between the coronary artery and the endocardial surface, which is likely to serve as an insulating layer and therefore limit the effect of myocardial heating by radiofrequency energy delivery, even when a long-electrode or irrigated-tip catheter is used.

## References

1. Cabrera JA, Sanchez-Quintana D, Farrè J et al. The inferior right atrial isthmus: further architectural insights for current and coming ablation technologies. J Cardiovasc Electrophysiol 2005; 16: 402-408.
2. Ouali S, Anselme F, Savoure A, Cribier A. Acute coronary occlusion during radiofrequency catheter ablation of typical atrial flutter. J Cardiovasc Electrophysiology 2002; 13: 1047-1049.

# Part IV

# Peculiar Anatomies

# Case 22
# Isolated Congenital Unilateral Absence of the Right Pulmonary Artery and Left Atrial Flutter: Are they Related?

## Case Presentation

This is a 51-year-old patient referred for episodes of atypical atrial flutter, with positive P waves in the inferior and precordial leads and negative in leads I and aVL (Fig. 1) at 290 ms cycle length. The arrhythmia recurred in spite of several sequential attempts with antiarrhythmic drugs (quinidine, propafenone, flecainide and amiodarone). The patient had episodes of hemoptisis during childhood, but no instrumental diagnostic procedure was performed at that time. While on sinus rhythm, the patient did not complain of any symptom and was in NYHA

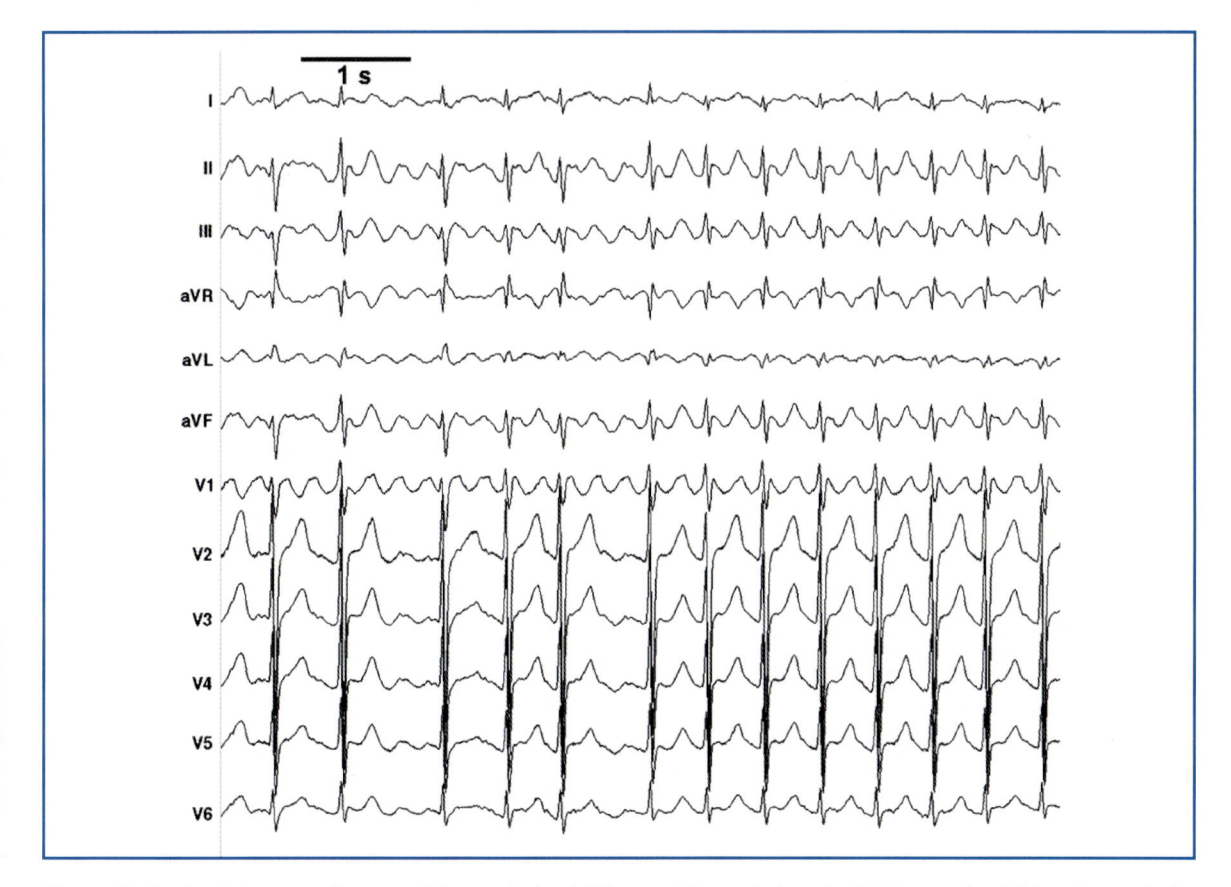

**Fig. 1.** Twelve-lead electrocardiogram of the atypical atrial flutter with a cycle length of 290 ms and variable atrioventricular conduction

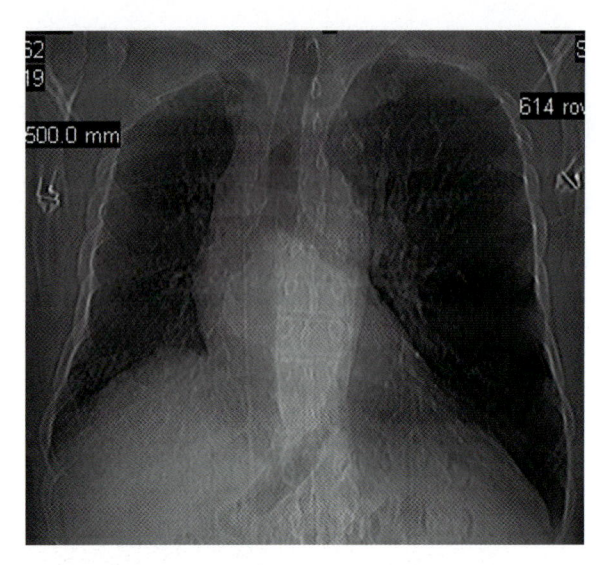

**Fig. 2.** Posteroanterior chest X-rays showing rightward displacement of the heart and asymmetric chest wall

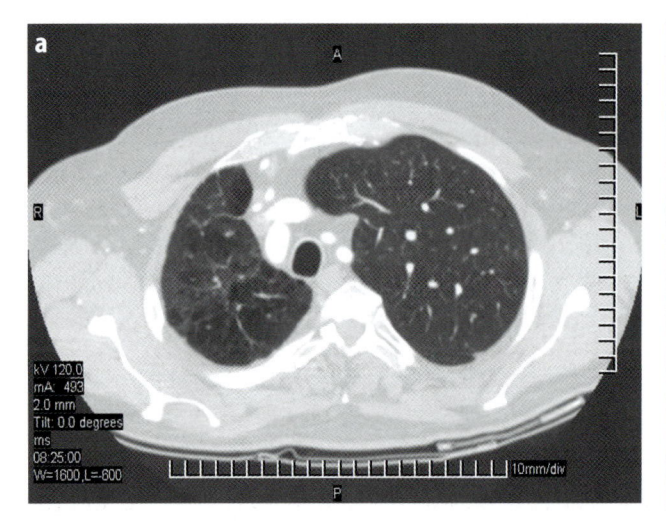

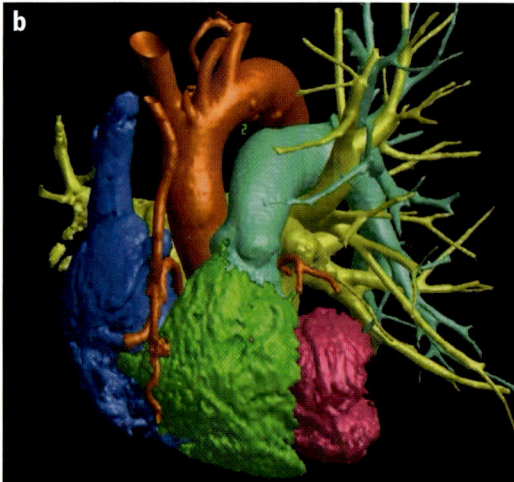

**Fig. 3a, b.** Transaxial image of the chest 16-slice computed tomography scan (**a**) and three-dimensional volume-rendering reconstruction of heart and great vessels in anteroposterior view (**b**). In **a**, *A* and *P* indicate anterior and posterior, respectively, and *R* and *L* right and left, respectively. The right lung is poorly expanded and dystrophic, with bollous cavities more evident in the posterior region. In **b**, the right atrium and superior vena cava are shown in *blue*, the right ventricle in *green*, the left ventricle in *violet*, the left atrium and pulmonary veins in *yellow*, the aorta in *orange* and the pulmonary artery with its left branch in *turquoise*. The absence of the right pulmonary artery branch is evident

class I. On admission, chest X-ray (Fig. 2) showed rightward displacement of the heart with an asymmetric chest wall. Echocardiography showed mild enlargement of both atria with minimal mitral regurgitation. A 16-slice computed tomography showed a poorly expanded and dystrophic right lung with evidence of several bollous cavities (Fig. 3a). Volume-rendering reconstruction clearly evidenced the absence of the right pulmonary artery (Fig. 3b). Reconstruction of the circulation in the right lung of this patient has been reported in detail elsewhere [1]. Briefly, the main collateral vessels to right lung were present, arising from a dilated right internal mammary and from the celiac trunk, but a ventilation-perfusion scintigraphy showed the absence of perfusion with almost normal ventilation in the right lung. Normal ventilation-perfusion was observed in the left lung. Three-dimensional reconstruction of the left atrium and pulmonary veins (Fig. 4) showed enlarged ostia of the left pulmonary veins, while the right pul-

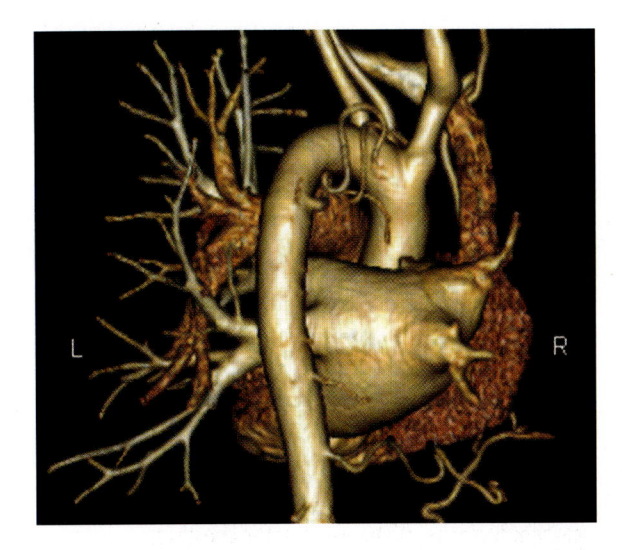

**Fig. 4.** Three-dimensional volume rendering image of the heart and great vessels in posteroanterior view. *L* and *R* indicate left and right, respectively. The absence of the right artery is again well evident, as is the difference in dimensions and branching between the left and right pulmonary veins

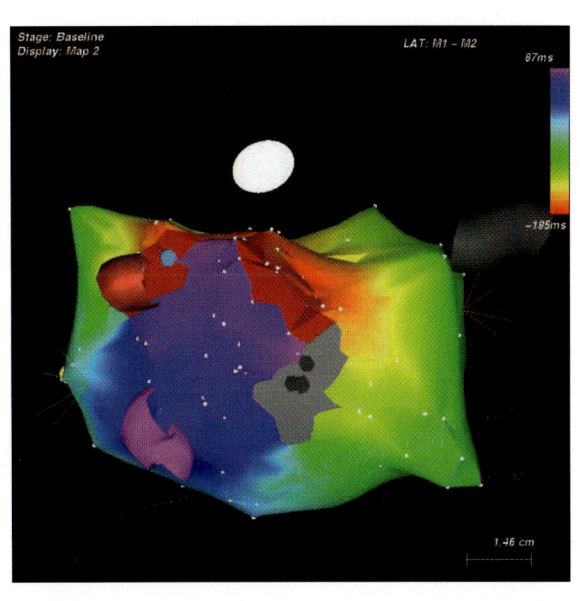

**Fig. 5.** Activation map of the left atrium during atypical atrial flutter in a cranial posteroanterior view. The *blue dot* indicates a site of double potentials; the *grey dots* indicate an electrically silent area in the posterior left atrial roof. The left and right superior pulmonary veins are shown as tubular icons, and the position of the right inferior pulmonary vein is shown by the points acquired in the proximal part of the vein

monary veins were of reduced diameter and had only minimal branching. The patient was admitted to the hospital during persistent recurrence of atrial flutter.

## Procedure

At the beginning of the procedure, the clinical tachycardia was present at 290 ms cycle length. Mapping was started, with a coronary sinus atriogram as the reference signal and the window of interest set as for macroreentry. Right atrial electroanatomic mapping clearly indicated the left origin of the arrhythmia. After transseptal puncture, mapping was continued in the left atrium until 97% of the tachycardia cycle length was reconstructed. The left atrial volume was 105 ml. The activation map (Fig. 5) showed that the tachycardia was sustained by a double-loop reentry, with a shared mid-diastolic isthmus located between an electrically silent area in the posterior wall and an area of block at the os of the left superior pulmonary vein. The first loop rotated clockwise around the electrically silent area, whereas the second loop had a counter-clockwise rotation around the os of the left superior pulmonary vein. Analysis of the bipolar voltage mapping (Fig. 6) during tachycardia showed the presence of very-low-amplitude potentials (< 0.2 mV) in the mid-diastolically activated isthmus, with the exception of a single point exhibiting a voltage of 1.1 mV. Sequential radiofrequency energy applications with an irrigated-tip catheter (maximum power 35 W, cut-off temperature 43°C, duration 60 s) along the mid-diastolic isthmus from the left superior pulmonary vein os to the electrically silent area prolonged tachycardia cycle length and eventually terminated the arrhythmia (Fig. 7), with local disappearance of electrical signals. Electrical stimulation using aggressive protocols induced no arrhythmia; therefore, the procedure was terminated. The subsequent 30-month follow-up was uneventful without any antiarrhythmic drugs.

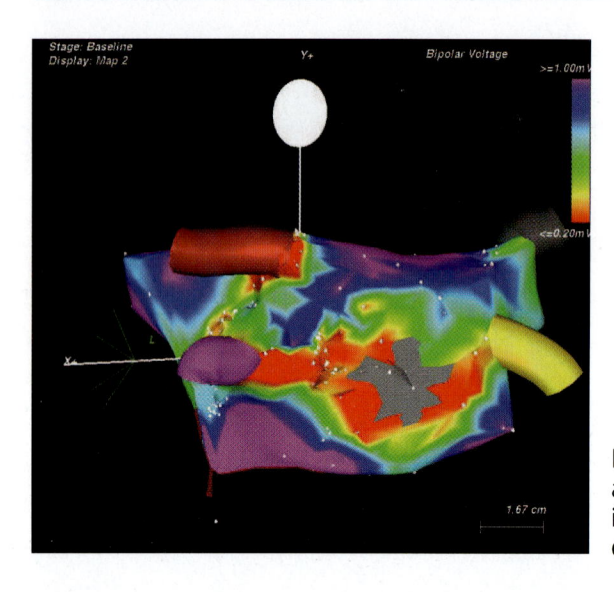

**Fig. 6.** Bipolar voltage mapping of the left atrium during atypical atrial flutter in posteroanterior view. Very low voltage is present around the posterior scar and in the area of the mid-diastolic isthmus

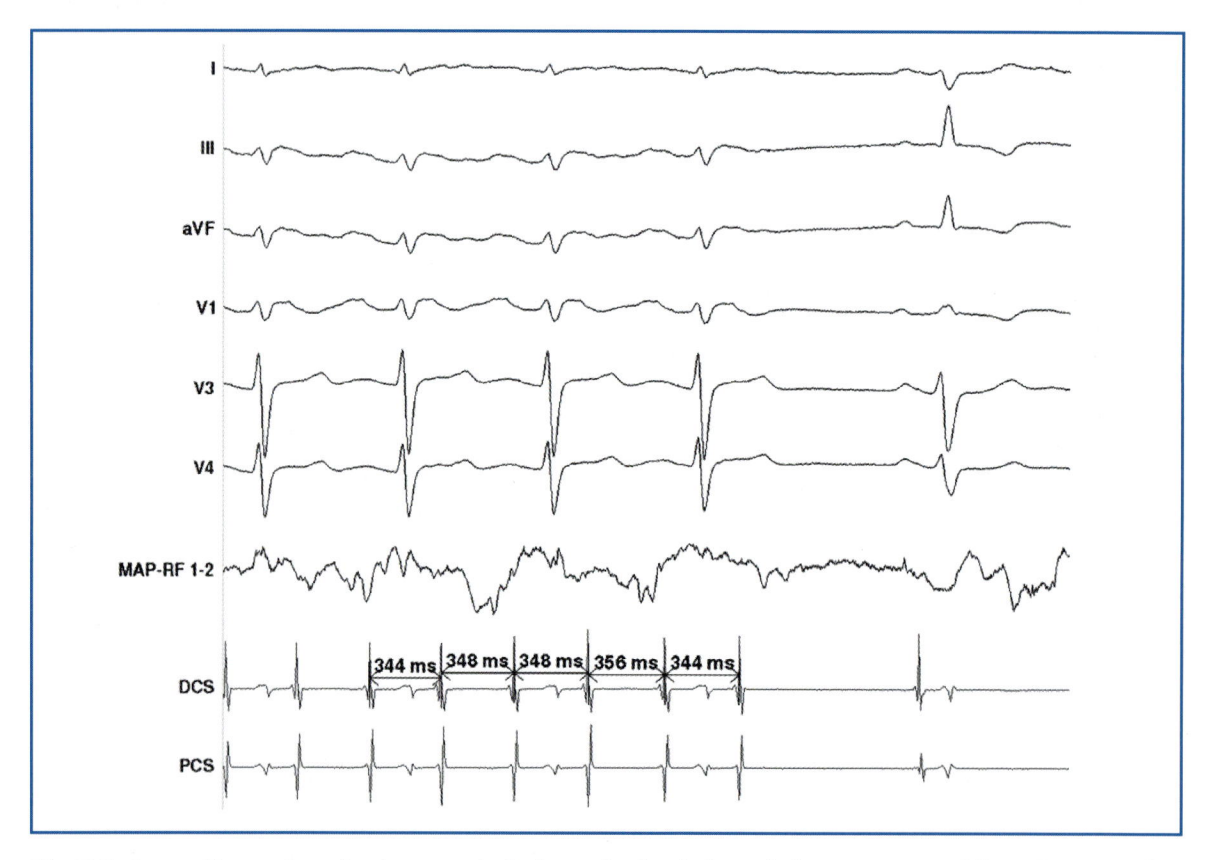

**Fig. 7.** Surface and intracavitary signals upon arrhythmia termination during radiofrequency energy delivery. From *top to bottom*, leads I, III, aVF, V1, V3, V4, bipolar signals from the distal electrode pair of the ablation catheter (MAP-RF 1-2) and bipolar signals from the distal (DCS) and proximal (PCS) coronary sinus are shown. During radiofrequency energy application in the mid-diastolic isthmus, the tachycardia cycle is prolonged and, eventually, the arrhythmia is terminated

## Commentary

Congenital unilateral absence of a pulmonary artery was first reported in 1868 [2] and its incidence, in the absence of other cardiac abnormalities, is 1/200,000 cases [3]. In Case 18, the absence of the right pulmonary artery was associated with a ventricular septal defect and subvalvular aortic stenosis. A recent review [4] of 108 cases of isolated unilateral absence of a pulmonary artery reported a 13% prevalence of asymptomatic patients and no incidence of palpitations among the referred symptoms. However, the considered population was younger, with a median age of 14 years (range 0.1–58 years) and a prevalence among infants (< 1 year of age) of 12%.

The relationship between an extracardiac abnormality, such as isolated absence of the right pulmonary artery, and a relatively uncommon arrhythmia, such as left atrial flutter, remains to be defined. In this patient, the absence of circulation in the right lung could have caused flow-overload in the left pulmonary veins, resulting in a jet lesion to the myocardium around their os and in the left atrium, where the flow from the left pulmonary veins encounters the posterior wall. Formation of this electrically silent area, combined with slow conduction in the adjacent area with very low amplitude potentials and mild left atrial enlargement, might have created optimal conditions for a stable reentrant circuit in the left atrium, which recurred frequently and was refractory to antiarrhythmic drug therapy.

*Acknowledgement. The images for this case were provided by Maurizio Del Greco, MD, Cardiology Department, S.Chiara Hospital, Trento, Italy, and Alessandro Cristoforetti, Department of Physics, University of Trento, Italy.*

# References

1. Del Greco M, Centonze M, Marini M et al. Three-dimensional reconstruction of the right lung circulation in a patient with isolated absence of the right pulmonary artery. Eur Heart J 2006; 27: 1281.
2. Pool PE, Vogel JHK, Blount SG. Congenital unilateral absence of a pulmonary artery. Am J Cardiol 1962; 10: 706-732.
3. Bouros D, Pare P, Panagou P et al. The varied manifestation of pulmonary artery agenesis in adulthood. Chest 1995; 108: 670-676.
4. Harkel ADJT, Blom NA, Ottenkamp J. Isolated unilateral absence of a pulmonary artery: a case report and review of the literature. Chest 2002; 122: 1471-1477.

# Case 23
# Left Atrial Ablation of Atrial Fibrillation in a Patient with Dextrocardia: the Complexities of an Inverted Anatomy

## Case Presentation

This is a 70-year-old female patient with atrial fibrillation and dextrocardia with situs visceris inversus. Over the last 10 years, the patient had experienced recurrent episodes of paroxysmal atrial fibrillation triggered by ectopies with "P on T" aspect. The arrhythmia recurred in spite of the administration of antiarrhythmic drugs. Other than the abnormal position, no relevant structural heart disease was documented by transthoracic echocardiogram. A pre-procedural transoesophageal echocardiogram showed no intracavitary thrombus. Contrast-enhanced computed tomography, in addition to three-dimensional reconstruction of the heart and of the pulmonary veins, allowed visualisation of the inverted position of the peripheral veins, with a rectilinear course of the axis of the left femoral-left iliac vein, inferior vena cava and right atrium. For this reason, transseptal catheterisation was unusually planned through the left femoral vein. Antiarrhythmic drug therapy was withdrawn 1 week before the procedure and the arrhythmia was persistent at the time of the procedure.

## Procedure

A multipolar catheter was positioned in the coronary sinus from the left internal jugular vein. A probe for intracardiac ehocardiography was inserted through the right femoral vein, whereas the mapping catheter was inserted through the left femoral vein. The right atrial anatomy was reconstructed, as shown in Figure 1a, b. Along with the inverted geometry of the right atrial chamber, the posterior displacement of the fossa ovalis, clearly identified and tagged (brown tag) with the help of intracardiac echocardiography, was unusual. Transseptal catheterisation was performed through the left femoral vein and, during withdrawal of the assembly from the superior vena cava, the needle indicator was positioned at 7 o'clock. Engagement of the fossa ovalis was confirmed by both a rightward "jump" and intracardiac echocardiography. Afterwards, the needle was advanced into the left atrium and its position was confirmed by both pressure recording and dye injection. After transseptal catheterisation was accomplished, a circular mapping catheter (Lasso 15, Biosense-Webster, USA) and the electroanatomic mapping/ablation catheter were inserted in the left atrium. Left atrial geometry was reconstructed; both atria are displayed in Figure 2a, b. As anticipated by computed tomography imaging, a common os of the "lateral" pulmonary veins was present, whereas early branching with multiple sub-branches was identified in the "medial" pulmonary veins. Electrophysiologically

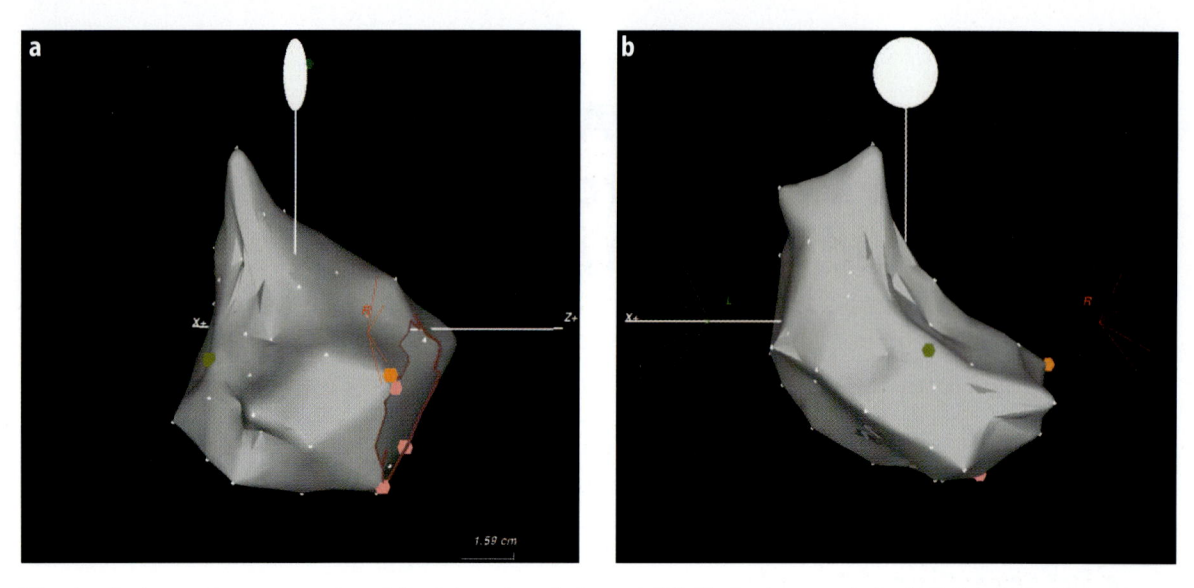

**Fig. 1a, b.** Anatomic reconstruction of the right atrium during atrial fibrillation in posteriorly tilted right lateral (**a**) and posteroanterior (**b**) views. The *orange dot* indicates the site of His-bundle recording. The *brown dot* indicates the center of the fossa ovalis, as also defined using intracardiac echocardiography. *Pink dots* indicate sites around the tricuspid annulus

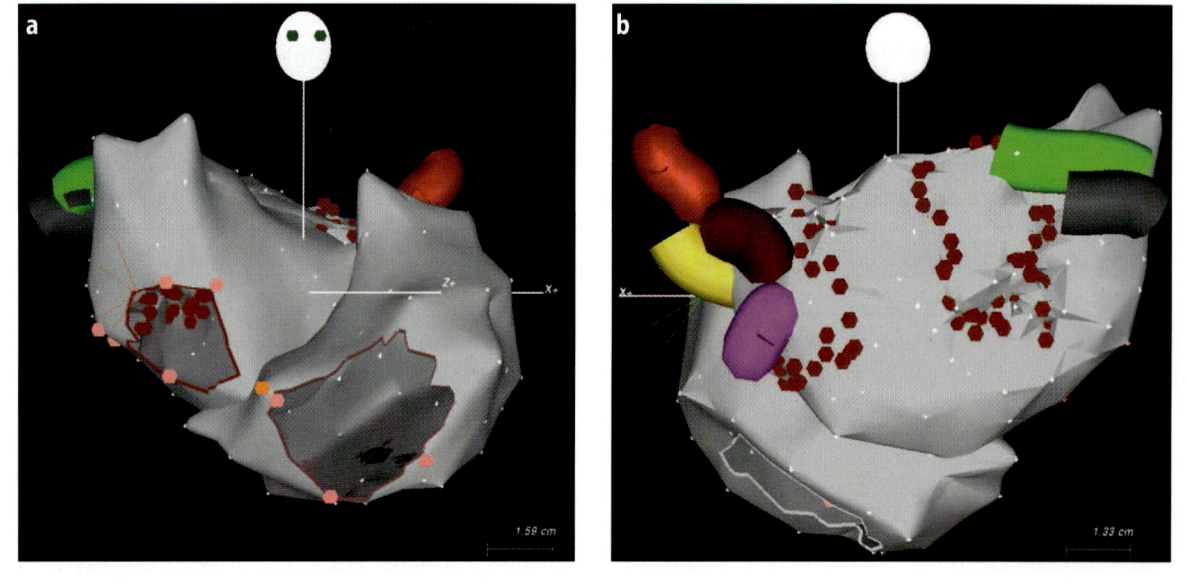

**Fig. 2a, b.** Anatomic reconstruction of both atria during atrial fibrillation in right anterior oblique (RAO) (**a**) and posteroanterior (**b**) views. The pulmonary veins are tagged by tubular icons; the *red dots* indicate the line of ablation. As shown in (**a**), in dextrocardia patients the RAO projection provides a mirror image of what is usually seen in left anterior oblique (LAO) view in normal hearts. The same applies to the LAO projection

guided antral ablation of the pulmonary veins was carried out by delivering sequential radiofrequency energy applications with an irrigated-tip catheter (maximum power 30 W, cut-off temperature 43°C, duration 60 s). After stable sinus rhythm had been restored by electrical cardioversion, bidirectional block of the atrium-vein conduction was assessed. During the 24-month follow-up, the patient was arrhythmia-free, initially on antiarrhythmic drug therapy, which was subsequently withdrawn.

## Commentary

In patients with dextrocardia, access to the left atrium to treat supraventricular arrhythmia may present serious difficulties. In this case, accurate reconstruction of the right atrium, precise localisation of the fossa ovalis with the help of intracardiac echocardiography and reconstruction of the left atrium with pulmonary-vein tagging were essential to safe transseptal catheterisation and to manipulating the roving catheter before and during ablation. It should be noted that, in patients with dextrocardia, fluoroscopy provides a mirror image of the normal anatomy, and the usual way of manipulating the catheter may not obtain the desired effect. Therefore, the actual catheter position has to be carefully monitored on the electroanatomic map, especially when pulmonary-vein ablation is performed. At the time of this procedure, the CartoMerge software was not available; therefore, imaging integration was not possible. This might have been of help, especially in the early phase of mapping.

*Acknowledgement.* The images for this case were provided by Maurizio Del Greco, MD, Cardiology Department, S.Chiara Hospital, Trento, Italy.

# Case 24
# Uncommon Anatomy of the Pulmonary Veins (Example 1): Common Trunk of the Inferior Pulmonary Veins

## Case Presentation

This a 66-year-old male patient with recurrent paroxysmal atrial fibrillation associated with hypertension, which was treated with beta-blockers. Previously, he underwent percutaneous revascularisation for angina pectoris. Over the last six months, the patient had complained of palpitations, which were documented by Holter monitoring as atrial fibrillation with fast ventricular response and initiated by left atrial ectopies. Transthoracic echocardiography showed a normal left ventricle with preserved systolic function and mild septal hypertrophy; the atria were normally sized and there were no signs of pulmonary hypertension. The chest X-ray was also normal. The patient never complained of dyspnea, either at rest or during effort. Since atrial fibrillation was not responsive to antiarrhythmic drug therapy, electrical isolation of the pulmonary vein was planned. In addition, a contrast-enhanced multi-slice computed tomography scan of the heart was performed with the patient in sinus rhythm.

## Procedure

Before the procedure, computed tomography scan data at 70% of diastole were imported into the electroanatomic system and segmented using the CartoMerge software to separate the thoracic structures and extract the three-dimensional anatomy of the left atrium and the proximal tract of the pulmonary veins. As shown in Figure 1a, b, the anatomy of the superior pulmonary veins was normal, although the os of the left superior pulmonary vein was more medial than expected, compared to the position of the left atrial appendage. Conversely, a large common trunk of the inferior pulmonary veins was evident in the posteromedial wall. The common trunk had a posteromedial orientation and directly gave origin to the right inferior vein, while the left inferior vein had an early take-off from the trunk, with a 90° angle and a lateral orientation. The imprint of the oesophagus and of the descending aorta on the left inferior vein, and branching of the latter into two parts were particularly evident. During the procedure, pulmonary-vein angiography was performed prior to ablation. Repeated attempts to subselectively catheterise the left inferior vein were fruitless, due to its position and take-off from the common trunk. Separate electroanatomic reconstructions of the left atrium and the proximal tract of the pulmonary veins were performed during sinus rhythm, with a coronary sinus atriogram as reference signal. Registration was done using a single point on the left atrial roof and the visual alignment/surface registration options. Superimposition of the computed tomography scan with the elec-

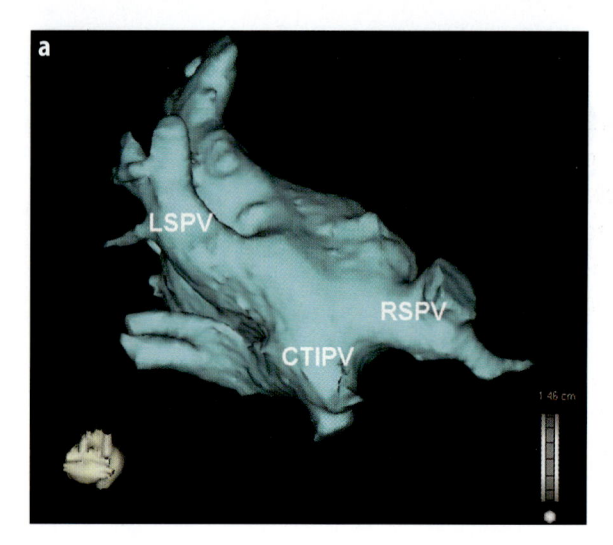

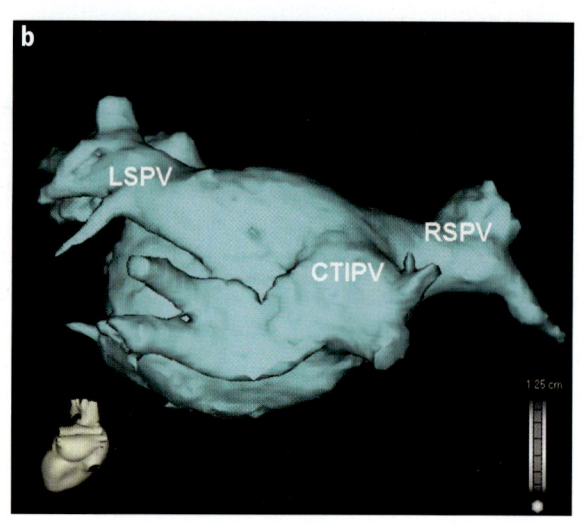

**Fig. 1a, b.** Three-dimensional imaging of multi-slice computed tomography scan acquisition in cranial right lateral (**a**) and posteroanterior (**b**) views. *CTIPV* Common trunk of the inferior pulmonary vein, *LSPV* left superior pulmonary vein, *RSPV* right superior pulmonary vein

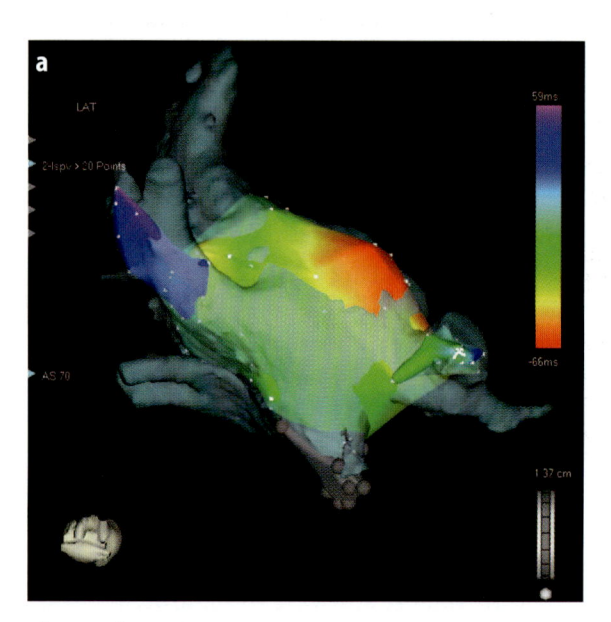

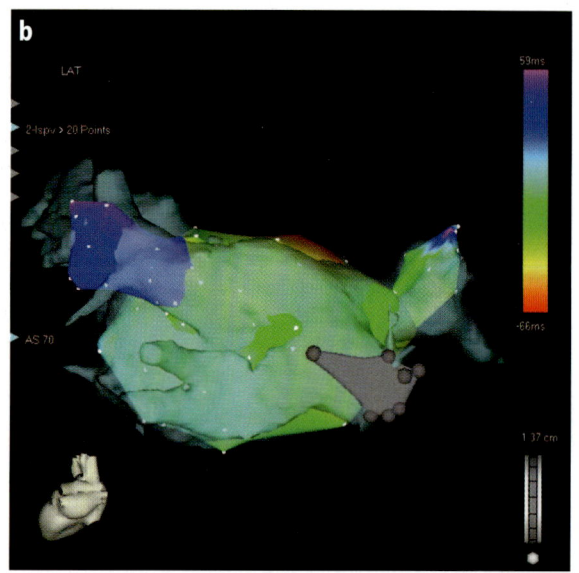

**Fig. 2a, b.** Superimposition of the activation electroanatomic map of the left atrium and proximal tract of the pulmonary veins on the computed tomography scan image in cranial right lateral (**a**) and posteroanterior (**b**) views. *Grey dots* indicate the absence of electrical activity inside the common trunk

troanatomic reconstruction (Fig. 2a, b) showed good alignment of the two three-dimensional images, with a mean distance between the two surfaces of 1.5±1.01 mm. Interestingly, mapping showed no electrical signal in the common inferior trunk, which therefore was annotated as electrically silent (grey area in Fig. 2a, b). The left inferior pulmonary vein, due to its anatomic peculiarity, could not be probed and mapped using a deflectable roving catheter. Electrical disconnection of the pulmonary veins at the venoatrial junction was successfully performed without complications using an irrigated-tip catheter (maximum power 30 W, cut-off temperature 43°C, duration 60 s) and a circular mapping catheter (Lasso Variable 2515, Biosense-Webster, USA). In a 12-month follow-up, the patient was arrhythmia free on beta-blocker therapy.

## Commentary

The lesson from anatomists [1] and radiologists [2] is that the pulmonary vein anatomy is highly variable. Nevertheless, a common trunk of the inferior pulmonary veins is a very unusual finding. Indeed, it represented the major pulmonary vein abnormality we encountered in the first 50 consecutive cases evaluated by computed tomography scan. Our observation [3] has been corroborated by other reports [4–6] describing variants of this pulmonary-vein abnormality. Its prevalence, although expected to be very low, is currently unknown.

If this asymptomatic abnormality had not been recognised beforehand, it could have prolonged the procedure and possibly compromised its safety in the fruitless attempt to identify the left inferior pulmonary vein os at its usual location. Currently, the wide range of anatomic variants in the pulmonary veins seems to justify the time and resources used for pre-procedural three-dimensional imaging.

## References

1. Ho SY, Cabrera JA, Tran VH Farrè J et al. Architecture of the pulmonary vains: relevance to radiofrequency ablation. Heart 2001; 86: 265-270.
2. Oh YW, Lee KY, Choi EJ et al. Assessment of pulmonary venous variation by multidetector row CT: clinical implication for catheter ablation techniques for atrial fibrillation. Eur J Radiol 2007. doi: 10.1016/j.eirad.2007.03.001.
3. Marazzi R, De Ponti R, Lumia D et al. Common trunk of the inferior pulmonary veins: an unexpected anatomical variant detected before ablation by multi-slice computed tomography. Europace 2007; 9: 121.
4. Dukkipati S, Holmvang G, Scozzaro M et al. An unusual confluence of the inferior pulmonary veins in a patient undergoing catheter ablation for atrial fibrillation. J Cardiovasc Electrophysiol 2006; 17: 1034.
5. Sra J, Malloy A, Shah H, Krum D. Common ostium of the inferior pulmonary veins in a patient undergoing left atrial ablation for atrial fibrillation. J Interv Card Electrophysiol 2006; 15: 203.
6. Shapiro M, Dodd JD, Brady TJ, Abbara S. Common pulmonary venous ostium of the right and left inferior pulmonary veins: an unusual pulmonary vein anomaly depicted with 64-slice cardiac computed tomography. J Cardiovasc Electrophysiol 2007; 18: 110.

# Case 25
# Uncommon Anatomy of the Pulmonary Veins (Example 2): the "Roof Pulmonary Vein"

## Case Presentation

This is a 50-year-old male patient with recurrent episodes of idiopathic paroxysmal atrial fibrillation refractory to medical therapy. During repeated 24-h Holter monitoring, long-lasting episodes of atrial fibrillation (up to 24 h) were initiated by P/T ectopies. He was then referred to our institution for ablation of atrial fibrillation. Transthoracic echocardiogram showed normal ventricular function and mild dilatation of the left atrium. Transoesophageal echocardiogram showed no intracavitary thrombi.

## Procedure

Before the procedure, the data set of the pre-acquired computer tomography scan was imported in the electroanatomic system and segmented, as described in Case 24. During segmentation, multiple branching of the pulmonary vein and the presence of a common os of the left pulmonary veins were noted. However, the most uncommon finding was a third right pulmonary vein, with a separate take-off from the medial left atrial roof (Fig. 1a, b). The direction of the course of this pulmonary vein was initially posterior and medial and then superior. Further off-line analysis showed that the diameter of this vessel measured 15 mm at the os but it quickly decreased to 9 mm. After the proximal tract, the course of the vein was similar to that of the right superior pulmonary vein, as it directed superomedially, draining from the right superior lobe. At the beginning of the procedure, the patient was in atrial fibrillation. After transseptal catheterisation, an attempt to restore sinus rhythm by DC-shock was made, but early recurrences of atrial fibrillation were repeatedly initiated by both the right and left pulmonary veins. Therefore, the left atrium and the pulmonary veins were anatomically reconstructed during atrial fibrillation. At this time, since the position of the os of the "roof vein" was not easily identified with the mapping catheter, no attempt to cannulate this vein was made. Registration of the computed tomography scan image, as described in the previous case, resulted in good superimposition of the two images (Fig. 2a, b), with a mean distance between the two surfaces, as automatically calculated by the system, of 1.79±1.2 mm. With the guidance of the endocardial and epicardial views obtained from the registered computed tomography scan image, the "roof vein" os could readily be accessed with the mapping catheter and the 20-pole circular mapping catheter (Lasso Variable 2515, Biosense-Webster, USA) could be positioned at the venoatrial junction (Fig. 3). The proximal part of the "roof vein" was then reconstructed and 22 sites were

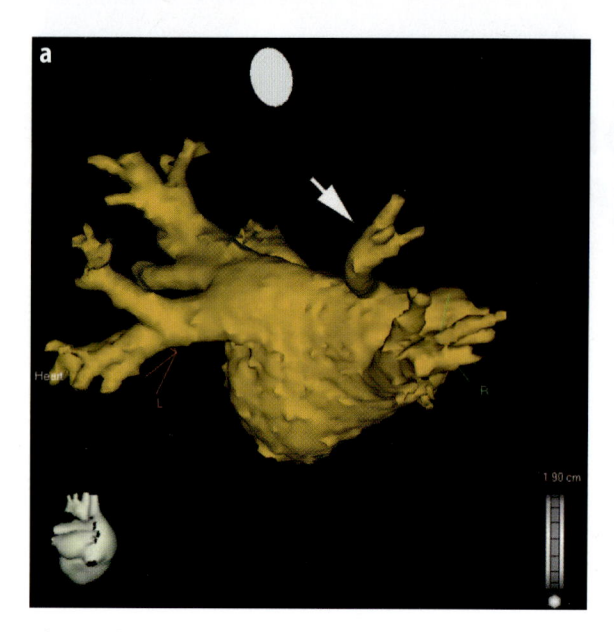

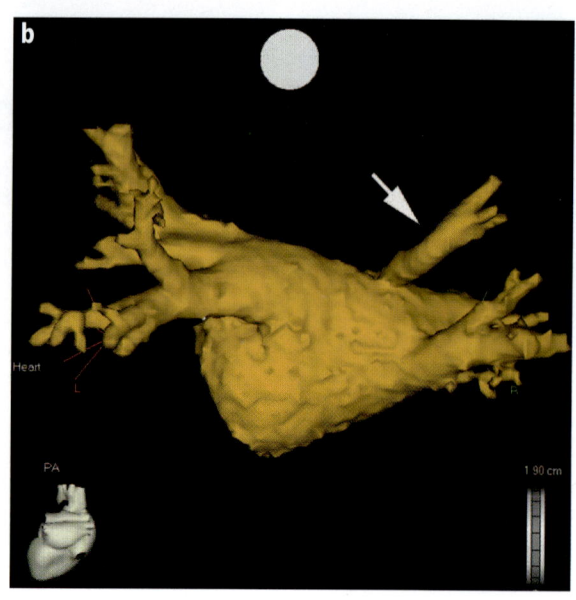

**Fig. 1a, b.** Three-dimensional computed tomography image of the left atrium and pulmonary veins in caudal right lateral (**a**) and posteroanterior (**b**) views. The "roof pulmonary vein" is indicated by the *arrow*

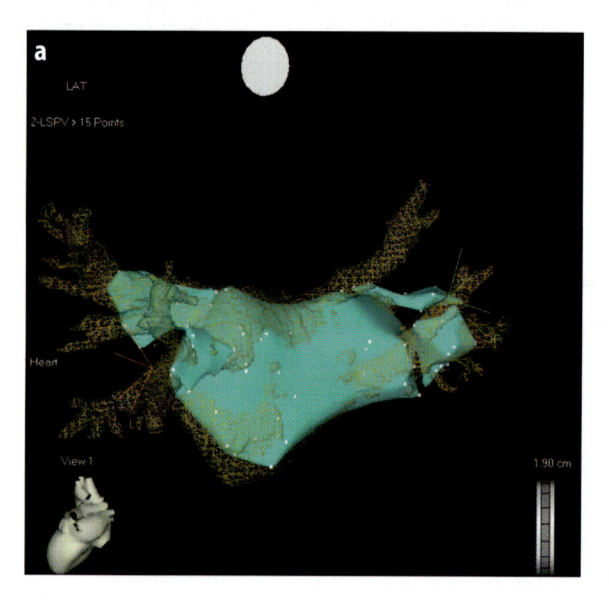

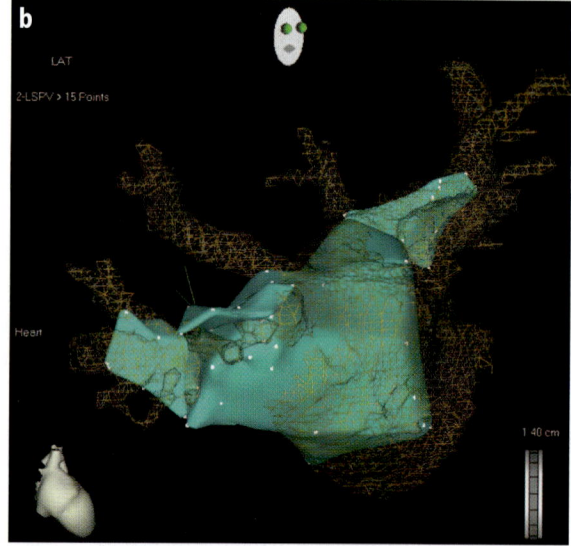

**Fig. 2.** Three-dimensional computed tomography image of the left atrium and pulmonary veins, displayed as a mesh and superimposed on the electroanatomic reconstruction of the left atrium and pulmonary veins. Posteroanterior (**a**) and right anterior oblique (RAO) (**b**) views are shown

acquired (Fig. 4a, b). As shown in Figure 5, at the os and inside the "roof vein" atrial activity during atrial fibrillation was very fast and highly fragmented, together suggesting very short refractoriness. Electrical disconnection was obtained by circumferential ostial ablation, delivering sequential radiofrequency energy applications with an irrigated-tip catheter (maximum power 30 W, maximum temperature 43°C, duration 60 s), as shown in Figure 6a. After electrical disconnection of the pulmonary veins, stable sinus rhythm resumed spontaneously. Postablation venography evidenced no variation of the diameter of the four pulmonary veins or of the "roof

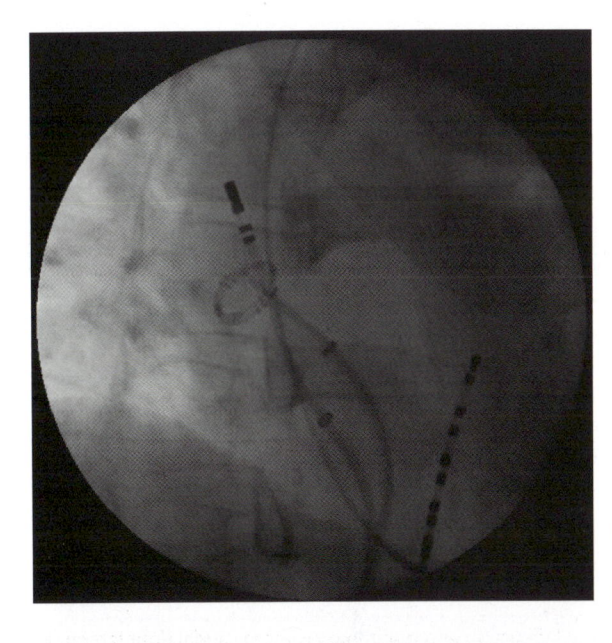

**Fig. 3.** Fluoroscopic image in 30° RAO view, showing the position of the circular mapping catheter at the os of the "roof pulmonary vein", while the mapping catheter is inside the vein

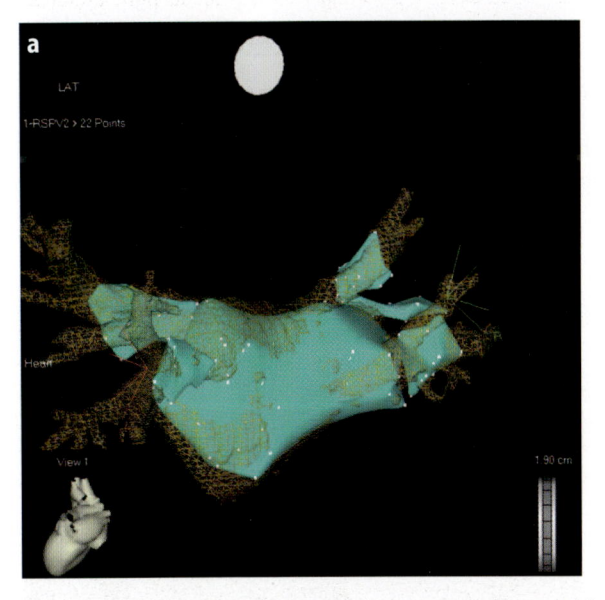

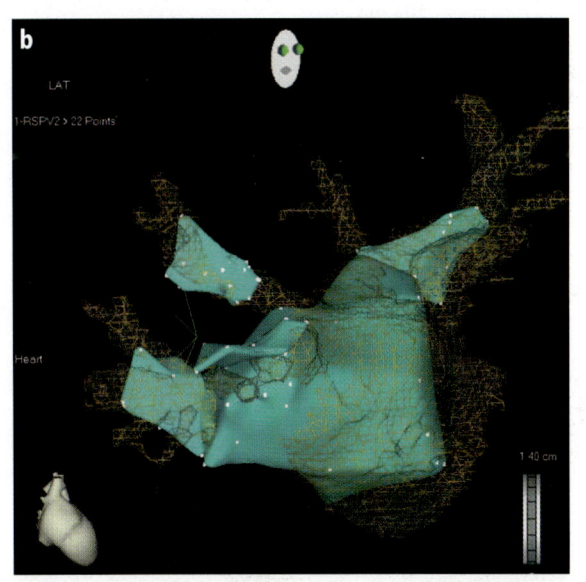

**Fig. 4.** Three-dimensional computed tomography image of the left atrium and pulmonary veins, displayed as a mesh and superimposed on the electroanatomic reconstruction of the left atrium and pulmonary veins, once the "roof pulmonary vein" had been reconstructed. Posteroanterior (**a**) and RAO (**b**) views are shown

vein" (Fig. 6b). During follow-up, the patient had atrial fibrillation recurrences during the first month after ablation. These disappeared in the following months and the patient is now off antiarrhythmic drugs.

## Commentary

Additional pulmonary veins are usually located between the superior and inferior pulmonary vein oses, draining from the right middle lobe or, more rarely, the left lingular segment (1). However, in this patient, the "roof pulmonary vein" had an independent course, with an orifice located in the medial left atrial roof, well-separated from the oses of the right pulmonary veins. As

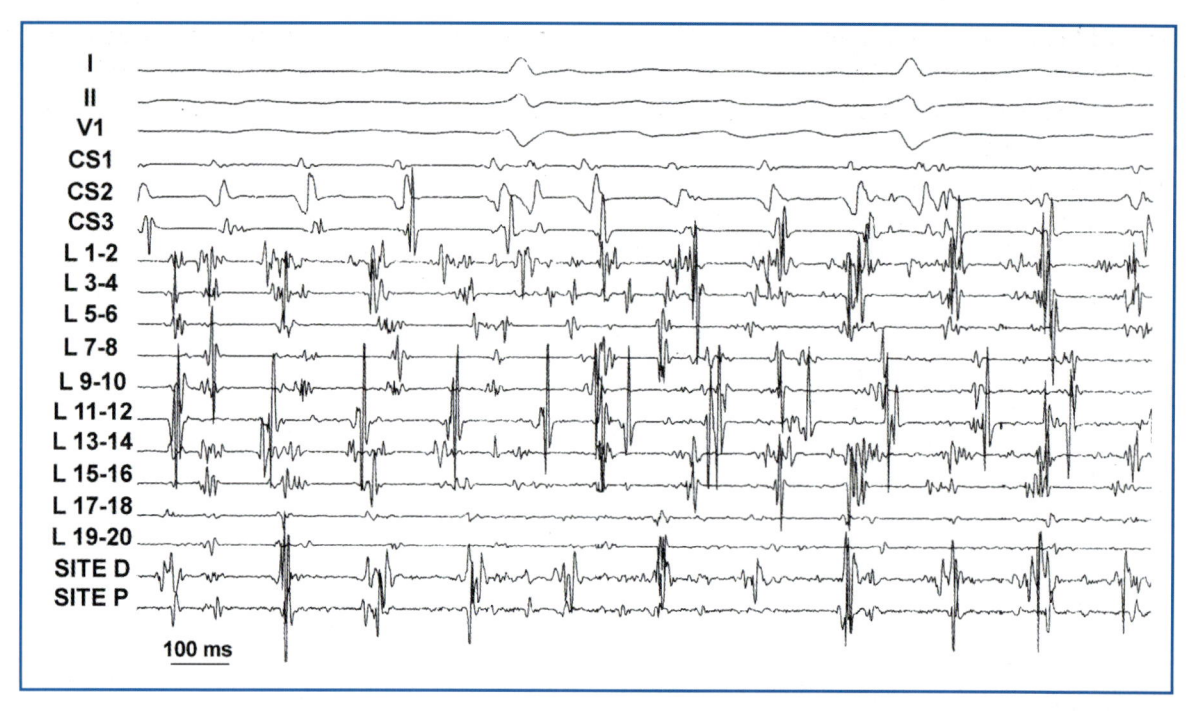

**Fig. 5.** Surface and intracavitary signals during atrial fibrillation, showing fast fragmented electrical activity inside the "roof pulmonary vein". From *top to bottom*, tracings are displayed as follows: lead I, II, V1, bipolar recordings of the coronary sinus catheter from distal to proximal (CS1–3), bipolar recordings from the 20-pole circular mapping catheter positioned at the os of the "roof pulmonary vein" (L1–2 to L19–20) and bipolar recordings from the distal (SITE D) and proximal (SITE P) electrode pairs of the mapping catheter positioned inside the vein

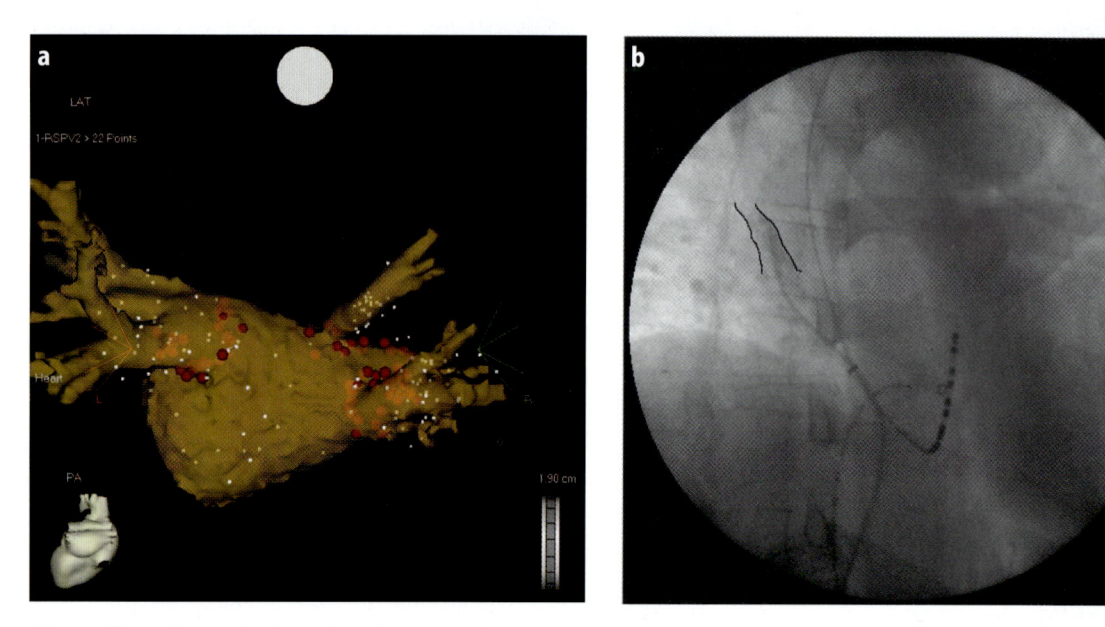

**Fig. 6.** Three-dimensional computed tomography image after ablation in a posteroanterior view (a) and postablation angiography of the "roof pulmonary vein" in a 30° RAO fluoroscopic view (b). In **a**, the *red dots* indicate the site of ablation around the pulmonary vein orifices. In **b**, an angiography catheter is in the "roof pulmonary vein" and dye injection shows no stenosis following radiofrequency delivery at its os

in Case 24, it is likely that this abnormality would have remained undiagnosed if pre-procedural three-dimensional imaging had not been performed. It is difficult to assess the contribution of electrical disconnection of this vein in the clinical success. The decision to also target this vein was based on the evidence of a very fast and highly fragmented electrical activity at the os and inside this vein. Safe cannulation of the vein and ostial ablation were rendered possible only by imaging integration with the computed tomography image. A recent report [1] indicated that recurrences of atrial fibrillation after successful isolation of four pulmonary veins may be related to foci in the additional pulmonary veins, not electrically disconnected in the previous ablation procedure. According to this study, disconnection of additional pulmonary veins is safe and effective in treating atrial fibrillation.

In this and in other cases (Cases 5, 17 and 24), the computed tomography image was registered by electroanatomic reconstruction of the left atrium and of the proximal part of the pulmonary veins. These are reconstructed with gentle positioning of the mapping catheter to avoid distortion of their anatomy. In our experience [2], this method allows more accurate alignment of the ostium of each pulmonary vein than if only the left atrium is considered. This is of crucial importance for ablation using imaging integration, sparing as much fluoroscopy time as possible while radiofrequency energy is delivered.

## References

1. Oh YW, Lee KY, Choi EJ et al. Assessment of pulmonary venous variation by multidetector row CT: clinical implication for catheter ablation techniques for atrial fibrillation. Eur J Radiol 2007. doi: 10.1016/j.eirad.2007.03.001.
2. De Ponti R, Marazzi R, Caravati F et al. Integration of computed tomography imaging and electroanatomic mapping to support electrophysiologically based procedures for ablation of atrial fibrillation. J Cardiovasc Med 2006; 7: 884-885.

Printed in Italy in May 2008